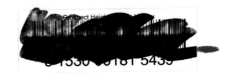

DATE DUE

# WOMEN DOCTORS GUIDE to
## *Health & Healing*

Oxmoor
House.

**Oxmoor House, Inc.**
Editor-in-Chief: Nancy F. Wyatt
Senior Health Editor: Sandy McDowell
Art Director: Cynthia R. Cooper
Copy Chief: Catherine R. Scholl

*Health*
Editor, Vice President: Doug Crichton
Executive Editor: Lisa Delaney
Design Director: Paul Carstensen
Managing Editor: Candace H. Schlosser

## *Women Doctors Guide to Health & Healing*

Contributing Development Editor: Debra L. Gordon
Managing Editor: Patricia Wilens
Copy Editor: L. Amanda Owens
Contributing Copy Editor: Laura A. Maher
Editorial Assistant: McCharen Pratt
Senior Designer: Emily Albright Parrish
Publishing Systems Administrator: Rick Tucker
Director, Production and Distribution: Phillip Lee
Books Production Manager: Larry Hunter
Production Assistant: Faye Porter Bonner
Interns: Rebecca Behan, Sarah Jackson

*Women Doctors Guide to Health & Healing*
© 2003 by Oxmoor House, Inc.
Book Division of Southern Progress Corporation
P.O. Box 2463, Birmingham, Alabama 35201

Published by Oxmoor House, Inc.

Library of Congress Control Number: 2003-107880
Hardcover ISBN: 0-8487-2576-X
Printed in United States of America

Softcover ISBN: 0-8487-2857-2
First Printing 2003

To order additional publications, call 800-765-6400
For more books to enrich your life, visit **oxmoorhouse.com**

## MEDICAL REVIEWERS

Alice Chang, M.D.
Division of General Medicine
Harvard Medical School
Editor, InteliHealth.com

Jesse Lynn Hanley, M.D.
Medical Director
Malibu Health and
Rehabilitation Center

## SPECIALTY MEDICAL REVIEWERS

Barbara Bartlik, M.D.
Weill Cornell Medical Center
New York-Presbyterian Hospital

Jane L. Frederick, M.D., F.A.C.O.G.
Huntington Reproductive Center
Medical Group

Susan Kaye, M.D.
Chief of Family Practice
Overlook Hospital

Kavita Kongara, M.D.
Director, Gastrointestinal Diagnostic
   Motility Center
Director, Women's Support Center
   for Gastroenterology Disorders
Winthrop University Hospital

Audrey Gottlieb Kunin, M.D.
President, DERMAdoctor.com
Department of Dermatology
University of Kansas Medical School

Catherine MacLean, M.D., Ph.D.
Division of Rheumatology
Geffen School of Medicine
University of California at Los Angeles

Jeanne Marrazzo, M.D.
Medical Director, Seattle STD/HIV
   Prevention and Training Center
University of Washington at Seattle

Adelaide Nardone, M.D.
Medical Consultant, Vagisil Women's
   Health Center

Melba Iris Ovalle, M.D.
Medical Director, Osteoporosis and
   Metabolic Bone Disease Center
Evanston Northwestern Healthcare

Alicia M. Weissman, M.D.
Department of Family Medicine
University of Iowa College of Medicine
   and Hospitals

## CONTRIBUTING WRITERS AND FACT CHECKERS

Alisa Bauman
Jennifer Goldsmith Cerra
Matthew Hoffman
Laura Metcalf

Deborah Mitchell
Linda Mooney
Peggy Noonan
Bebe Raupe

Elizabeth Shimer
Anita Small
Carol Sorgen
Holly Swanson

# Introduction

*Women Doctors Guide to Health & Healing* had been in production for nearly a year when an interesting study published in the *Journal of the American Medical Association* hit the news. "Female Physicians Spend More Time with Patients," read the headlines. The article, an analysis of more than 26 studies conducted over the past 34 years, found that female doctors engage in more positive social and emotionally focused talk than their male counterparts.

This news came as no surprise to the writers and editors working on this book. After interviewing hundreds of top female medical professionals about everything from atherosclerosis to yeast infections, we know that female doctors have a unique perspective on all aspects of a woman's health.

Women doctors seem to intuitively understand the special stresses that their female patients live with, from handling full-time jobs to caring for aging parents and kids, all while also functioning as the family CEO, cook, chauffeur, gardener, and accountant. Because they, too, are women, female doctors understand how women cope with these stresses and target their advice to fit women's busy lives.

Luckily, there are now plenty of women doctors. Women currently constitute one-fourth of all physicians practicing in the United States. Their numbers are growing, with women now applying to medical school at nearly the same rate as men. The figures are even higher in the field of obstetrics and gynecology, a specialty in which 71 percent of residents are women.

That's encouraging, because we need all the women doctors we can get. The growing field of gender-based medicine, which looks at health differences between women and men, is making one surprising discovery after another. We've learned how differently some drugs work in women than in men ... how a heart attack can be quite a different experience for a woman ... as well as how certain tests are best performed on women at certain times of the month.

"In every system of the body, from the hairs on our heads to the way our hearts beat, we are finding there are significant, unique sex-based differences in human physiology," writes Marianne J. Legato, M.D., in *Eve's Rib: The New Science of Gender-Specific Medicine and How It Can Save Your Life.*

In short, women's physical and emotional health differs significantly from that of men. So who better to talk to women about their health than women doctors?

We also know that you want to see—and hear from—women doctors. When we queried subscribers to *Health* magazine about their personal preferences, 38 percent said they preferred a female doctor, compared to only 9 percent who said they preferred a male. If the medical problem was so-called female-related, 57 percent wanted to be treated by a woman.

Why? Eighty-one percent said a woman could better identify with their experiences, while 80 percent also felt "more comfortable sharing my experience with a woman." And 59 percent said, "I feel that I'm taken more seriously by a woman."

Not only did we limit our experts to females, but also we tapped women doctors as medical reviewers to ensure that the information is fresh and helpful, as well as correct. Our lead advisor is Alice Chang, M.D., an associate physician in the division of general medicine at Harvard Medical School and an editor at Harvard Medical School's InteliHealth.com consumer health Web site. All references to complementary and alternative medicine were vetted by Jesse Lynn Hanley, M.D., who calls herself a "woman's woman" and practices the kind of medicine that integrates the complementary with the traditional. Dr. Hanley is the medical director of the Malibu Health and Rehabilitation Center. You might want to take special note of the natural and alternative health tips in the "Mother Nature, M.D." sidebars.

Throughout *Women Doctors Guide to Health & Healing,* you'll find the kind of action-packed tips and thoughtful explanations you've come to expect from *Health* magazine. Think of this book as an ongoing, informative conversation with your own personal female doctor. Written by women, for women, with women in mind.

To your health!

Debra L. Gordon
Contributing Development Editor

# Contents at a Glance

# Contents

# 4 Digestive System .................69

## *Pipeline and Lifeline*

# 11 Immune System ......................197
## *Beating What's Bugging You*

# 12 Life Crises ...........................218
## *Getting the Better of Turns for the Worse*

# 15 Mind and Emotions ..............276
## Smart and Sensitive
## Advice for the Inner You

# 16 Mouth and Teeth ...................308
## Preserving a Sparkling Smile

# 17 Nails ............................................... 323
## *Hands-on Help Is Here*

# 18 Pain ............................................... 330
## *It's Time for Relief*

# 1 Bones and Joints

chapter

## Preserving a Strong Foundation

*Bones are living, growing tissue.
To continue their pain-free support,
feed and nurture them every day.*

What comes to mind when you hear the word *bone*? Something you give
your dog to chew on? The color of your favorite shoes? If you've been told
you have osteoporosis or arthritis, *bone* takes on a new meaning. Suddenly,
bones matter. Of course, they've always mattered. Bones make up your
skeleton, the foundation upon which your body is supported, and they protect your internal organs. But your bones tend to be out of sight, out
of mind. That is, until a bone breaks, or your joints hurt, or you begin to
shrink as your spine compresses.

The lowdown on bones is this: They are a living, growing, always-
changing substance. You need to feed and nurture them—something too
many women forget. "Our lifestyles are not optimal for bone health,"
says *Bess Dawson-Hughes, M.D.,* of the Calcium and Bone Metabolism
Laboratory at Tufts University in Boston. "There's no question about that."

Nevertheless, there are steps you can take to protect your bones and
preserve their strength.

### OSTEOPOROSIS: IT'S NOT INEVITABLE

Once upon a time, acquiring a bent-over "dowager's hump" was considered
an unavoidable part of growing older. Fortunately, our understanding of
osteoporosis has improved in recent years, as have therapies for this progressive condition. These treatments may turn around what has become an
epidemic among American women.

Osteoporosis is the medical term for eroded bones—bones that are thin
and weak. The erosion starts at the cellular level with changes in collagen,

20

a protein that forms the matrix units, a kind of scaffolding that supports the minerals and chemicals that comprise bone, says **Melba Iris Ovalle, M.D.,** medical director of the Osteoporosis and Metabolic Bone Disease Center at Evanston Northwestern Healthcare and clinical instructor at Northwestern University's Feinberg School of Medicine in Chicago. Calcium plays a major role in strengthening and hardening these matrix units. Without calcium, bones lose mass and strength, becoming increasingly fragile and susceptible to fractures.

*Whatever your age or state of health, take action* now *to stop and reverse bone loss.*—Bess Dawson-Hughes, M.D.

An estimated 44 million Americans are at risk of or have osteoporosis. Of these, approximately 34 million have osteopenia, meaning they have low bone mass, which places them at increased risk for osteoporosis. Of the around 10 million who have full-blown osteoporosis, or low bone density, about 8 million are women. And these estimates are probably low because many people are not screened for osteoporosis.

Osteoporosis is a silent disease: Women often don't realize they have a problem until they break a wrist or hip. In fact, osteoporosis leads to more than 1.5 million fractures each year, and half of all women ages 50 and older will experience an osteoporosis-related fracture during their lifetimes.

"The prevalence of osteoporosis is increasing at an astronomical rate," warns **Bess Dawson-Hughes, M.D.,** of the Calcium and Bone Metabolism Laboratory at Tufts University in Boston. "Between now and 2020, we antici-pate a 40-percent increase in the prevalence of low bone mass and osteoporosis. We all have to deal with it and not wait until we see the manifestations of it." Whatever your age or state of health, you need to take action *now* to stop and reverse bone loss, she urges. You can prevent breaks and fractures with care, yet many women remain in denial about their weakening bones. "There's a strong belief among women of all age groups that it will never happen to them," says **Laura Tosi, M.D.,** associate professor of orthopaedic surgery and pediatrics at George Washington University School of Medicine and Health Sciences in Washington, D.C. "Or they believe there will be a cure soon, so why bother? When it comes to the health of bones, grabbing the attention of the public is very difficult."

## BUILDING AND BREAKING BONE

Bone breakdown and loss are natural and inevitable aspects of aging, but deterioration to the point of osteoporosis is neither natural nor inevitable. Loss of bone mass is a condition that develops over time and requires the interaction of several factors, including hormones, nutrition, heredity, and environment.

The foundation of bone health is laid early in life: You accumulate 98 percent of your bone mass by the time you are age 20. During these formative years, it's crucial to get enough dietary calcium and exercise if you want to escape osteoporosis later in life.

Until you reach about age 30, your body builds and stores bone efficiently. Then bone breakdown slowly begins to exceed buildup. The rate of bone loss accelerates as you move into menopause, with a slower rate of loss in later years. Still, for the rest of your life, you continue to lose about 1 percent of your bone mass each year.

## *Adolescent girls need calcium to build bone health for life.*—Laura Tosi, M.D.

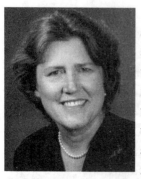

*Think of your bones as a sand castle, says Laura Tosi, M.D. You need a strong foundation while you're young to be able to resist the erosive tide of menopause.*

Dr. Tosi likens the bone life cycle to building a sand castle. "Between ages 10 and 14, a girl acquires about 50 percent of the bone she's going to have," she says. If she doesn't get enough calcium from dairy or other sources, her castle may be small, with thin walls. "Through your 20s and 30s, the waves start coming in, but your castle holds for a while," continues Dr. Tosi. "But when you hit menopause, the tide starts to wear your castle away. If you're not very tall or strong, you're going to wear away fast."

When that happens, women reach what's called the fracture threshold. This is the point at which bone mineral is low enough that a simple fall—or even pushing open a heavy door—can shatter a bone. "The goal is to help women build their sand castles strong so that they never hit the fracture threshold," says Dr. Tosi.

## THE STRIKES AGAINST YOU

Osteoporosis is largely preventable, though some risk factors are beyond your control. For example, no one has found a way to stop the aging process. But with a little effort, you can modify those risk factors that can be changed and reduce those that can't. These are some factors you can't change.

- Gender: Face it, ladies, 80 percent of people with osteoporosis are women. Women tend to have a lower bone mass than men when they're young, which means they have less bone to lose before they get into trouble. And since estrogen is a bone-building hormone, once women hit menopause and estrogen production slows, bone destruction gets the upper hand.
- Age: The ability to absorb and use calcium and other bone-building nutrients declines with age. So the older you are, the longer you may have been living with a deficiency of these vital nutrients.
- Race: Osteoporosis was once considered a disease of Caucasians, but research now tells a different story. The National Osteoporosis Risk Assessment (NORA), a two-year study that assessed more than 200,000 postmenopausal women, announced its findings in 2001: Women of Asian or Hispanic heritage are at the same high risk for osteoporosis as Caucasians, while African-Americans have the least risk. After menopause, however, all women lose bone at the same rate.
- Menopause: Estrogen plays a vital role in building bone, so the decline in estrogen that accompanies menopause sets the stage for osteoporosis. Women who experience early menopause (typically before age 45) or surgical menopause (removal of the uterus and both ovaries) are at the highest risk for osteoporosis because they're thrown into menopause prematurely and suddenly.
- Family and personal history: If your mother has or had osteoporosis or vertebral fractures, you're likely to have low bone mass and are at risk for similar problems. Also, experiencing a fracture early in life can mean you're more likely to develop osteoporosis, since it suggests your bones are weak to begin with.
- Disease and surgery: Some medical conditions can contribute to loss of bone mass. These include diabetes, Cushing's disease, anorexia nervosa, bulimia, and malabsorption (poor absorption and utilization of nutrients). Surgeries that alter hormone or nutrient absorption—such as thyroidectomy, gastrectomy, and intestinal bypass—can also lead to bone loss.

"Eating a well-balanced diet is the best way to feed your bones," says Dr. Dawson-Hughes. "I prefer that to a lousy diet and a lot of supplements. There are combinations of nutrients in foods that we don't know how to reproduce in pills."

*Get vitamin D from salmon and tuna to help your bones absorb calcium efficiently.*—Bess Dawson-Hughes, M.D.

As you design your bone-healthy diet, make sure you hit these essentials.

**Consider calcium.** "There's a big shortage of calcium in the American diet," says Dr. Dawson-Hughes. This nationwide deficiency is due to a significant decline in consumption of dairy products and other calcium-rich foods. These are the government's recommendations for calcium for women.

- Ages 9 to 18 years: 1,300 milligrams
- Ages 19 to 50: 1,000 to 1,200 milligrams (Pregnant or breast-feeding women should increase their intake to 1,200 milligrams.)
- Ages 51 and older: 1,500 milligrams

One quick way to boost your calcium consumption is to increase the amount of low- and nonfat dairy foods you eat. Most Americans get 75 percent of their calcium from milk, cheese, yogurt, and ice cream. "You can increase calcium intake with nondairy foods, but you have to work harder," says Dr. Dawson-Hughes. Good nondairy sources include soybeans, fortified tofu, legumes, beans, and cruciferous vegetables, such as broccoli, cabbage, and cauliflower. Calcium-enriched orange juice has even more of this bone-builder than fortified soy and rice milks, which contain about the same amount of calcium as cow's milk. (For tips on supplements and how to calculate your daily dietary calcium intake, see "Counting on Calcium," page 28.)

**Get nutrients from the sun.** Vitamin D helps your bones absorb calcium. You need 400 to 800 International Units (IUs) of vitamin D each day to help calcium get into your bones. "An increasing number of studies show that you can reduce your risk of fracture just by increasing your vitamin-D intake," says Dr. Tosi. The primary natural source of vitamin D is sunshine. Just 15 minutes of direct sunshine on your face and hands may be all it takes for your body to manufacture its daily needs. Go easy on sunscreens when you're getting your dose of D, says Dr. Dawon-Hughes. They can completely block the benefits of vitamin D, so give yourself about 10 minutes sunscreen-free before slathering the stuff on, she suggests. Other sources of vitamin D include most dairy products; cold-water fish, such as salmon and tuna; and multivitamins, which typically contain 200 to 400 IUs.

**Manage your magnesium.** This mineral is essential for bone health and—good news, here—most women get plenty in their diets. "Magnesium is present in so many foods, it's hard to avoid it in the diet," says Dr. Dawson-Hughes. Magnesium-rich foods include whole grains, dark green vegetables, bananas, almonds, figs, nuts, and seeds. If you take calcium supplements, don't mix them with magnesium supplements or take calcium-magnesium combination supplements. "It doesn't make sense because they compete for the same absorption mechanisms," says Dr. Dawson-Hughes. "If you flood your system with magnesium, you might hinder calcium absorption."

**Check your vitamin K.** "Bones need a structure for calcium to attach to, and vitamin K plays an important role in forming that structure," says *Beth Kitchin, M.S., R.D.,* assistant professor in the department of nutrition sciences at the University of Alabama at Birmingham and director of the

## DEXA SCAN: A PAIN-FREE BONE DENSITY TEST

*Screening for osteoporosis is swift and painless. You don't even have to take off your clothes.*

A bone density test may be the easiest medical procedure you'll ever experience. You don't have to forgo breakfast or wriggle out of your panty hose. The test is completely painless—in fact, it doesn't even hurt in your checkbook, since it's covered by most insurance plans, including Medicare. You just lie on a table while a machine scans your body from overhead. Five minutes later, you're on your way.

Called a dual-energy X-ray absorptiometry, or DEXA scan, the "test" is actually an X-ray that provides detailed information about your bone density. It is often used to assess your hip and spine, which are most susceptible to bone loss and fracture.

Most doctors recommend that a woman should have a DEXA scan once she reaches menopause to get a baseline reading of her bone status. "This baseline is a snapshot of where you are," says *Marie Savard, M.D.,* a Philadelphia internist and author of *How to Save Your Own Life.*

"The scan doesn't tell you if you are losing bone mass quickly or that anything serious is going to happen." But declining levels of estrogen can cause a woman to lose 2 to 3 percent of bone mass during the first five years of menopause. Therefore, Dr. Savard says, a DEXA scan should be repeated every two years for comparison to track your bone health.

EatRight Information Service at the Osteoporosis Prevention and Treatment Clinic. You produce some vitamin K in your intestines, but most comes from your diet. The recommended daily intake of vitamin K is 65 to 80 micrograms. It's most abundant in green and leafy vegetables, egg yolks, alfalfa, and safflower and soybean oils. Small amounts of vitamin K can be found in some multivitamins and mineral supplements, but don't rush out to buy some pills. "I've not seen any data saying people are deficient in vitamin K," says Kitchin. Women who take blood thinners, such as Coumadin (warfarin), should talk to their doctors before taking vitamin-K supplements or eating too many foods rich in vitamin K, as the vitamin interferes with the effects of those drugs.

*Eating a balanced diet is the best way to feed your bones. Foods provide benefits that can't be duplicated by supplements.*—Bess Dawson-Hughes, M.D.

**Mix in minerals.** The best means of getting valuable nutrients is food. In reality, though, few people eat a nutritious diet. To help ensure you get what you need for bone health, consider taking a multivitamin-mineral or mineral-complex supplement that contains 2 milligrams boron, 10 to 15 milligrams manganese, 20 to 40 milligrams zinc, and 1 to 2 milligrams copper, advises *Leslie Axelrod, N.D., L.Ac.,* associate professor at the Southwest College of Naturopathic Medicine in Tempe, Arizona. These minerals, along with calcium and magnesium, are important components in the formation of bones and maintenance of their health. Be careful not to take more than the recommended amount of zinc because too much can suppress your immune system, warns Dr. Axelrod.

**BONE-ROBBERS** Some foods actually rob your body of calcium and, therefore, should be consumed in moderation. Be on the lookout for these thieves.
- Protein: The debate continues over how much protein you need to maintain health—or whether it actually causes harm to your bones. Until there's a definitive answer, moderation seems to be the key.

"It's excessive consumption of animal protein that may be harmful to bone because the protein contains certain amino acids that can contribute to bone loss," says Kitchin. She suggests that women eat no more than about 0.38 grams protein per pound of body weight, which means a 120-pound woman needs about 46 grams protein a day. Examples of high-protein foods include:

> — Chicken, canned, 5 ounces: 31 grams
> — 2% cottage cheese, 1 cup: 31 grams
> — White beans, 1 cup: 19 grams
> — Lentils, 1 cup: 18 grams

• Salt: As your body processes salt, calcium is sucked out of your bloodstream. "So the more salt in your diet, the more calcium in your urine," says Dr. Dawson-Hughes. To replace that blood-based calcium, your body steals stored calcium from your bones. "Americans consume 5 to 10 times more salt than we need," says Dr. Dawson-Hughes, which means we send a lot of calcium down the toilet. The Food and Drug Administration recommends that people consume no more than 2,400 milligrams sodium per day, and Kitchen warns her clients not to exceed 3,000 milligrams daily. "That can be difficult because salt is in so many products," she says. Read package labels to help avoid high-sodium foods. You can also lower your salt intake by not adding salt to your food when cooking or eating. Use herbs and spices instead.

## *For a bone-healthy diet, limit your consumption of protein, salt, and caffeine.—Beth Kitchin, M.S., R.D.*

• Caffeine: "Caffeine steals calcium from your body because it is a diuretic and causes you to excrete calcium in your urine," says Kitchin. But you might not have to forgo the java yet. Until more is known about how caffeine contributes to calcium loss, Kitchin recommends a woman limit her caffeine intake to 200 milligrams per day. One 6-ounce cup of coffee contains about 100 milligrams caffeine, 6 ounces of most types of tea have around 70 milligrams, and 12 ounces of most soft drinks contain about 50 milligrams.

## COUNTING ON CALCIUM

*Always choose dietary sources of calcium over supplements.*

### FOOD SOURCES

These foods are excellent sources of calcium:

| | | |
|---|---|---|
| Cereal (General Mills Total) | ³/₄ cup | 1,000 milligrams |
| Cereal (General Mills Corn Flakes) | 1¹/₃ cups | 1,000 milligrams |
| Ricotta cheese (part skim) | 1 cup | 669 milligrams |
| Cornmeal (self-rising, enriched, yellow) | 1 cup | 483 milligrams |
| Yogurt (plain, skim milk) | 8 ounces | 452 milligrams |
| Collards (frozen), cooked without salt | 1 cup | 357 milligrams |
| Sardines (Atlantic, canned in oil) | 3 ounces | 325 milligrams |
| Milk (nonfat or skim) | 1 cup | 301 milligrams |
| Spinach (frozen), cooked without salt | 1 cup | 277 milligrams |
| Soybeans, cooked without salt | 1 cup | 261 milligrams |
| Provolone cheese | 1 ounce | 214 milligrams |
| Cheddar cheese | 1 ounce | 204 milligrams |
| Cereal (General Mills Basic 4) | 1 cup | 196 milligrams |
| Beans, white, canned | 1 cup | 191 milligrams |
| Kale (frozen), cooked without salt | 1 cup | 179 milligrams |
| Molasses (blackstrap) | 1 tablespoon | 172 milligrams |
| Oats, instant | 1 packet | 163 milligrams |
| Bok choy, cooked without salt | 1 cup | 158 milligrams |
| Cottage cheese (low-fat or 1% milkfat) | 1 cup | 138 milligrams |
| Tofu (firm, prepared with calcium sulfate and magnesium chloride) | ¹/₄ block | 131 milligrams |
| English muffin (plain) | one | 99 milligrams |
| Broccoli (frozen), cooked without salt | 1 cup | 94 milligrams |

For a more complete list, go to www.nal.usda.gov/fnic/foodcomp/Data and click on "Nutrient lists."

## PRACTICE HEALTHY HABITS

Little things mean a lot. This is particularly true when it comes to the health of your bones. Here's a heads up on some habits you can change today to make a beneficial difference in your bones tomorrow.

**Put out the smoke.** Now you have yet another reason to quit smoking. "There's great data showing that a fracture won't heal properly if you smoke," says Dr. Tosi. Smoking reduces the blood supply to bones, and

## SUPPLEMENT SOURCES

If you need a calcium supplement, take this advice from **Bess Dawson-Hughes, M.D.,** of Tufts University in Boston.

**Choose the form most convenient for you.** The two most commonly used supplements are calcium carbonate and calcium citrate. To get consistent absorption, you must take a carbonate supplement with food, since digestion generates the stomach acid necessary for its absorption. You can take citrate at any time, however, since it doesn't require stomach acid to be absorbed.

**Consider Tums.** This chewable antacid contains 300 milligrams calcium carbonate per tablet. It can be a handy way for some women to get supplemental calcium, but it does not contain the vitamin D needed to aid in the absorption of the calcium.

**Avoid oyster shell-calcium.** Steer clear of these supplements unless they are refined to remove contaminants, such as lead. Also avoid dolomite and natural bone sources because they may also have heavy-metal contamination.

## ADD IT UP

Now that you know about the two factors that make up your calcium intake, you need to calculate the amount of dietary calcium you take in. Read nutrition labels to determine the calcium content in individual foods you eat. Then choose a supplement to make up the difference to reach your recommended daily requirement.

In the example below, the total dietary calcium intake for the day is 810 milligrams. Depending on her age and corresponding daily requirement, an adult woman would need to supplement with 250 to 500 milligrams calcium. But she could avoid the supplement by adding 1 cup yogurt, which can provide up to 400 milligrams of additional calcium.

| Food | No. Servings Per Day | Calcium Per Serving (milligrams) | Total Calcium (milligrams) |
|---|---|---|---|
| Cereal (Basic 4) | 1 | 196 | 258 |
| Nonfat milk | 1 | 301 | 301 |
| Broccoli | 1 | 94 | 94 |
| Provolone cheese | $1/2$ | 214 | 107 |
| English muffin | $1/2$ | 99 | 50 |

Total calcium for the day 810

nicotine intake impairs absorption of calcium and slows production of bone-forming cells, all of which increase the risk of fractures.

**Monitor your meds.** Drugs are often-overlooked contributors to the development of osteoporosis. If you take medicines to treat such chronic ailments as rheumatoid arthritis, seizure disorders, gastrointestinal problems, or thyroid conditions, you can be causing significant damage to bone. "So many women are on thyroid medications," says Dr. Axelrod. "Long-term use of these drugs is a risk factor for osteoporosis, especially if the medications are not monitored carefully and women are given slightly too high doses, which is fairly common." Other bone-damaging medicines include glucocorticosteroids (used for asthma and arthritis), anticonvulsants, heparin, antacids that contain aluminum, methotrexate (used for arthritis), and the immunosuppressant cyclosporine. Talk to your doctor about any prescription or over-the-counter drugs you take that may be contributing to bone loss. If you use any of the drugs mentioned here, ask your doctor if you can switch to a comparable but less bone-damaging medication.

## *Long-term use of some arthritis and thyroid medications can be harmful to bones.*—Laura Tosi, M.D.

**Stimulate your bones.** We've been told how important it is to enhance bone health with weight-bearing aerobic exercise. These are the activities in which your legs support most of your body weight, such as walking, jogging, dancing, running, and playing tennis. The action of your feet hitting the ground stimulates bone cells, which helps strengthen bone. You should get at least 30 minutes of weight-bearing aerobic exercise, three times a week.

But don't stop there. For premenopausal women who don't have osteoporosis, the best exercise program includes high-impact aerobic exercise. All women need strength training, says Miriam E. Nelson, Ph.D., director of the Center for Physical Fitness at the Gerald J. and Dorothy R. Friedman School of Nutrition Science and Policy at Tufts University, and author of *Strong Women, Strong Bones*. These are some highlights from Dr. Nelson's program.

- Strength training: Using light weights takes you a long way toward building strong bones and helps tone muscles, improve balance and coordination, and give you more energy. Start slowly, with light weights (or no weights at all) and the easiest version of the exercises described. Your goal is three exercise sessions a week. After a few weeks, you should be able to increase the weight to make the exercises more challenging. Start out with pairs of 1- and 3-pound dumbbells, and perhaps one heavier set. Also try ankle weights, which are strap-on cuffs that hold various weighted bars. All are available at sporting-goods, discount, and department stores. In her book, Dr. Nelson recommends a series of 12 or more strength-building exercises. For example, this seated overhead press strengthens the bones and muscles of the shoulders and upper spine, and helps improve posture:

— Sit toward the edge of an armless chair, with your feet flat on the floor about hip-width apart. Hold one dumbbell in each hand. Bend your elbows to bring the weights up to shoulder height, with weights parallel to the floor. Your palms should be facing toward you, and your wrists should be straight.

— Keeping your palms facing you, slowly extend your arms to raise the dumbbells slightly in front of but over your head until your elbows are only slightly bent.

— Hold for two seconds, then slowly return to the starting position. Take a deep breath and repeat the exercise seven times, for a total of 8 repetitions.

• High-impact exercise: The jumping jacks you used to do in gym class were on the right track: This type of exercise is proven to significantly improve your hipbones in just a few months. Two minutes per day of vertical jumping is an efficient way to improve bone mass. However, this exercise is hard on the joints, so Dr. Nelson warns that only pre-menopausal women who do not have osteoporosis should go for high impact. Also, don't do high-impact exercises if you have balance problems or a history of ankle, knee, or back complaints.

*If you have osteoporosis, work with a physical therapist to learn neutral spine techniques that reduce your risk of fracture.—Beth Kitchin, M.S., R.D.*

**Neutralize your spine.** If you already have osteoporosis, you should only exercise under the guidance of an instructor who takes your condition into consideration. "When people with osteoporosis do a lot of bending and twisting of the spine, it increases the risk of vertebral fractures," says Kitchin.

She recommends a program that incorporates the concept of a neutral spine, which teaches you how to avoid bending and twisting while performing everyday functions. Kitchin worked with a physical therapist to develop a program called TYBONE, which stands for Tone Your Bones Osteoporosis Nutrition and Exercise. "We train women in neutral spine, helping them with balance, strength, and posture," she says. "We teach them how to sit and stand in neutral spine, how to do gardening, housework, even gym workouts."

Although many physical therapists are familiar with the concept of neutral-spine training, many physicians are not. "Women need to ask their doctors for a referral to a physical therapist who can teach neutral-spine techniques," says Kitchin. Although you should have a professional show you specific ways to move using these techniques, these are some practical steps you can take at home to adapt your environment.

- Keep items you use most frequently on waist-level shelves so you don't have to reach up or down to get them.
- Place heavy items on moveable carts so you don't have to carry them.
- Get extensions or longer handles on brooms and mops so you won't have to bend over while cleaning.

## TREATING OSTEOPOROSIS

It's only been in the past decade or so that drugs have been available to prevent and treat osteoporosis. A doctor may prescribe one of these drugs to a woman who doesn't have the disease if her bone density test shows bone loss or she has certain risk factors for the disease, such as a family history of osteoporosis. And women with osteoporosis who have had fractures routinely receive such prescriptions, says Dr. Ovalle.

Preserve your bones with healthy habits, recommends Melba Iris Ovalle, M.D. If you already have osteoporosis, try a bisphosphonate drug, such as Fosamax, to build up your bones.

There are four main categories of osteoporosis medications: bisphosphonates, hormone replacement therapy (HRT), designer estrogens (SERMs), and calcitonin. All are antiresorptive drugs, meaning they slow or stop special cells on the surface of bones from dissolving bone tissue, while allowing bone formation to continue.

- Bisphosphonates: The synthetic bone salts Actonel (risedronate) and Fosamax (alendronate) are the most powerful weapons women have against osteoporosis. They can increase bone mass by 4 percent or more per year, says Dr. Ovalle. Research shows that if you increase bone density by just 5 percent, you reduce your risk of fractures by about 40 percent.

These drugs are considered safe, except for women with kidney problems. "Bisphosphonates literally just go to bone, strengthen bone architecture, and increase bone mass," says Dr. Ovalle. They are best used to prevent fractures in women who are already diagnosed with osteoporosis. Other women should start with the healthy habits listed previously to reduce their risk.

- Hormone replacement therapy: With HRT, the lower the dose, the better, says Dr. Ovalle. Just 0.3 milligrams HRT—about half the dose doctors usually prescribe—work to prevent bone loss and build 2 to 3 percent more bone mass a year. However, some women may require a higher dose of 0.625 milligrams, especially if they already have osteoporosis.

## SHOULD I SEE A DOCTOR?

*There are guidelines for how often you should get a Pap smear and have your teeth cleaned. But when should you see a doctor about your bones?*

"At the very least, most women should talk to their doctors about osteoporosis as they become menopausal," says *Kim Thornton, M.D.*, a reproductive endocrinologist and assistant professor in the department of obstetrics, gynecology, and reproductive biology at Beth Israel Deaconess Medical Center at Harvard Medical School in Boston.

These circumstances and factors should also send you to your doctor:

**Certain drugs:** "Some medications place you at high risk of developing osteoporosis. These include thyroid drugs, corticosteroids, or anticonvulsants," explains Dr. Thornton. If you take these drugs and your doctor hasn't talked to you about your increased risk of osteoporosis, make an appointment for having that discussion right away.

**Certain medical conditions:** Ovarian failure, hyperthyroidism, or any condition for which the treatment is a long-term course of steroids can increase your risk of osteoporosis. Make sure your doctor knows about this history.

**Present or past history of eating disorders:** Regardless of age, women who have a history of anorexia nervosa or bulimia should see a doctor about their bone health. Studies show that these eating disorders place women at serious risk of bone loss.

**Abnormal cessation of menstrual periods:** "Women who don't have normal menstrual periods should learn why," says Dr. Thornton.

**Other risk factors:** If you are small-boned, are losing height, have a family history of osteoporosis, or are a smoker, consider having your bone-mineral density checked before you become menopausal.

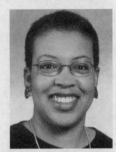

*Some medical conditions and medications increase your risk of osteoporosis, regardless of your age, warns Kim Thornton, M.D. Talk to your doctor about your bone health.*

Yet HRT is unlikely to be the first treatment your doctor recommends for osteoporosis. That's because in 2002 the Women's Health Initiative, the largest trial looking at women and HRT use, identified a higher risk of breast cancer associated with using HRT for several years. The study also determined that HRT does not prevent heart disease and, in fact, can slightly increase the risk for stroke and heart attacks. As a result, more physicians will be trying other therapies before HRT to prevent and treat osteoporosis, says **Alice Chang, M.D.,** an instructor at Harvard Medical School. If you are taking HRT for the health of your bones, Dr. Chang advises you to discuss the potential risks and benefits with your physician and ask whether you should switch to a nonhormonal therapy.

- Designer estrogens: Drugs in this category, called selective estrogen receptor modulators (SERMs), include Nolvadex (tamoxifen) and Evista

## ONE WOMAN'S STORY: OSTEOPOROSIS

*At 63, Martha Gore didn't understand why she couldn't stand up straight anymore. "You're aging," her doctor said. End of story? Not for her.*

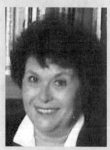

*Martha Gore safeguards her bone health by taking a once-weekly dose of nonhormonal Fosamax.*

Martha Gore had been blessed with good posture all her life. So when her husband, Vic, noticed her slouch—and she couldn't get a satisfactory explanation for its cause from her primary doctor—Gore sought a second opinion. The first time she met with her new physician, Gore expressed concern about her posture. "He had me stand up, then he told me I had osteoporosis."

The Gores knew nothing about the disease. "We never connected people who were bent over with osteoporosis. We thought that was caused by arthritis." In hindsight, Gore sees her risk factors clearly: early menstruation and menopause, an older sister with the disease, and a brother who was bent over in his 60s.

When her first DEXA bone density test showed serious osteoporosis and "bones that looked like Swiss cheese," Gore's doctor insisted that she take hormones. But three courses of hormone therapy left her with rashes and other distressing side effects. And even in the late '80s, there were indications that hormone therapy posed a breast-cancer risk. Gore had had enough. Armed with a degree in library science and a natural penchant for research, she put her skepticism to work for herself.

She learned about Fosamax (alendronate), nonhormonal medication designed for the prevention and treatment of osteoporosis. After taking the drug for seven years, Gore's bone density has improved about 3 percent a year. She and her doctor are thrilled with the results.

(raloxifene). Tamoxifen is used primarily to treat breast cancer, but while studying the drug's effectiveness against that disease, researchers discovered that it also helps preserve bone. Scientists later developed raloxifene, the first SERM approved by the U.S. Food and Drug Administration for the prevention and treatment of osteoporosis. You should not take SERMs if you're premenopausal—they'll put you into menopause—or if you're taking HRT.

- Calcitonin: This medication is a synthetic form of a natural hormone secreted by the thyroid gland. It stops the loss of bone by blocking the activity of osteoclasts, which are the cells that digest bone matrix. Doctors prescribe calcitonin for women who are five or more years past menopause. It is available by injection or as a convenient nasal spray, with the brand name Miacalcin.

"I had a bad fall in 2001, and I didn't break a thing," she says. "That says a lot for the treatment." That same year, Gore was able to change her dosage of Fosamax from once-a-day to a newly released once-a-week formulation.

Gore makes good use of the approximate 30 minutes she must remain upright after taking Fosamax. For example, during that time, you may find her mopping the kitchen floor, using a specially designed bent handle that allows her to stand straight and avoid placing stress on her back as she cleans.

She's made additional adjustments to help prevent falls. "I don't reach up high. I rearranged my kitchen so that everything is at about my eye level or below. I don't use a stove; I cook on a hot plate and use an eye-level portable oven so that I don't have to lean down to lift anything out. I have a rolling table on which I place heavier items so that I don't have to carry them to the table," says Gore. And she acknowledges that she's got a lot going for her in another way: "If you have a really understanding, cooperative husband, it's a lot easier when you're dealing with something like this."

Doctors laughed at Gore when she began taking 500 milligrams calcium a day about 20 years ago. And although she still developed osteoporosis, Gore believes the condition could have been worse without the supplements. "Maybe if I'd been taking 1,000 or 1,500 milligrams, it would have made a greater difference," she says.

Gore now takes a higher dose of calcium, plus magnesium and potassium, every day. She gets her vitamin D the natural way: from sunshine. "I read on my patio every day for 20 minutes," says Gore. She also walks or uses her treadmill regularly, doesn't smoke, and watches her salt intake.

Her wish for women who read this? "I hope they realize that osteoporosis isn't just an aging thing," says Gore. "Osteoporosis has a psychological effect on women who are caught up in staying young—it's an affront to their perception of who they are. I didn't go through that because I never had a problem with aging. But that's why so many women don't deal with it until it's so late."

## ARTHRITIS: WHEN YOUR JOINTS ARE OUT OF SORTS

"I have a touch of arthritis in my hands." "That pain in my hip? The doctor says it's arthritis." "Whenever I complain to my doctor about aching, painful joints, he says it's arthritis." You hear it all the time: someone complaining about aches and pains in her hands or neck or hip, and it being blamed on arthritis. Is arthritis a convenient scapegoat or legitimate diagnosis?

*Arthritis* is a general term for more than 100 conditions, all of which share one trait: painful joints. The Centers for Disease Control and Prevention estimate that 43 million Americans have some form of arthritis, making it

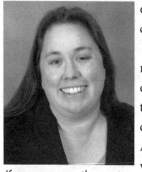

*If you use an over-the-counter ointment to relieve the aches of osteoarthritis, be careful not to add heat treatments—the combination can burn your skin, says Deborah Jane Power, D.O.*

one of the most prevalent diseases and the leading cause of disability in the United States.

The most common forms are osteoarthritis and rheumatoid arthritis. Osteoarthritis is a degenerative disease that usually results from wear and tear on the joints. Rheumatoid arthritis, a systemic chronic disorder, is typically more severe and debilitating. And—as luck would have it—both forms affect women more often than men.

Why women? No one knows for sure, says *Deborah Jane Power, D.O.*, clinical assistant professor of medicine at the Arizona Arthritis Center at University of Arizona Health Sciences Center in Tucson. "Some say there's a hormonal connection, but that doesn't explain osteoarthritis that occurs in postmenopausal years," she says. Another theory targets biomechanical differences. Simply put, men and women are built differently: Women have wider hips, which place more stress where the femurs (the long upper leg bones) meet the knee joints.

The reason why more women have rheumatoid arthritis is less debated. It is an autoimmune condition—one in which the body attacks its own cells—and the vast majority of autoimmune conditions affect more women than men.

### OSTEOARTHRITIS: WHAT'S GOING ON IN THERE?

Experts generally agree that if you live long enough, you'll get osteoarthritis, even if you don't have any symptoms, says Dr. Power. That's because this form of arthritis is typically the result of certain joints—usually the knees, hips, fingers, and spine—wearing out like a favorite pair of jeans. But that doesn't mean that osteoarthritis affects only the elderly. People in their 20s and 30s can also get the disease, especially if they have subjected their joints to a lot of stress by being athletes or dancers, or if arthritis runs in their family. Osteoarthritis occurs most often in the knees, hips, fingers, or spine.

You can better understand osteoarthritis if you know what joints are and how they work. A joint is the point at which two or more bones meet. To prevent them from rubbing together, the ends of each bone are covered with protective cartilage, a strong tissue composed of a protein called collagen. Synovial fluid acts as a lubricant to help the joints move smoothly, bathing the joints like oil does an engine.

When long-term use of joints damages cartilage, the result is osteoarthritis. Pieces of cartilage break off into the synovial fluid. As cartilage wears away, the ends of the bones rub together, causing stiffness and pain in the joints. Main factors causing osteoarthritis include the following.

- Family history: "If a parent had significant osteoarthritis—say, with knobby knuckles—it's likely you'll develop the same condition," says Dr. Power. If you're double jointed or have knock-knees or bow legs, you're also more likely to develop the disease.

- Injury: The injuries you suffered in youth may return to haunt you in middle age. "Then you have osteoarthritis in a joint that you sprained back in high school gymnastics," says Dr. Power. "Usually, injuries cause arthritis to develop sooner. It's secondary arthritis due to the trauma and not what would naturally progress due to the wear and tear of aging."

**LIVING WITH OSTEOARTHRITIS** "Osteoarthritis is a chronic disease, so it should be dealt with in an ongoing way, with lifestyle changes and other self-care measures," says *Marie Savard, M.D.,* a Philadelphia internist and author of *How to Save Your Own Life.* Use medication sparingly and with caution, she says. Why? Because arthritis usually affects older women who may already have high blood pressure, kidney problems, or other medical conditions, and using arthritis drugs can make those conditions worse.

*Take the natural supplements glucosamine and chondroitin to help ease the pain and stiffness of osteoarthritis, says Marie Savard, M.D.*

Make these lifestyle changes to help ease the pain of arthritis.

**Lose excess pounds.** For every pound you gain, your knees bear an additional 2 to 3 pounds. "Many people who have osteoarthritis in their knees are significantly overweight," says Dr. Power. Your hips also suffer because they have to withstand two times more pressure per pound added. If excess weight is a cause, losing weight can be a remedy. "Reducing weight can help reduce the pain of osteoarthritis," says *Catherine MacLean, M.D., Ph.D.,* assistant professor of medicine in the division of rheumatology at the Geffen School of Medicine at the University of California at Los Angeles. (For advice on losing weight, see "Weight Control," page 478.)

*If you're overweight, shed those extra pounds to ease your arthritis pain.*
—*Catherine MacLean, M.D., Ph.D.*

**Exercise regularly.** People with osteoarthritis who exercise regularly have less pain and better function, the ability to perform normal activities, says Dr. MacLean.

**Avoid exercise-related injuries.** Before exercising or participating in any sport, warm up with 5 to 10 minutes of stretching, which increases your blood flow and heart rate, warms and stretches your muscles, and reduces the risk of additional injury to a joint. After exercising, take five minutes to cool down with easy stretching.

**TREATMENT OPTIONS** If lifestyle changes don't relieve osteoarthritis pain, Dr. Savard has her patients try the natural supplements glucosamine and chondroitin, which can be purchased separately or in a combination product. Glucosamine is an amino sugar that helps in formation and repair of cartilage; chondroitin is part of a protein that gives cartilage its elasticity.

"Several studies have demonstrated a small reduction in pain from taking these supplements," says Dr. MacLean. A large study, sponsored by the National Institutes of Health, is currently underway.

Dr. Savard recommends taking at least 500 milligrams glucosamine and 400 milligrams chondroitin, three times a day, until you feel better. Expect it to take a while to work, however: four to six weeks at the earliest, and up to three months for some individuals. "When using glucosamine and chondroitin, people generally feel less stiffness and pain when moving and going about their daily living," says Dr. Savard. There is no data on the superiority of one brand over another.

There are other treatment options in the osteoarthritis drug arsenal. Keep this expert advice in mind when you consider painkillers.

**Make your first choice acetaminophen.** For mild to moderate osteoarthritis, acetaminophen is the best choice, says Dr. MacLean. "It is the drug with the fewest side effects, and it is just as effective as nonsteroidal anti-inflammatory drugs (NSAIDs), such as aspirin, ibuprofen, and naproxen." And since some patients with severe osteoarthritis respond to this drug, it should always be tried before other medications.

**Next, try NSAIDs.** These drugs can work to reduce pain. But make sure you and your doctor keep tabs on possible and potentially dangerous side effects, such as stomach bleeding and ulcers, says Dr. MacLean.

Your doctor may also want to prescribe a new class of NSAIDs called COX-2 inhibitors. Their pain-relieving powers are the same as other NSAIDs, but they have fewer gastrointestinal side effects, says Dr. MacLean. Drugs in this category include Bextra (valdecoxib), Celebrex (celecoxib), and Vioxx (rofecoxib). She recommends that people with osteoarthritis who have had gastric bleeding or an ulcer, or are older than 75, be treated with a COX-2 inhibitor. Or they may take a traditional NSAID along with a proton pump inhibitor (PPI), a medication that reduces stomach acid, thereby reducing the risk of further gastrointestinal injury. They may take misoprostil instead of a PPI, but it may cause diarrhea. For people who take an aspirin daily for cardiovascular protection and are also at risk for gastrointestinal bleeding (that is, people who have had gastric bleeding or an ulcer, or are over age 75), she recommends taking a PPI or misoprostil along with both COX-2 inhibitors and traditional NSAIDs.

**Consider stronger medications.** If acetaminophen or NSAIDs don't work for you, your doctor may prescribe low-strength narcotics, such as Darvocet (propoxyphene) or acetaminophen with codeine, says Dr. Power.

**Rub on relief.** Capsaicin is a chemical component of cayenne peppers that can bring relief when rubbed over the painful area. Over-the-counter brands include Capzasin-P and Zostrix. Don't use these ointments with heat treatments, advises Dr. Power. The combination can burn your skin. And wash your hands after applying so you don't get any of the ointment into your eyes.

**Try an intravenous painkiller.** Injecting glucocorticoid drugs, such as cortisone and cortisol, into the affected joints can help ease pain and inflammation, says Dr. Power. Results vary: Some patients get relief from pain for up to six months, others for just a few weeks. Side effects can include a temporary increase in blood sugar and risk of infection, as well as dimpling of the skin, pain, or bleeding at the injection site. These medications can also cause the pain and inflammation to worsen for a day before improving. This is known as a steroid flare-up. If you experience a flare, ice the area, advises Dr. Power.

Other forms of injection include the following.

- Viscosupplementation: This relatively new treatment also involves injections into the affected joint. The substance injected is hyaluronic acid, a natural substance found in the body that makes synovial fluid thick and sticky. Some studies show that viscosupplementation is beneficial; others show it worked no better than placebo. This therapy works best for patients who still have some cartilage and is generally used only when other therapies don't work, says Dr. Power.
- Acupuncture: While not an injection in the traditional sense, the insertion of small, thin needles into points in the body is thought to control the flow of energy throughout the system. There is strong evidence that acupuncture relieves arthritic pain, says Dr. Power.

### RHEUMATOID: THE OTHER ARTHRITIS

Rheumatoid arthritis has evidently plagued people since the dawn of time. Indications of the disease have been discovered in skeletons dating from 6500 to 450 B.C. An Icelandic doctor described its symptoms in 1782, noting that they affected women more often than men.

We've learned more about the condition since then. Today, rheumatoid arthritis is classified as a systemic autoimmune disease, meaning the body attacks various parts of itself—primarily the joints, but also the eyes, skin, lungs, and heart. For reasons not fully understood, when you have rheumatoid arthritis, your immune system attacks the cells inside your joint capsule, identifying certain markers on your joint's cells as foreign material. During the attack, white blood cells race to attack the site, causing inflammation of the joint lining, a condition known as synovitis. The result is a red, warm, swollen, and painful joint. This inflammation also stimulates your synovial membranes to grow and reproduce abnormally, making the liquid thicker than usual and keeping the joint swollen.

Over time, inflammation and abnormal synovial cells damage the bone and cartilage; muscles, tendons, and ligaments around the joint become weak. As the disease progresses, deformities can develop in the joints.

While experts know a lot about what happens during the rheumatoid arthritis process, they're still fuzzy on the why. "Genetics definitely has something to do with rheumatoid arthritis, but we don't know the whole cause or what the trigger is," says **Audrey M. Nelson, M.D.,** former professor of internal medicine at the Mayo Medical School in Rochester, Minnesota. And although more women than men get the disease, hormones don't seem to be the cause. "No one has been able to show the link," says Dr. Nelson. "It's not estrogen because rheumatoid arthritis can appear before or after menopause."

## IS IT OSTEOARTHRITIS OR RHEUMATOID ARTHRITIS?

*Many people are confused by these two terms. So here's a quick look at the similarities and the differences between the two conditions.*

### OSTEOARTHRITIS
- Usually begins after age 40.
- Usually takes many years to develop.
- Affects only a few joints, typically the knees, hips, fingers, feet, or spine. Rarely affects the ankles, elbows, or wrists. May affect joints on both sides of the body.
- Joints become painful with use, so pain may worsen during the day.
- Swelling, inflammation may develop over time.

### RHEUMATOID ARTHRITIS
- Usually appears between ages 15 and 50.
- Symptoms may develop suddenly, over a few weeks or months.
- Pain and stiffness are often worse in the morning and last at least an hour. Movement and use of the joint often help symptoms improve.
- Swelling occurs in at least one joint, often with swelling of a symmetrical joint area. For instance, if a knuckle on the right hand is affected, so is a knuckle on the left hand.
- Motion causes pain in at least one joint.
- Joints are often more red, swollen, or warm than in osteoarthritis.
- X-rays may provide evidence of rheumatoid arthritis after the disease has been present for several years.
- Pea-sized nodules may form under the skin on the back of the arm below the elbow, at the base of the skull, at the Achilles tendon, or at other so-called pressure points throughout the body. These painless lumps are caused by inflammation of blood vessels and appear in about 20 to 25 percent of people with rheumatoid arthritis.
- Results are positive on a rheumatoid factor test. Rheumatoid factor is a substance often found in the blood of people who have the condition, although its absence doesn't rule out rheumatoid arthritis. In the first year of the disease, about 60 percent of people with rheumatoid arthritis test positive for the rheumatoid factor. In subsequent years, the number increases to about 80 percent.

Some experts believe that stress may play a role. "There are many cases in which someone in the family dies or there's a long illness and the caregiver breaks out with rheumatoid arthritis," notes Dr. Power. Yet, so far, no one's been able to prove that stress triggers the disease.

**TREATING RHEUMATOID ARTHRITIS** Years ago, early treatment of rheumatoid arthritis typically included NSAIDs and acetaminophen. Today, the focus is on disease-modifying antirheumatic drugs (DMARDs), says Dr. Nelson. Some of the more common DMARDs are Azulfidine (sulfasalazine), Plaquenil (hydroxychloroquine), and Rheumatrex (methotrexate). These medications not only relieve the pain and inflammation of rheumatoid arthritis, but also help slow the progression of the disease. "The consensus is that it's important to treat rheumatoid arthritis aggressively with DMARDs right away to try to slow the damage because most of the damage is done in the first couple of years of the disease," explains Dr. Nelson.

If you have severe pain, your doctor is likely to add to your DMARDs, since they take several months to work. These drugs are often used with NSAIDs, as well as small amounts of glucocorticoid steroids, such as prednisone, says Dr. Nelson. Doctors sometimes prescribe all three DMARDs together, since studies show they have an additive effect. If your doctor recommends Rheumatrex, she'll also likely suggest you take 1 gram folic acid every day. "Folic acid helps protect against some of the drug's side effects, especially canker sores and potential liver problems," says Dr. Nelson.

Some patients, however, don't respond well—or at all—to DMARDs. Then other medications are considered.

**Ask about TNF blockers.** New research indicates that people with rheumatoid arthritis may benefit from drugs that block the immune system protein known as tumor necrosis factor (TNF), which is involved in inflammation and tissue damage. These drugs include the following.

- Enbrel (etanercept): "Enbrel has been shown to slow the progression of joint destruction," says Dr. Power. "Some people argue that it should be a first-choice medication because, if you can prevent the destruction, why wait?" One reason may be the price: The twice-weekly self-injections of Enbrel add up to about $15,000 per year, and most insurance companies won't cover use of the drug until patients have tried more traditional medications. And Medicare doesn't cover *any* outpatient drug.

- Remicade (infliximab): This TNF blocker is given intravenously. It's even more expensive than Enbrel: up to $25,000 per year, depending on the dosage. Medicare will cover the cost of this drug because it is administered in a hospital or doctor's office.

Finding the right medications—and monitoring them—is a job best left to a rheumatologist. "They should not be prescribed by doctors who are not rheumatologists because use of these drugs requires knowledge of their nuances: when to prescribe them, when to change them, and the latest in side effects. No one recipe fits everyone," says Dr. Nelson. For example, both Enbrel and Remicade suppress the immune system, increasing the risk of infections. "We screen for tuberculosis before placing anyone on these drugs," since they may reactivate it in anyone who has had the disease, says Dr. Power.

**Try omega-3 fatty acids.** A British study reports that supplementing the diet with omega-3 fatty acids can reduce both the degree of morning stiffness and the number of painful joints. This nutrient is found primarily in cold-water fish, such as salmon and tuna. *Leslie Axelrod, N.D., L.Ac.,* associate professor at the Southwest College of Naturopathic Medicine in Tempe, Arizona, recommends 3 grams fish-oil supplements a day. If you want to avoid the fishy aftertaste that is a possible side effect with fish-oil supplements, get your omega-3s with 2 to 3 tablespoons flaxseed oil a day, she says.

## MOTHER NATURE, M.D.: RHEUMATOID ARTHRITIS

*Making changes in your diet may enable you to manage rheumatoid arthritis naturally.*

More than two dozen studies have found evidence that symptoms of rheumatoid arthritis can be relieved by adhering to a vegan diet, which excludes any animal products, such as milk, meat, fowl, cheese, and eggs. "Up to 70 percent of cases of rheumatoid arthritis are caused by food," says *Mary McDougall,* co-author of a scientific study on relieving rheumatoid arthritis through diet and the recipe developer for the McDougall Program for Women. Here's why.

In some people, animal proteins slip through the intestinal wall into the bloodstream. Dairy proteins found in milk products are a particular problem. The body perceives these proteins as foreign bodies and makes antibodies to attack them. These antibodies then can form clumps that get stuck in joint tissue, causing pain and inflammation. Because the amino acids in the joints are similar to those of animal proteins, the antibodies also attack the joints.

According to McDougall and other researchers, the best remedy is to completely eliminate dairy and other animal proteins from the diet. About 70 percent of people with rheumatoid arthritis experience good results within three to four days after they stop eating animal proteins, says McDougall. More dramatic benefits become apparent within two weeks.

# 2 Brain
## chapter
## Keeping Your Wits About You

*You can't turn back the clock, but there's evidence that sound lifestyle choices can help you maintain a healthy brain as you age.*

Alzheimer's and Parkinson's diseases are the most common degenerative ailments affecting the nervous system. Researchers continue to make progress in identifying the causes of these conditions and in refining treatments.

Both illnesses are linked to age-related changes in the brain. A healthful diet and lifelong commitment to physical and mental activity can help your brain stay young. Many self-care strategies exist for coping with the symptoms of these diseases and—with luck—preventing future problems.

## ALZHEIMER'S DISEASE: BEYOND FORGETFULNESS

Every day, you hear women joking about having senior moments—those annoying memory lapses that seem to occur more frequently as we get older. A little forgetfulness is a normal side effect of aging. But a serious decline in mental function can be a sign of Alzheimer's, a condition in which abnormal proteins accumulate in the brain, reducing the cells' ability to communicate.

No one knows what causes Alzheimer's disease, although genetic factors are certainly involved. Diet, exercise, and various lifestyle decisions also seem to play a role. So does gender: The majority of Alzheimer's patients are female. Because women live longer than men, they may be more likely to develop age-related problems, says *Marilyn Albert, Ph.D.,* director of the Gerontology Research Unit at Massachusetts General Hospital and professor of psychiatry and neurology at Harvard Medical School.

Medications currently available can slow the progression of Alzheimer's, but they can't stop it. In recent years, however, doctors have identified a variety of tactics that may reverse some problems—or even prevent mental decline from starting.

Experts recommend these lifestyle choices to keep Alzheimer's disease at bay.

**Take antioxidants.** Every second of every day, cells in your body transform oxygen into dangerous molecules called free radicals, which damage tissues throughout the body, including in the brain. Evidence suggests that free radicals play a key role in the development of Alzheimer's. Antioxidant nutrients, such as vitamins E and C, neutralize free radicals and may prevent some damage. Antioxidants are found in all plant foods, as well as in nutritional supplements.

- Vitamin E: "We know that vitamin E slows the course of Alzheimer's disease," says Dr. Albert. She advises women to take a daily dose of 400 to 800 International Units (IUs) vitamin E. Supplements are generally safe unless you are a woman who takes aspirin or blood-thinning medications every day—supplements strengthen the effects of those medications, creating a risk of bleeding. So it's a good idea to talk with your doctor before taking vitamin E.
- Vitamin C: This antioxidant enhances the effects of vitamin E in the body. As a bonus, studies have found that vitamin C enables Alzheimer's medications to reach the brain more readily. You can take supplements that contain 500 to 1,000 milligrams vitamin C, but many fruits and vegetables provide healthful amounts of it.

### SHOULD I SEE A DOCTOR?

*It's normal to suspect the worst when you realize you can't remember phone numbers or people's names. But in most cases, forgetfulness has more to do with normal aging than with the onset of a serious illness.*

Albuquerque neurologist *Jill Marjama-Lyons, M.D.,* cautions that any decline in mental function is potentially a cause for concern. Talk to your doctor if any of these warning signs apply:

- Forgetfulness is accompanied with physical changes, such as fatigue.
- Memory lapses are more frequent or are getting more severe. "With Alzheimer's disease, there's a worsening of symptoms over time," says Dr. Marjama-Lyons.
- Forgetfulness interferes with routine functioning. Anemia or low levels of vitamin $B_{12}$ or thyroid hormone can cause mental abilities to decline. Even if you feel fine apart from occasional memory lapses, you may want to see a doctor to rule out other problems—and to gain peace of mind.

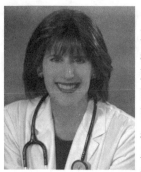

*A high-fat diet may contribute to age-related mental changes. Eat fresh fruits, vegetables, and fish to help keep your brain healthy, advises Susan Lark, M.D.*

**Get the fat out.** Studies suggest that people who load up on high-fat foods are more likely to develop age-related mental changes than those who dine on leaner cuisine. Dietary fat can accumulate in the brain's blood vessels, reducing blood flow and possibly causing mental decline, says *Susan Lark, M.D.,* author of *The Chemistry of Success: Six Secrets of Peak Performance.* And if you're eating a lot of fatty foods, you're probably consuming too few protective plant foods. Doctors usually advise women to limit fat intake to 30 percent of total calories, but less is even better, says Dr. Lark. (For more information on how to limit your fat intake, see page 487.)

**Dine on fish and flax.** Fish is loaded with essential fatty acids (EFAs), which inhibit the body's production of prostaglandins, the biochemicals that increase cell-damaging inflammation in the brain. So feast on such fatty fish as salmon and mackerel, which are high in EFAs. Or take EFA supplements, such as flaxseed oil (1 to 2 tablespoons daily) or ground flaxseed (4 to 6 tablespoons daily). You can use flaxseed oil as the base for a tasty vinaigrette on greens or a vegetable salad. Mix 2 tablespoons flaxseed oil with an equal amount of lemon juice or wine vinegar. Add some honey and aromatic herbs, such as rosemary or oregano, and mix well. If you choose to get your EFAs from ground flaxseed, simply sprinkle 1 to 2 tablespoons over cereal or blend it with fruit and low-fat milk to make a nutritious smoothie.

**Stub out that cigarette.** Smoking unleashes vast amounts of tissue-damaging free radicals. Anyone with a family history of Alzheimer's—or who already suffers from the disease—should quit smoking to discourage future damage, warns Dr. Albert.

**Ask about NSAIDs.** Along with ibuprofen, naproxen, and other nonsteroidal anti-inflammatory drugs (NSAIDs), aspirin appears to reduce the risk of Alzheimer's disease. This is probably due to aspirin's ability to reduce inflammation in the brain, says Dr. Albert. Research is still in the early stages, but studies suggest that people who take aspirin and similar drugs may be at least 40 percent less likely to develop Alzheimer's. There may be a greater reduction in risk with NSAID use for longer than two years. Since NSAIDs may cause stomach upset or other side effects, your doctor is unlikely to recommend them solely to prevent this condition, adds Dr. Albert. But if you already take an NSAID for easing arthritis or preventing heart attack, you may be getting an important brain bonus.

**Consider taking estrogen.** "Brain research and cognitive studies over several decades show that estradiol (the main type of estrogen produced by the ovaries) plays an important role in maintaining and improving memory," says menopause specialist *Elizabeth Lee Vliet, M.D.,* of Dallas and Tucson, author of *Screaming to Be Heard: Hormone Connections Women Suspect and Doctors Still Ignore* and *It's My Ovaries, Stupid!* "I find women describe more improvement in memory and other symptoms when they restore the form of estradiol their bodies always made. They show the greatest benefits when therapy starts early in menopause, before damage occurs."

Many women are confused about estrogen because of recent headlines about the Women's Health Initiative (WHI) study, which indicated that hormone therapy may have an *adverse* effect on memory. "It's important to put this study in perspective," says Dr. Vliet. "Women in the study took either Premarin—an estrogen derived from the urine of pregnant horses (CEE)—or Prempro, a combination of CEE and synthetic progestin. These are not the same hormones our bodies make before menopause and don't have the same beneficial effects, as the WHI clearly showed. I don't see any reason to keep using horse-derived products."

Another problem is that WHI participants were older than the average age of menopause (about 50) when most women would normally start taking estrogen for its protective effects on brain cells. "The average age of the WHI women was about 65," explains Dr. Vliet. "Many had high blood pressure, high cholesterol, or diabetes—all of which increase risk of brain damage and later Alzheimer's. Using nonhuman forms of hormones in a group of elderly women with existing health problems is a critical flaw in the study. We know that once brain cells start to wither and damage is done, we can't overcome that very well by adding hormones later, especially if they are ones so different from what our body makes."

Because there are dangers associated with hormone replacement therapy (HRT) after menopause, preventing Alzheimer's should not be the only reason you take supplemental estrogen. (For more information on HRT, see page 251.)

**Exercise daily.** Regular workouts increase the flow of blood and oxygen to the brain. Activity also enhances the production of natural compounds called trophic factors, which improve the brain's ability to repair damage. You don't have to live at the gym to get beneficial amounts of brain-protecting exercise, says Dr. Albert. Walking as little as a mile a day, going up and down stairs, or lifting packages all have the power to empower your mind. Be active on a daily basis to give your brain the boost it needs to stay healthy.

*The brain needs exercise, just like other parts of your body. Use it or lose it.—Jill Marjama-Lyons, M.D.*

**Challenge your mind.** Do crossword puzzles, play word games, read challenging books, or listen to lectures. "Your brain is like other parts of your body," says *Jill Marjama-Lyons, M.D.,* an Albuquerque neurologist. "If you don't use it, you lose it." Research performed on laboratory animals shows that connections between brain cells increase when subjects are put in stimulating environments. The same is evidently true for humans. A study of 678 nuns, for example, found that the women with the most education and greatest language abilities were less likely to develop Alzheimer's disease.

**Knock out stress.** This is easier said than done, of course—especially for women who work in addition to managing busy families. But emotional pressure increases levels of the stress hormones that impair the brain, says Dr. Albert. Everyone controls and reacts to stress differently. Long walks may help you stem rising tension, as can yoga and meditation. Or simply set aside time for a luxurious soak in the tub. (See "Stress-Busters," page 283.)

**Treat the blues.** Evidence shows that depression contributes to shrinkage in areas of the brain that control memory, reports Dr. Albert. Indications of depression and Alzheimer's can appear similar, leading to delays in getting correct diagnosis and treatment. Symptoms of both include disturbed sleep, loss of energy, lack of interest in normal activities, or changes in appetite or weight. Women are more likely than men to experience depression, so see a doctor immediately if you suspect you might be suffering from it. Bring along a complete list of medications you take. A number of common drugs, such as those used to treat high blood pressure, can cause depression in some people.

**Look into pregnenolone.** This hormone is converted into major sex hormones, including testosterone in men and estrogen, progesterone, and testosterone in women. Your body's production of pregnenolone declines by as much as 60 percent between ages 35 and 75, resulting in a corresponding drop in estrogen—which, in turn, may cause memory problems. Taking a supplement of pregnenolone can help boost hormone levels and appears to improve thinking and recall, says Dr. Lark. She recommends 5 to 10 milligrams pregnenolone daily for women in their 40s; 10 to 15 milligrams for postmenopausal women between ages 50 and 65; and 10 to 20 milligrams for women over age 65. Women taking progesterone as part of a hormone replacement program may require a lower dose of supplemental pregnenolone, because the hormone is converted into progesterone. Pregnenolone is not a traditional therapy and, although preliminary evidence suggests that it is safe, further

## MOTHER NATURE, M.D.: ALZHEIMER'S DISEASE

*The herb ginkgo biloba has been thought to improve brain function. But does research support this assertion? Yes and no.*

A two-year study on the benefits of ginkgo biloba created a stir when the results were published in the August 2002 *Journal of the American Medical Association*. The research seemed to refute the claims of ginkgo supporters, concluding "ginkgo provides no measurable benefit in memory … to adults with healthy cognitive function."

Seems clear-cut. But hold on a minute, warns *Susan Lark, M.D.,* author of *The Chemistry of Success: Six Secrets of Peak Performance.* The key words in the conclusion may be "adults with healthy cognitive function."

"The people tested were normal—they didn't have memory loss," explains Dr. Lark. "The results showed no improvement because the subjects didn't have a problem in the first place."

So does ginkgo help to restore memory loss? Or prevent continued deterioration of mental function? The scientific jury is still out, and more trials are under way. A small study conducted in 1997 concluded that ginkgo "may be of some help in treating the symptoms of Alzheimer's disease and vascular dementia," but it also stated that ginkgo biloba was certainly not a cure for either condition.

Nevertheless, ginkgo biloba gets an enthusiastic endorsement in many sectors of the medical community. "Studies show ginkgo is beneficial if you already have Alzheimer's disease," says *Marilyn Albert, Ph.D.,* director of the Gerontology Research Unit at Massachusetts General Hospital and professor of psychiatry and neurology at Harvard Medical School.

While the efficacy of over-the-counter products may be exaggerated by advertising hype, most scientists agree that ginkgo biloba is a powerful antioxidant that blocks the effects of free radicals. It improves blood flow to the brain and boosts production of neurotransmitters, the chemicals that help brain cells communicate.

If you are experiencing memory lapses or simply want to take steps to keep your brain healthy, consider taking 40 milligrams ginkgo three times daily, suggests Dr. Lark. Ginkgo biloba is safe, she says, and its side effects are rare.

Be sure to let your doctor know if you're using this herb because it may increase the risk of bleeding, especially if you're also taking blood-thinning medications.

studies are needed to determine its long-term effects. Pregnenolone—or any other supplement—should be taken *only* with the approval of your doctor.

**Consider taking DHEA.** Short for the tongue-twisting chemical name dehydroepiandrosterone, DHEA is another hormone that is transformed into estrogen or testosterone. It's not clear how DHEA works, but one small study found that people who took it daily showed significant improvements on memory tests. Premenopausal women produce all the estrogen their bodies need, but Dr. Lark advises those who have reached menopause to consider taking 5 to 15 milligrams DHEA daily. DHEA can interact with some medications and may have side effects, so always consult with your doctor before taking this over-the-counter hormone.

## PARKINSON'S: THE SLOWLY ENCROACHING DISEASE

The initial symptoms of Parkinson's disease are so subtle that you may not even realize there's a problem. The first sign may be a slight shaking in your hands or even in just a single finger. Little by little, the tremors become more pronounced and can spread to affect your whole arm, your opposite side, or other parts of your body, such as the leg or chin. That said, as many as one-

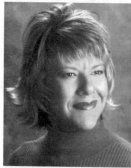

third of Parkinson's patients don't experience tremors at all, says *Jill Marjama-Lyons, M.D.,* a neurologist and Parkinson's specialist in Albuquerque.

As the disease progresses, your body movements can become slowed and less coordinated. Eventually, you may have serious difficulty with limb and facial movement, talking, and swallowing.

Doctors aren't sure what causes the condition, but this much is known: Parkinson's occurs when certain brain cells die. These are the cells that produce dopamine, a chemical that enables cells to communicate with each other. By the time a woman develops the motor symptoms of Parkinson's, up to 60 percent of her dopamine-producing cells have already died,

*Eating a healthy diet and taking vitamins B and C are important tools for preventing and treating Parkinson's, says neurologist Jill Marjama-Lyons, M.D.*

says Dr. Marjama-Lyons. As these cells continue to die and dopamine activity declines, your muscles are less able to make smooth, controlled movements.

Parkinson's disease can be genetic, however, experts believe the condition stems from multiple factors, both environmental and genetic.

Estrogen may play a role in protecting some women from Parkinson's. More men are diagnosed with the condition than women. And it occurs less frequently in postmenopausal women who take hormone supplements, compared to those who do not, says Dr. Marjama-Lyons. "There are effective therapies that allow people with Parkinson's to control motor symptoms and to live high-quality, independent lives," says Dr. Marjama-Lyons. "It is crucial to work with a neurologist who specializes in Parkinson's treatments and is up-to-date on the latest research and techniques."

Medication can either replace dopamine in the brain or help the existing dopamine work more efficiently. A more aggressive treatment is the surgical placement of electrodes into the brain, a procedure called deep brain stimulation. This procedure is beneficial to patients with disabling symptoms that are not sufficiently controlled by medication.

*When you have Parkinson's disease, immobility can lead to fatal injury. Exercise is key to staying fit.*
—*Katrina Gwinn-Hardy, M.D.*

A study is currently under way to explore whether certain drugs are helpful in slowing the progress of Parkinson's. Both commonplace and experimental drugs are included in the test, which is being conducted by the National Institute of Neurological Disorders and Stroke (NINDS) at the National Institutes of Health in Bethesda, Maryland. "Such a study is very much needed," says **Katrina Gwinn-Hardy, M.D.**, a neurologist and principal investigator in the Division of Neurogenetics at NINDS. "We have known treatments for symptoms, but this study may help us discover how to help people preserve the health of the nervous system."

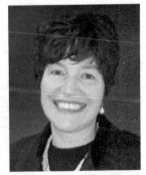

*Consult a physical therapist who can help you develop—and stick with—an exercise program that may enable you to stave off the effects of Parkinson's, says Katrina Gwinn-Hardy, M.D.*

NINDS is also spearheading research aimed at improving treatment for nonmotor complications of Parkinson's and side effects of prescribed medications. These include sleep problems, depression, cognitive impairment, and involuntary movement, which are often the most discouraging effects of the disease.

Together, research and existing therapies offer great hope for the future of Parkinson's treatment. "Most people with Parkinson's can live long, active lives," says Dr. Gwinn-Hardy. "They may die *with* the disease, but they won't die *from* it if they take care of themselves."

Here's what our experts advise to help you cope with Parkinson's disease.

**Exercise regularly.** Energy levels are unpredictable in women with Parkinson's, but don't let fatigue hold you back. "People who exercise do so much better," says Dr. Gwinn-Hardy. "They maintain their flexibility and have fewer falls—and it's the falls from lack of walking ability that often cause people to die because of this disease." Daily workouts are key to staying mobile. Try stretching and taking walks. Or simply make the deliberate decision to avoid elevators and to climb stairs instead.

**Work with a physical therapist.** If you're exceptionally self-motivated, it's fine to create your own exercise program and stick with it. Most people do much better with the help of a physical therapist for six months to a year. "The therapists I work with were able to get one of my patients out of a wheelchair and walking again," adds Dr. Gwinn-Hardy. "It makes such a difference if you have a dedicated physical therapist who will work with you."

**Eat a balanced diet.** This means consuming fruits and vegetables every day and limiting total daily fat consumption to about 30 percent of your total calories. Broccoli, spinach, grapefruit, and other plant foods that are loaded with vitamin C, beta-carotene, and other antioxidants may help curtail nerve-cell damage caused by free radicals, says Dr. Marjama-Lyons. Free radicals are suspected to play a role in the development of Parkinson's.

**Take B-complex supplements.** The family of B vitamins, which includes thiamin and vitamins $B_6$ and $B_{12}$, are essential for nerve health. "I advise any woman with Parkinson's to take a multivitamin that contains all the B vitamins, such as Centrum Silver," says Dr. Marjama-Lyons.

**Up your vitamin C.** In addition to its protective role as an antioxidant, vitamin C helps the body repair damaged tissues. Get the recommended 60 milligrams daily by eating vitamin C–rich citrus or other fruits and vegetables. For extra insurance, you may want to take a daily supplement that contains 500 to 1,000 milligrams vitamin C.

**Dine on fiber-rich foods.** A good way to prevent constipation, a frequent symptom of Parkinson's disease, is to eat plenty of legumes, whole grains, and other fiber-rich plant foods, says Dr. Marjama-Lyons. Fiber absorbs water in the intestines, which promotes regularity and makes bowel movements more comfortable.

**Drink, drink, drink.** Along with adding fiber to your diet, this simple approach goes a long way toward keeping you regular. Most women don't swig nearly enough water, in part because their bodies' thirst mechanism becomes less sensitive with age. Take in at least eight 8-ounce glasses of liquid daily, advises Dr. Marjama-Lyons. In addition to water, juice and sports drinks are good choices that provide vitamins and electrolytes, the elements and compounds necessary to maintain the body's metabolism. Sodium, potassium, and calcium are examples of electrolytes that could be found in a fortified beverage.

**Check out antidepressants.** Depression is a common and potentially debilitating consequence of coping with Parkinson's disease, says Dr. Gwinn-Hardy. Dozens of medications can alleviate symptoms of depression. A few may have an unexpected bonus: Researchers at Boston Medical Center discovered that some antidepressants may slow degeneration of valuable dopamine-containing neurons in the brain. As with other drugs that affect the central nervous system, antidepressants readily cross the blood-brain barrier, which makes them potentially useful for treating Parkinson's.

# 3 Breasts
## Beyond Mothers and Lovers

*Babies see food. Men see sex. Doctors see disease. Businessmen see dollar signs ... psychoanalysts place them at the center of the unconscious, as if they were unchanging monoliths.*

—Marilyn Yalom, *A History of the Breast*

Enough already! Your breasts belong to you, and what's important is how *you* feel about them. Unfortunately, if you're like most women, you think they're too big or too small, or you fret that they sag too much. And when you're not worrying about how they look, you worry about what's going on underneath: Could you have breast cancer?

Mental-health professionals say that how you feel about your breasts is a good indication of your level of self-esteem and self-worth. And because of the critical position breasts play in your role as a woman, you need to take care of them.

## BREAST CHANGES AND DISCOMFORT: TOO TENDER?

Female breasts are a work in progress. Their development begins in the womb, when cells become specialized for specific tasks, says *Marisa Weiss, M.D.,* a breast radiation oncologist in the Philadelphia area and president of Breastcancer.org. Some of those fetal cells then go forth and make breast glandular tissue.

Then they wait. Breast growth doesn't begin until about age 11, when estrogen levels rise, triggering hormone receptors in the breasts that send a signal to fast-track milk-gland growth. That's when a girl's breasts blossom, taking on a size, shape, and firmness that depend more on her hormones and heredity than on any gravity-defying bra or breast-increasing exercises.

Once menstruation begins, breast problems can also begin. Here's an overview of some of the most common ones.

- Cyclic fibrocystic changes, also erroneously called fibrocystic breast disease, which involves fluid-filled lumps called breast cysts
- Fibroadenomas: firm, rubbery, usually benign lumps

## CYCLIC FIBROCYSTIC CHANGES: EBB AND FLOW OF FLUID-FILLED LUMPS

"It's like a reminder: 'Attention, your period is on its way,' " says Daria Smith, a 38-year-old teacher in New Jersey, describing her monthly breast discomfort. Smith's problem is not unique. About half of all women experience symptoms of cyclic breast glandular changes, called fibrocystic changes, during their reproductive years.

Blood and other bodily fluids can accumulate in breast tissue throughout the menstrual cycle, especially in the two weeks before menstruation. The result may be swelling, tenderness, pain, and lumpiness—all typical responses to the hormonal changes that occur in a woman's body.

Why some women experience more severe symptoms than others is no mystery. "That's because breasts have structures called lobules and ducts, glands that respond to hormonal changes in the body," explains Dr. Weiss. "Some women's breast tissue responds more than others. Some have more estrogen receptors, some may have more sensitive receptors, while some women simply have more estrogen in their bodies."

Some women develop cysts, fluid-filled sacs that feel like lumps, in their breasts. Unlike cancerous growths, the cysts characteristic of fibrocystic breasts are usually in both breasts, are tender, and can move somewhat within the breast tissue when touched. Often these cysts grow larger just before your period in response to changes in your levels of the hormones estrogen and progesterone. In fact, the swelling can be so significant that some women need a larger bra just before their periods, says Dr. Weiss.

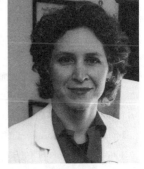

*A breast cyst is rarely malignant, says Marisa Weiss, M.D. Nevertheless, have your doctor check it out to know for sure.*

If you or your doctor discover a lump, it's important to make sure it's harmless. To do this, your doctor will examine your breast and may perform an ultrasound to see if the lump is a fluid-filled cyst or solid mass. If the ultrasound indicates the presence of a cyst—and it isn't bothering you—your doctor may just watch it closely to see if it stays the same, gets smaller, or goes away in a few cycles. She may ease a painful cyst by inserting a needle to remove the fluid, which collapses the cyst. That aspiration process can also be used as a diagnostic tool to distinguish cysts from other problems.

Breast cysts are almost never malignant, says Dr. Weiss. In fact, there's only a 1-percent chance that a cyst is cancerous. And having cysts doesn't increase your risk of getting breast cancer. Still, cystic lumps can be confused with cancerous lumps. "If you're a woman who has a lot of cysts, you should follow them over time," advises Dr. Weiss. "If one gets bigger, then you can have an ultrasound or needle aspiration to make sure it's okay."

## IMPLANTS: CHANGING YOUR BREASTS

*If you're not satisfied with the breasts you have, you can ask a plastic surgeon to give you the breasts you want. But there's a lot to consider before you go under the knife.*

In 2000, nearly 190,000 breast-augmentation procedures (not including reconstruction) were performed in the United States. About 94 percent of the women received saline implants, which consist of a silicone rubber shell filled with varying amounts of a saltwater solution. The remaining 6 percent received silicone-gel implants.

Silicone-gel implants are available only through clinical trials for women who meet strict criteria. Most are implanted in women who choose postmastectomy implants. The Food and Drug Administration called for a moratorium on the use of silicone-gel implants after defects were found. Thousands of women sued several implant manufacturers because their implants leaked, claiming the released silicone was responsible for autoimmune diseases, such as rheumatoid arthritis and lupus.

Most women who have their breasts enlarged are pleased with the results: They feel sexier and more self-confident. If you are considering breast implants, you're more likely to be satisfied if you carefully weigh the facts beforehand. Use your preoperative consultations to be sure you know what you want and understand the options and risks, says *Sharon Ann Clark, M.D.,* a plastic surgeon in San Mateo, California, and spokesperson for the American Society of Plastic Surgeons.

Think about these issues before making a decision.

**How big is too big?** "Women should stay within what's anatomically reasonable," says Dr. Clark. "Sizing is critical. Many women have misconceptions about what size they can comfortably handle." They need to consider if their skin can stretch enough to accommodate the breasts they want and, if they're athletic, how their performance will be affected. To help women experience what bigger breasts feel like, Dr. Clark encourages patients to experiment with models in her office. She says some patients buy a bra in the desired size and fill it with something, such as shoulder pads or water balloons, to simulate larger breasts.

"It's a lot easier to go from a smaller to a bigger implant," says Dr. Clark. If you originally get a big implant and decide later that you want

Consider these expert recommendations on coping with the discomfort of breast cysts.

**Pop a pill.** Over-the-counter medications, such as aspirin, ibuprofen, and acetaminophen, can offer relief from pain and inflammation, and are usually safe when taken as directed, says Philadelphia internist *Marie Savard, M.D.,* author of *How to Save Your Own Life.*

**Get hormone help.** "Believe it or not, such hormones as those in oral contraceptives can help because they provide for more balanced estrogen and progestin levels," says Dr. Savard. This is especially true for women with irregular menstrual cycles.

a smaller one, it's very hard to make the pocket smaller. "If the pocket is larger than the implant, then when the woman lies down, the implant will slide to the side, and there will be a wide depression between her breasts," explains Dr. Clark.

**Make an incision decision.** There's more than one way to put in a breast implant, and you can choose where the incision will be.

- Belly-button method: In this method, the surgeon makes an incision in your belly button and uses an endoscope (a flexible lighted tube) to maneuver below the skin to the breast area to insert the implant.
- Under the armpit: This approach sometimes uses an endoscope. An incision is made in each armpit, so there are no scars on the breasts.
- Areola and base-of-the-nipple incisions: These allow surgeons a great deal of control over implant placement. The scar is visible, but it tends to heal well.
- Inframammary-fold incisions: These incisions are made just above the fold of the underside of the breast. Surgeons have the most control when using this method, but the scar is visible. This approach is most often chosen by women who don't want an incision near the areola,

usually because they are concerned about their nipples and breast-feeding issues and less concerned with a scar underneath. When women have very small breasts, this method can be difficult because it's harder to predict where the fold will end up after the implant is in, says Dr. Clark.

**Consider the follow-up care.** According to a 1997 study, complications arising from silicone or saline implants require follow-up surgery within five years in approximately 12 percent of breast augmentations and about 33 percent of post-mastectomy implants.

**Mammograms: Still required.** Once you have breast implants, inform the mammographic technician that you have them so she can use the proper technique when imaging your breasts.

**It's a life-changing decision.** "Fat cells are fluffy," says Dr. Clark. "Once you put an implant in, you can't take it out and be exactly the same." That's because implants press against fatty tissue and compress it.

**Please yourself.** Choose what is pretty for you, a size that is flattering to you and your lifestyle. The decision is yours, not your partner's or a friend's.

**Use hot compresses.** Get relief with applications of a hot compress soaked in herbal oils. Available at health-food stores and from online suppliers, herbal oils typically have an olive-oil base and are soothing, as well as therapeutic. *Gloria Schwartz, N.D.,* of the Integrative Health Center in Ashland, Oregon, recommends poke-root oil for breast lumps. To make a compress, soak a soft cloth or washcloth in hot water with several drops of oil, then wring it out. Apply the moist cloth to your breast for 5 to 10 minutes. You can apply a compress several times a day. If you use castor oil or poke-root oil, make sure you wipe off your nipple before nursing, as the oil can give your baby diarrhea. Don't ever take herbal oils internally without consulting an experienced herbalist or naturopathic doctor, says Dr. Schwartz.

**Pass the peas, please.** Cold compresses, even a bag of frozen peas, can also help relieve breast pain, says Dr. Savard.

> *To ease painful breast cysts, apply a soft cloth soaked in hot water and herbal oil.*—Gloria Schwartz, N.D.

### FIBROADENOMAS: RECOGNIZING OTHER (USUALLY) BENIGN LUMPS

"It felt like a marble, rolling around near my nipple," says a 43-year-old woman, describing what she found while doing a breast self-examination. "I told myself it was probably nothing, but I called my doctor." It turned out to be a fibroadenoma, which is a firm, rubbery tumor that is usually benign.

When you discover any breast lump, your doctor will first examine it manually. If she suspects that it's just a cyst, she will try to prove it with ultrasound or by aspiration of the cystic fluid. If ultrasound shows that the lump is solid or aspiration yields no fluid, then it is probably not a cyst. Further evaluation is needed to make sure the lump is benign, like a fibroadenoma.

Fibroadenomas can be seen on a mammogram or ultrasound but cannot be diagnosed without a biopsy. To be certain that a solid lump is benign, your doctor may perform a core biopsy, in which she inserts a needle into the lump to collect several small tissue samples for analysis. This procedure is done under local anesthesia at an outpatient facility.

Or your doctor may recommend a Mammotome biopsy, a procedure that is performed either in a doctor's office or outpatient facility. With this type of biopsy, the doctor uses either ultrasound imaging or a computer to locate the suspect area, then inserts a needle to remove a tissue sample for examination. The small incision is closed with a bandage. A Mammotome biopsy is three times more accurate than a core biopsy, says **Susan Kaye, M.D.**, chief of family practice at the Overlook Hospital in Summit, New Jersey.

Which test or procedure your doctor chooses depends on the breast abnormality and the technology available in your area, explains Dr. Weiss.

## MOTHER NATURE, M.D.: TREATING FIBROCYSTIC BREASTS

*Diet and lifestyle choices may help you avoid some breast lumpiness every month.*

Naturopathic physician **Gloria Schwartz, N.D.**, of the Integrative Health Center in Ashland, Oregon, has a theory: "Much of the problem with fibrocystic breasts involves poor liver function." This prevents your body from breaking down and disposing of estrogen. In other words, your estrogen levels remain too high. Not surprisingly, high estrogen levels are also a trademark of other breast conditions, including breast cancer.

One of the secrets to treating fibrocystic breasts, says Dr. Schwartz, is to improve your liver function with diet. These are her recommendations for natural methods that may help:

**Cut out caffeine.** That includes coffee, tea, colas, and, yes, chocolate. Green tea is okay, as well as caffeine-free herbal teas. In one study, reducing caffeine decreased or eliminated fibrocystic symptoms in 61 percent of participants.

**Encourage elimination.** "There seems to be a correlation between chronic constipation and fibrocystic breasts," says Dr. Schwartz. So fill your diet with fiber-rich foods, such as whole-grain breads, pastas, and breakfast cereals; fresh fruits and vegetables; and such legumes as peas and beans. You should eat five or more servings of fruits and vegetables, as well as several of grains, cereals, and legumes daily.

**Don't shake the salt.** Excess salt promotes water retention, which leads to tender breasts by causing breast tissue to swell, putting pressure on surrounding tissue. Instead of salt, use herbs, spices, and lemon juice to flavor your food. Be wary of processed foods, which tend to be high in salt, warns Philadelphia internist **Marie Savard, M.D.**, author of *How to Save Your Own Life*.

**Trim the fat.** Some studies have found that a low-fat diet significantly reduces breast tenderness, swelling, and lumpiness in women.

**Try B6.** Vitamin B6 has a diuretic effect, enabling your body to rid itself of excess fluid, which can be the cause of swelling and tenderness in fibrocystic breasts. Dr. Schwartz recommends you take 50 to 100 milligrams vitamin B6 daily when your breasts are sore. Use B6 and other nutritional supplements only with the approval and supervision of your physician.

**Relieve pain with magnesium.** Dr. Schwartz reports success using magnesium to relieve breast pain in her patients. She recommends taking 400 milligrams when your breasts ache. If you experience diarrhea, cut the dosage in half.

Should you be concerned about a fibroadenoma? "It's just an exaggerated gland that has responded to hormones," says Dr. Weiss. She calls these tumors clinically insignificant and says they usually don't need to be treated or removed if the fibroadenoma diagnosis is certain.

## BREAST CANCER: EVERY WOMAN'S NIGHTMARE

Every three minutes, another American woman is diagnosed with breast cancer. Skin cancer is the only type that affects more women, and lung cancer is the only type that kills more women. In the United States, breast cancer claims the lives of more than a hundred women a day.

The enemy is the uncontrolled growth of damaged cells in the breast. The damaged cells multiply and form cancer. Breast cancers that stay only in the breast tissue are referred to as *in situ,* meaning in place. Most cancers of this type can be cured, but other forms of breast cancer are invasive. They can spread regionally to lymph nodes or other parts of the body, a process known as metastatis. Cancers require more vigorous treatment if they have spread.

Reasons for the cell damage that leads to tumors range from inherited genetic abnormalities to environmental toxins and, perhaps, even food choices. Estrogen also plays a significant role. Hormone-related risk factors for breast cancer include onset of menstruation at a relatively early age, getting pregnant later than age 30, reaching menopause at a relatively late age, or being overweight. That's why it's key to know what you can and can't control in terms of preventing breast cancer.

### ACCEPTING RISK FACTORS YOU *CAN'T* DO ANYTHING ABOUT

Did your mother ever tell you that you had to play the cards you're dealt? Well, that's partly correct when it comes to breast cancer. There are some factors that may increase the odds of getting breast cancer, but nothing is guaranteed. Having these risks doesn't mean you'll get cancer, nor does having none mean you won't get it. These are some of those risk factors over which you simply have no control.

- Age: About 77 percent of all breast-cancer cases in women occur when they are older than age 50. Nineteen percent are found in women in their 40s.
- Gender: More than 99 percent of breast-cancer cases are in women, but men can get the disease.

- Family history: Your chance of getting breast cancer is two times greater if your sister, mother, or daughter has the disease, compared with a woman whose relatives don't have it. That risk increases to five times greater if you have two of these relatives with breast cancer. Women who have a female fraternal twin have more than double the normal risk of developing breast cancer after menopause, according to a Mayo Clinic Cancer Center study. Investigators believe elevated hormone levels in fraternal twin pregnancies may increase risk for adults who were exposed to them in the womb. (The study found that, statistically, identical twins had no greater risk than singletons.)

## SHOULD I SEE A DOCTOR?

*Every woman should see a doctor for an annual checkup. But there are warning signs you can look for.*

These symptoms are red flags of potential breast disease that should send you to your physician, says **Marisa Weiss, M.D.,** a breast radiation oncologist and president of Breastcancer.org.

**Any abnormal, persistent lump:** Whether you find a lump during a shower or regular breast self-exam, have your doctor check it out as soon as possible. More than 80 percent of lumps turn out to be benign. But if it is cancerous, isn't it better to catch it early when you have the best chance to beat it?

**Any unusual, persistent pain:** This would be pain that is not related to fluctuations in your menstrual cycle. For example, if your breasts are normally a little tender before your period, it's not cause for concern. But if you experience a new kind of pain that persists, contact your physician.

**Any change in appearance:** Contact your doctor if one or both breasts display any of the following changes.
- A change in the size or shape of the breast
- Ridges or pitting of the skin that make it look like the skin of an orange

- Unusual, persistent rash around the nipple that can't be explained by nursing, clothing or soap irritation, or other causes
- A change in one or both nipples; for example, if your nipples are normally everted (stick out) and one or both become inverted
- A change in the look or feel of the skin of the breast, areola, or nipple (for example, warm, swollen, red, or scaly). This could include pink skin or open sores that don't heal. To be safe, see your doctor.

**Any nipple discharge not related to breast feeding:** Clear or milky secretions from both breasts are usually benign. A brown or red discharge may indicate an infection, benign tumor, and, in some cases, cancer. Your doctor may check the fluid for cancerous cells. Or she may do a ductogram, a type of mammogram that can reveal a growth inside the milk duct.

**Enlarged axillary (underarm) lymph nodes:** Enlarged lymph nodes on only one side may be due to trauma (even shaving) or infection, but it can sometimes be a sign of cancer.

- Early menstruation: Women who begin menstruating before age 12 are more likely to develop breast cancer than those who start later. That's because estrogen flows through their bodies longer, and breast tissue is especially vulnerable to estrogen exposure during adolescence.
- Late menopause: Women who go through menopause after age 55 also have estrogen circulating in their bodies longer, increasing their risk of breast cancer. Studies have found that women who experienced menopause before age 45 had half the breast-cancer risk of those who went through it after age 55.
- Race: Although Caucasian women have a higher risk of developing breast cancer than other ethnic groups, African-American women are 67 percent more likely to die of the disease than Caucasians. There are many theories about the causes of this difference, but nothing concrete. "It may be related to socioeconomic factors," says *Sue Joslyn, Ph.D.,* an epidemiologist at the University of Northern Iowa. "Another reason may be biological or tumor differences. African-Americans are much more likely to have 'hormone receptor negative tumors,' which are more aggressive, harder to treat, and more likely to recur." Breast cancer in African-Americans is typically detected in late stages, which may partially explain their higher mortality. Yet, in studies in which breast cancers in both African-American and Caucasian women were detected at the same stage, African-Americans still had a higher mortality, says Dr. Joslyn. Studies to uncover the reasons for these findings are under way.

## TAKING CONTROL OF RISK FACTORS YOU *CAN* DO SOMETHING ABOUT

To get a complete understanding of your risk for breast cancer, you have to look beyond such uncontrollable factors as age and family history. Diet, exercise, alcohol and tobacco use, hormone use, and weight are all risk factors you can do something about.

**Make breast-healthy food choices.** Experts agree that eating a healthier diet may be able to reduce your risk of breast cancer. What should you eat? *Marisa Weiss, M.D.,* a breast radiation oncologist in the Philadelphia area and president of Breastcancer.org., offers women the following advice.

- Choose organically grown fresh foods over processed foods. Limit your consumption of canned, frozen, and boxed foods that contain preservatives and artificial colorings and flavorings.

## ONE WOMAN'S STORY: BREAST CANCER

*An Arizona woman takes life in stride before and after her mastectomy.*

Hazel Masters is, as her friends say, one tough old broad. She earned that honorary title in December 1996, when the then-62-year-old underwent a so-called drive-through mastectomy. She entered the operating room at 8 a.m., returned home barely three hours later, and hiked five miles the next day. Tough broad, indeed.

The road leading up to that hike was a short one. A month earlier, Masters had seen her doctor for a routine gynecological exam. "The only pain I expected was in receiving the bill," she says. But that changed during her breast exam.

"I looked into my doctor's eyes, and her expression wasn't what I was used to seeing," Masters recalls. "She said, 'I feel a lump.' She took my hand and placed it on my breast. I felt the lump. I must confess I'd never given myself a breast self-exam."

Masters cried as she dressed in the tiny, sterile room. "What's to happen to me now?" she wondered. But she decided the question as she drove home that day: If it was cancer, she would do all she could to rid herself of it.

Masters certainly didn't fit the profile of a typical breast-cancer victim. She'd lived the model of a healthy life for decades: She didn't drink or smoke, had been a vegetarian for more than 30 years, got 8 to 10 hours of sleep every night, and exercised every day.

When the news came that she had cancer, she quickly decided on a mastectomy. "I've never regretted my hasty decision," she says. She had the breast removed on December 19, 1996.

The next day, Masters donned a baggy shirt and sweatpants, tucked the drainage tube and small plastic container used to collect the draining fluids under her clothes, and hiked one of Tucson's scenic trails.

In December 2002, Hazel celebrated six years of freedom from breast cancer. She never needed radiation or chemotherapy, but she did take tamoxifen, an antiestrogen drug many women take after a bout with breast cancer.

"I can truthfully say I was never angry about having breast cancer," says Masters. "Frightened, yes, but I never asked, 'Why me?'"

Her advice to women who are diagnosed with breast cancer: "It's not a death sentence. Strive toward a positive attitude, which I think is the most important thing. Take responsibility for yourself. Humor plays a big part in the healing process. Support groups are a must (she belongs to two). And never give up."

At age 68, Masters continues to live a healthy lifestyle, including exercising several hours a day, six days a week, just as she did before the surgery. "My oncologist says the reason I recovered so well is because I exercise," she explains.

Whenever Masters talks to others about breast cancer and her experiences, she meets women who say that they don't need to have a mammogram because there's no cancer in their families. That's when she gives them her "tough love" message. "I tell them somebody can be the first to have it in any family. And it could be them."

- Choose the majority of your foods from the plant kingdom: fruits, vegetables, and whole grains. These are generally low in fat and sugars but high in fiber.
- Avoid most dairy fats. Instead, eat nonfat or low-fat dairy products. Dr. Weiss reminds women that pesticides and hormones are concentrated in animal fat, so it's best to consume as little as possible.
- Substitute soy protein for animal proteins, says Dr. Weiss. Commercial meat and poultry may be from livestock subjected to supplemental hormones. Dr. Weiss suggests that you substitute organic vegetable proteins or buy only products that are certified hormone-free and raised on pesticide-free feeds, especially if you have had breast cancer.
- Avoid foods that contain added sugars, salt, or fat.

Why can these foods reduce your risk of breast cancer? Researchers don't have all the answers, but studies suggest that phytonutrients (plant-based chemicals) and antioxidants, found primarily in fruits and vegetables, have cancer-fighting powers. Fiber helps eliminate estrogen from the body (remember, too much estrogen is a factor in breast cancer). Pesticides, hormones, and other additives in meat and dairy products have cancer-causing abilities.

> *To reduce your risk of breast cancer, avoid processed foods in favor of fresh foods that are low in fat and high in fiber.*—Marisa Weiss, M.D.

Need we say more? Well, we will anyway. Results of a huge study (involving 35 countries) published in the January 2002 issue of *Cancer,* the journal of the American Cancer Society, show that a high percentage of daily calories from animal foods correlates strongly with an increased risk of death from breast cancer. A high percentage of calories from fruits and vegetables has an equally strong link to a decreased risk of death.

**Get a good workout.** Here's yet another reason to get off the couch. Three female Canadian researchers found that women who were lifelong exercisers had a 42-percent lower risk of breast cancer than women who were never active. It's never too late to start: They also found that women who started exercising after menopause had a 40-percent lower risk of breast cancer.

The study showed that frequency and duration of exercise are more important than intensity. The researchers recommend a daily regimen of one hour of brisk walking or two hours of moderate activity, such as heavy housework, gardening, or childcare. The recommendation for women who are more active in their jobs, such as waitresses, is a 30-minute brisk walk every day. Other studies show that the benefits of exercise are greatest in women who keep their weight proportionate to their height.

## A WOMAN'S RIGHT TO THE *RIGHT* TREATMENT: MAMMOGRAMS

*Consider these contradictory headlines:* "Mammograms Don't Save Lives" *and* "Mammograms Reduce Breast Cancer Deaths by 30 Percent." *Which should you believe?*

"Mammogram studies are complicated, and trying to evaluate them is very hard to do," says *Susan Harvey, M.D.,* assistant professor of radiology at the University of Vermont College of Medicine and author of a study on effective ways to use mammograms to detect breast cancer. "Some studies have been misrepresented by journalists. You can use statistics in different ways," she says. "That doesn't mean they're inaccurate: It's simply spin." And depending on how you spin the results, you can find studies that support the use of screening mammography and others that seem to refute it.

"I can't fathom not doing mammography," says Dr. Harvey. "It seems a huge step back to just wait until you can feel the breast cancer." Women should view mammography as a tool, just like breast self-examination (BSE) and a breast exam by a health professional are tools, she says. Used together, these approaches offer women the best chance of detecting breast cancer if it's there.

However, many women don't do BSE, and a mammogram may be the only screening tool they use. Dr. Harvey advises women to follow the American Cancer Society's guidelines: Women age 40 and older should have a mammogram and physical examination by a health-care professional annually. But this recommendation is controversial, says *Susan Kaye, M.D.,* chief of family practice at the Overlook Hospital in Summit, New Jersey. She recommends mammograms and a physical examination every other year for women in their 40s who do not have a high risk for breast cancer, with annual exams starting at age 50.

You can also ask your doctor to have your mammogram read more than once. At the University of Vermont, Dr. Harvey found that double reading of all screening mammograms increased breast cancer–detection rates nearly 8 percent.

Double reading of mammographic views is common outside the United States. In Europe, for example, one mammographic view is taken and double-read, but screenings are typically done every two to three years. In the United States, four views are taken annually and read once.

Double readings are not common in the United States, but you can request it. For now, you will likely be asked to pay for that service, warns Dr. Harvey. But the cost of such a reading is worthwhile, especially if it picks up a missed cancer.

**Quit smoking.** The role of smoking as an independent factor in breast cancer is controversial. One recent study suggests an increased risk of breast cancer in women who were heavy smokers for a long time. The highest risk was for women who had smoked at least 20 cigarettes a day for 40 years or more. Similarly, the Nurses' Health Study (a 25-year study of more than 120,000 women) showed a modest increase in risk for women who started smoking before age 17. Studies have shown that smoking increases the risk of developing and dying of other cancers, as well as heart disease and stroke. So it's healthier for you to quit.

**Skip that second drink.** The exact impact of alcohol consumption on breast cancer is unknown. While some studies suggest alcohol increases a woman's risk of breast cancer, others say it provides no additional risk. In a follow-up of the Framingham Study, in which more than five thousand women were followed for up to 40 years, researchers concluded that "light consumption (two to three drinks per week) of alcohol or any type of alcoholic beverage is not associated with increased breast cancer risk." Dr. Weiss tells her patients to limit alcohol consumption to no more than five drinks per week.

**Reconsider HRT.** Controversy surrounds the safety and effectiveness of hormone replacement therapy (HRT) and its connection to breast cancer. In January 2000, the Breast Cancer Detection Demonstration Project—which followed 46,000 women—found that a combination of estrogen and progestin (the typical HRT mix) may increase the risk of breast cancer beyond that of estrogen use alone. (Doctors can't prescribe estrogen alone, unless you've had a hysterectomy, because it significantly increases your risk of uterine cancer.) More recently, the Women's Health Initiative study of the health benefits of estrogen and progestin was canceled because scientists found a slightly higher incidence of breast cancer among women taking that form of HRT.

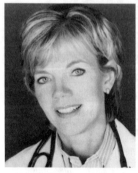

*Worries about breast-cancer risks don't have to eliminate HRT as a tool for managing symptoms of menopause, says Marie Savard, M.D. Short-term use at a low dose can be a good choice, she says.*

Wonder if hormone therapy is right for you? There are no easy answers. Philadelphia internist *Marie Savard, M.D.,* author of *How to Save Your Own Life,* believes that women and their physicians have forgotten what HRT was originally designed to do: relieve symptoms of menopause.

"If you're having symptoms that affect the quality of your life, then that should be key in your mind when thinking about hormones," she says. "We know they're effective for that purpose. But we're talking about short-term use, perhaps only a year, and taking as little as possible for as brief a time as possible." She believes many women could do fine on half the dose doctors typically prescribe. Find a doctor who will work with you to tweak your dosing, until you find the lowest dose that works

## EXAMINING YOUR OWN BREASTS

*When it comes to detecting breast cancer, a woman has to play a major role by carefully inspecting her breasts at least once a month.*

All the time you need to do a breast self-examination (BSE) is about 10 minutes once a month, preferably a week after your period ends. That's when hormone levels are low and your breasts less apt to be swollen and sore.

The American Cancer Society offers these easy guidelines for a self-exam:

• Lie down and place a pillow under your right shoulder. Raise your right arm above your head.

• Place the finger pads of the three middle fingers of your left hand on your right breast. Press firmly. (You may want to talk to your doctor or a nurse to help you decide how hard you should press. She can help you do a breast self-exam in her office so that you'll feel more comfortable and confident when you do it at home.)

• Move your fingers around your breast in a regular pattern. There are three common patterns from which to choose: 1) circular, in which you start at the nipple and move your fingers around in an ever-expanding circle, like a snail-shell pattern; 2) wedge, in which you start at the nipple each time, then move toward the outer edge of your breast in a sunburst pattern; or 3) up and down, in which you begin at the top of your breast, work down to the bottom, then move over about $1/2$ inch and work back up your breast. Each pattern is repeated until the entire breast has been examined. Always be sure to examine the tissue under your nipple as well.

• To examine your left breast, move the pillow under your left shoulder and use the same pattern to repeat the procedure.

• Stand for the rest of the examination. Place your right arm behind your head and use the finger pads on the middle three fingers of your left hand to repeat the chosen examination pattern on your right breast. When you're done, place your left arm behind your head and examine your left breast in the same manner. Some women do the standing part of the examination in the shower—it can be easier to feel any abnormalities in the breast when the skin is soapy and wet.

• While standing in front of a mirror, do a quick visual check of your breasts for any dimpling, redness, swelling, or changes in the nipple.

If you detect any lumps or other abnormalities during your examination, contact your doctor immediately.

for you, she suggests. (For more on menopause and hormone replacement therapy, see page 251.)

**Lose weight.** Being overweight increases your risk for breast cancer. A Harvard study of more than 95,000 women found that women who gain 22 to 44 pounds after age 18 have a 40-percent increased risk of developing breast cancer after menopause. The link between weight and breast cancer is estrogen. Abdominal fat cells produce estrogen, even after your ovaries shut down after menopause, so women who have a lot of weight around their abdomen tend to have higher levels of estrogen.

## SURVIVE AND THRIVE: TREATMENTS THAT WORK

Every year, more than 203,000 women are told, "You have breast cancer." After the shock, disbelief, anger, and fear move in, it's time to bring in hope.

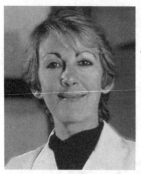

"Breast-cancer treatment today is very promising and is progressing very well," says *Carla I. Falkson, M.D.,* professor of medicine and medical director of the Breast Health Center at the University of Alabama at Birmingham's Comprehensive Cancer Center. "There are new things on the horizon all the time."

*Try to stay hopeful if you get a diagnosis of breast cancer, says Carla I. Falkson, M.D. Treatments are improving all the time.*

Surgery, radiation, chemotherapy, and hormone therapy are the most common treatments for breast cancer. Often, women and their doctors find that a combination of these therapies provides the best results. But each woman's treatment regimen is highly individualized and depends on such factors as age, severity of the cancer, type of breast cancer, other medical conditions, specialized test results, and the woman's own wishes.

For more information on current treatment options, visit the American Cancer Society's Website at www.cancer.org.

# 4 Digestive System
## Pipeline and Lifeline

*To eat is human; to digest, divine.*
—Mark Twain, American writer and humorist

You have to wonder about the wacky relationship we have with our digestive system. A good chunk of our day concerns food: earning money to buy it, shopping for it, preparing it—or finding others to prepare it for us—and, finally, ingesting it. After that, it's all downhill … literally.

Digestion begins when saliva jump-starts the process of breaking down foods to convert nutrients into the fuel that keeps the human machine running. It takes about 12 to 24 hours for food to travel the route we are all so familiar with, from mouth to esophagus to stomach to small intestine to large intestine to rectum to anus. Trouble is, things in the gut don't always go smoothly.

If your digestive system is off kilter, nothing else in your body is going to work the way it should. "The digestive system is really a second nervous system," says *Elizabeth Lipski, Ph.D., C.N.N.,* a clinical nutritionist in Asheville, North Carolina, and author of *Digestive Wellness*. And while we may think of neurotransmitters—chemicals that transmit messages to the brain—as existing only in our brains, there are many more in our digestive systems. So when women get stressed, they often feel it first right in their guts, says Dr. Lipski. That's why this chapter offers help with such common digestive problems as constipation and gas, as well as more serious conditions, such as inflammatory bowel disease and colon cancer.

## IRRITABLE BOWEL SYNDROME: CALMING AN UPSET GUT

The most common digestive problem women cope with is irritable bowel syndrome (IBS). Women are at least three times more likely to have this condition than men.

With IBS, your intestinal muscles don't contract properly. Instead of your intestines moving food through your intestines at a steady pace, they can push it through too hard and fast, causing gas, bloating, and diarrhea. Or they may slog it through too slowly, resulting in constipation. You can have cramps and diarrhea one day, with bloating and constipation the next. Mucus in the stool is also a common sign of IBS. Diagnosis can be a challenge and is based on having such chronic symptoms, explains *Charlene M. Prather, M.D.,* director of the Gastrointestinal Motility Center and associate professor of Internal Medicine at St. Louis University School of Medicine. There is no specific test for IBS.

The causes are varied, says Dr. Prather. Stress plays a role. So does overeating or eating foods that produce gas, such as beans, raw vegetables, coffee, chocolate, and fatty foods, as well as carbonated beverages. These can all make symptoms worse by distending the bowel, which causes abdominal pain. Additionally, about 4 in 10 people with IBS are lactose-intolerant, meaning they can't digest lactose, a sugar in dairy products.

Although IBS can be annoying and—as it's name implies—make you irritable, it can be prevented and relieved by diet and lifestyle changes. Follow the advice for managing constipation (see page 90), diarrhea (see page 93), or gas (see page 95), as well as these tips.

**Educate yourself.** Informed patients fare better, says *Lisa Ganjhu, D.O.,* assistant professor of clinical medicine at Columbia University College of Physicians and Surgeons in New York City. "Take control of the disorder and don't let it overcome you," she says, noting that there are many good IBS support groups and organizations online, such as the one run by the American Gastroenterological Association at www.gastro.org.

**Keep a diet diary.** "Sometimes, it's not what you ate an hour ago, but what you ate 12 hours ago that might be giving you symptoms," says Dr. Prather. To identify your triggers, record everything you put in your mouth for a week, including foods, beverages, mints, even gum. (Sweeteners, such as fructose, sorbitol, and mannitol, can cause symptoms in sensitive people.) Also chart any symptoms that occur—and the times that they occur—so that you can identify any links between the food and symptoms.

**Try an elimination diet.** Try eliminating known IBS-triggers—citrus fruits and juices, such wheat products as breads and pastas, dairy products, shellfish, nuts, soy foods, alcohol, and coffee and tea (both decaf and regular)—from your diet for one week. During that week, stick to foods that you're sure

## ONE WOMAN'S STORY: IRRITABLE BOWEL SYNDROME

*Heavy menstrual periods and cramps were a misery for one Florida woman until she discovered the true reason for her pain.*

From the time Joyce K. Reynolds, now a 56-year-old business coach in Fort Lauderdale, Florida, started menstruating at age 10, she had very heavy periods accompanied with bad cramps. The cramps got worse as she grew older. In fact, the pain sometimes sent her to the emergency room.

Doctors recommended taking painkillers, but apart from some minor relief from Motrin, an anti-inflammatory medicine, they didn't help. Stronger drugs might have dented the pain, but Reynolds didn't want to take anything that might cloud her thinking. Only her strong will kept the cramping episodes from controlling her life during the day. "I was such a controlled, Type-A dedicated worker that I wouldn't allow that to interfere with my work," she says. But willpower only delayed the inevitable. By evening, the pain she'd been holding back erupted, and she'd be in agony for hours, until finally getting relief when she had a bowel movement.

That important clue should have pointed Reynolds and her doctors toward the diagnosis of irritable bowel syndrome (IBS). "I didn't know that bowel activity was the cause of the pain. I just thought it was the result," she says.

Looking back, Reynolds realizes that although she did have menstrual cramps, "the majority of the pain and agony I went through was IBS." She believes that the stress associated with menstruation—she dreaded those heavy, painful periods—made her symptoms worse. Stress is a recognized IBS trigger, she learned, and IBS symptoms are usually worse at the start of a menstrual period.

The episodes continued even after Reynolds had a hysterectomy, which was supposed to cure her so-called menstrual problems. "Imagine my shock when I experienced the same cramping, all the same horrendous things," after the hysterectomy, she says. "Then, I was finally able to track it down."

Actually, the connection was suggested by Reynolds' sister, who had been diagnosed with IBS and was taking Levsin (hyoscyamine). Reynolds talked to her own doctor about the medication and got a prescription.

The medicine changed her world. "I started gaining confidence that I didn't have to be afraid of IBS," she says. And as long as she had those little pills with her, Reynolds remained free of attacks. She took yoga and tai chi classes to stretch and keep her body relaxed, and began to drink more water, which she believes helps her stay healthy.

Today, Reynolds is doing so well that she can't remember the last time she had an IBS attack. It still bothers her, though, that the medical profession didn't help her find the solution. "I encourage women to really be conscious of their own bodies, study their own symptoms, read, experiment, and follow their intuition," she says. "Frankly, we know a lot more about ourselves than any doctor could ever know."

don't trigger symptoms. These might include cooked vegetables, canned fruits, such nonwheat grains as rice and millet, and lean protein, such as chicken and fish, suggests **Susan L. Burke, M.S., R.D., C.D.E.,** director of nutrition services for eDiets.com. At the end of that week, reintroduce one possible trigger food or beverage at a time. If you remain symptom-free after three days, add that food or beverage to your okay list. Test each possible trigger in this manner. If a reintroduced food or beverage causes IBS symptoms, you'll know to avoid that food.

*There's a strong connection between your brain and gut. Finding ways to relax can make a huge difference in your symptoms.*—Lisa Ganjhu, D.O.

**Reduce stress.** "There is a very strong brain-gut axis," says Dr. Ganjhu. "Be aware of your body. Listen to it. Develop relaxation methods that work for you." Consider the patient who worked in a stressful job in the theater industry and had a 10-year history of abdominal pain and constipation: Her

## SHOULD I SEE A DOCTOR?

*Some digestive difficulties are benign and can be self-treated—or even ignored. But others can be signs of a serious illness.*

There are many different conditions that can cause problems in the digestive tract. See your doctor if you have any of these symptoms:
- Abdominal discomfort unrelated to eating
- Vomiting, weight loss, appetite loss
- Black, tarry stools
- Blood in vomit
- Severe pain in the upper right abdomen
- Indigestion, accompanied with shortness of breath, sweating, or pain that radiates to the jaw, neck, or arm
- Bloody diarrhea that lasts even a single day

- Diarrhea that lasts longer than a week; if you get dehydrated, have a fever, and severe abdominal pain with diarrhea
- A gallbladder attack with fever or pain that lasts longer than one to two hours
- Constipation or other changes in your bowel habits that persist for a few weeks
- Heartburn several times a week
- Flatulence that doesn't go away; if you're flatulent and feel full before you normally would; if you have pain, diarrhea, vomiting, weight loss, or other symptoms along with flatulence

pain would get worse around showtimes or deadlines. But her symptoms diminished when she started taking yoga. Another woman began walking for exercise and, with dietary changes, is now completely free of IBS-related constipation. IBS itself is stressful because it is unpredictable and its symptoms appear without warning, says Burke. Another management tip is to plan your day as far in advance as possible, allowing yourself time for activities so that you don't feel pressured or rushed. "You can't relieve yourself of stress 100 percent, but you can learn to cope with it," says Dr. Ganjhu.

**Be choosy about fiber.** The soluble and insoluble fiber in whole grains, vegetables, and fruits promote regularity, which is helpful for people with IBS who are constipation-prone. Many people with IBS, however, can't tolerate grains—not even bland oatmeal. If you have this problem, try other high-fiber options, such as pears, apples, bananas, strawberries, cooked beans, and ground flaxseed, says *Elizabeth Lipski, Ph.D., C.N.N.,* a clinical nutritionist in Asheville, North Carolina, and author of *Digestive Wellness.*

**Graze.** Switch from three large meals a day to six or more smaller, more frequent noshes. Smaller quantities are easier for your body to process and have less of an effect on your gastrointestinal tract, says Burke.

**Limit your fat intake.** A low-fat diet is also important because eating fat stimulates the colon and can cause pain after eating. Limit your portion sizes for fat in both animal and plant fats, advises Burke. This includes meats, poultry skin, vegetable oils, shortening, avocado, and whole-milk dairy products, such as milk, cheese, yogurt, and butter.

**Go for H₂0.** Drink at least eight 8-ounce glasses daily, says Burke. "You need water for digestion and elimination and to regulate metabolism," she explains. You'll also need water to move fiber through your system.

**Consider medications.** Certain medications can help treat diarrhea, control pain, or abort an attack of spasms, says *Alice Chang, M.D.,* an instructor at Harvard Medical School. These include certain antidepressants, such as Elavil (amitriptyline) and Norpramin (desipramine), as well as the antispasmodics Bentyl (dicyclomine) and hyoscyamine, which goes by numerous brand names including Levsin. Talk to your doctor about whether these medications are right for you, advises Dr. Chang.

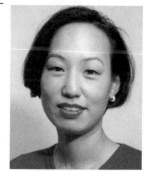

*Talk with your doctor about which medications will help control your IBS symptoms, advises Alice Chang, M.D.*

## INDIGESTION: YOUR STOMACH FIGHTS BACK

Indigestion is your basic upset stomach. In doctor lingo, it's also known as dyspepsia. The woman who has gastric or stomach discomfort may experience a variety of sensations, such as pain, gas, bloating, and nausea. It can be caused by eating too much, eating too fast, eating while stressed, eating too much fat, smoking, overindulging in alcohol, taking medicines that irritate the stomach, or just being tired and stressed.

To relieve indigestion, try these suggestions.

**Eat BRAT.** Until you feel better or can see your doctor, eat light and stick with easy-to-digest, low-fat, low-fiber foods, suggests *Lisa Ganjhu, D.O.,* assistant professor in clinical medicine at Columbia University College of Physicians and Surgeons in New York City. Try the BRAT diet, which takes its name from the foods it advocates: bananas, rice, applesauce, and dry (no butter or other spreads) toast.

*Try drinking ginger tea to soothe a stomachache. If you pick ginger ale instead, make sure it contains real ginger and not just artificial flavors.*
—*Elizabeth Lipski, Ph.D., C.N.N.*

**Go with ginger.** Health experts recommend using ginger to treat motion sickness, morning sickness, and nausea "because it works," says *Elizabeth Lipski, Ph.D., C.N.N.,* a clinical nutritionist in Asheville, North Carolina, and author of *Digestive Wellness.* You can take this natural nausea remedy in several ways: Chew fresh ginger from the produce rack (it is very spicy) or choose candied ginger for a more pleasant taste. Dr. Lipski suggests you brew up some ginger tea by pouring 1 cup boiling water over ½ teaspoon powdered ginger or two to three quarter-sized slices of fresh gingerroot; you can add peppermint to enhance the ginger's effect. Ginger capsules also work. Start with two capsules; if symptoms return, one to two capsules every four hours should do the trick, she says. Or drink ginger ale—just be sure the beverage you buy is made with real ginger, not artificial flavorings, or it won't have the same antinausea properties. If carbonated beverages make your stomach upset worse, let the ginger ale go flat before you drink it.

**Pick mint.** People have used mint to settle their upset stomachs since ancient times. You can chew fresh mint leaves, preferably from your own garden, suggests *Janet Gold,* a certified nutritionist in Lakewood, Colorado. Or you can drink one to two cups of peppermint tea to relieve stomach upset. To brew the tea, steep 1 teaspoon dried peppermint leaves in 1 cup boiling water for 10 minutes. Excellent organic teas are also available in bags, says Gold. Take note that many peppermint candies don't contain any real mint, so they may not help tame the turmoil in your tummy.

**Crunch on crackers.** Plain dry crackers or similar dry foods may be easier on your stomach than liquids because they soak up acids and reduce stomach upset. Choose whole-grain, no-sugar-added products, suggests Gold. A good choice is crispbread, which is a coarse, crackerlike product available at health-food stores that is excellent at soaking up offending substances in the stomach.

## HEARTBURN: FIRE DOWN BELOW

When the acid in your stomach backs up into your esophagus, you've got heartburn. The intense burning pain starts below your breastbone and sometimes radiates up to your throat. Experts estimate 40 percent of Americans suffer from heartburn at least once a month. It strikes pregnant women particularly hard; in fact, half of all pregnant women complain of heartburn during later stages of their pregnancies. (For more information, see page 363. The tips suggested to ease heartburn during pregnancy will also help when you're not.)

To prevent heartburn, experts recommend you take these steps, as well as those suggested for soothing ulcers (see page 80).

**Pass on peppermint.** Although peppermint can soothe an upset stomach, it is not recommended for people with heartburn, says *Lisa Ganjhu, D.O.,* assistant professor in clinical medicine at Columbia University College of Physicians and Surgeons. That includes mint-flavored antacids. Mint relaxes the lower esophageal sphincter (LES), a muscle that's supposed to stay closed—except when you're eating—to keep strong stomach acids from washing up into the esophagus.

*Peppermint may soothe an upset stomach, but it can aggravate heartburn. So avoid mint-flavored antacids.*—Lisa Ganjhu, D.O.

**Avoid known triggers.** Steer clear of foods that are known to trigger heartburn, suggests *Yvonne Romero, M.D.,* an esophagologist and assistant professor at the Mayo Medical School in Rochester, Minnesota. These include chocolate; coffee; tea; colas; mints; gum; alcoholic beverages; tobacco; such acidic foods as citrus fruits and juices; such spicy foods as chili and curry; onions; tomato products; and fatty, greasy, and fried foods. You may not have a problem with all of these foods.

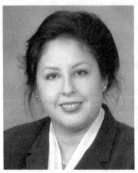

*It could be a bedtime snack that's causing your heartburn, says Yvonne Romero, M.D. Have your last bite to eat two to four hours before you go to bed.*

**Bend when empty.** You can make heartburn worse by bending over, lying down too soon after eating, wearing tight clothes, or otherwise putting pressure on your stomach when it's full, says Dr. Romero. She advises you to allow at least two to four hours after a meal before you go to bed.

**Lose weight.** Being overweight can put enough pressure on the stomach to push acid out. Picture your stomach as a balloon filled with water, then loosely tied shut. When you squeeze the balloon, you push some of the liquid out. If you take off those excess pounds, you take away the squeeze effect, says *Elizabeth Lipski, Ph.D., C.N.N.,* a clinical nutritionist in Asheville, North Carolina.

**Raise your bed.** Elevating the head of your bed can relieve nighttime heartburn, says Dr. Lipski. She recommends putting a 6-inch wooden beam under the head of your bed. It sounds uncomfortable, she says, "but the difference is barely noticeable, and the heartburn improves." Another alternative is to use a wedge between your mattress and box spring. Wedges are available at drugstores.

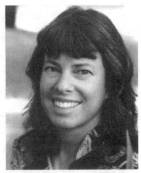

Drink a little cabbage juice every day to keep heartburn under control, suggests Elizabeth Lipski, Ph.D., C.N.N.

**Check your medicines.** Some medicines can cause or aggravate heartburn. These include birth control pills, progesterone, Valium (diazepam), nitroglycerine, and theophylline, notes Dr. Lipski. Aspirin, ibuprofen, naproxen, and other over-the-counter and prescription nonsteroidal anti-inflammatory drugs, as well as cholesterol-reducing statin drugs (including Lipitor, Pravachol, and Zocor), can also fuel heartburn fires.

> *It may sound uncomfortable, but a 6-inch beam placed under the head of your bed is barely noticeable—except for the relief it makes to heartburn.*
> —*Elizabeth Lipski, Ph.D., C.N.N.*

**Quit smoking.** As if you needed yet another reason to quit! Tobacco inhibits saliva, which helps buffer stomach acid, says Dr. Romero. It's also thought to stimulate stomach-acid production, while at the same time relaxing the esophageal sphincter, the muscle that normally prevents stomach acid from leaking out into the esophagus.

**Try cabbage juice.** Cabbage is high in glutamine, an amino acid (a component of protein) that helps the digestive system heal. "It may also contain other beneficial substances we haven't discovered yet," says Dr. Lipski. For this alternative treatment, she says ¼ cup cabbage juice each day is enough to provide a good benefit. Dr. Lipski says most people get relief within minutes. Since cabbage juice has a strong flavor, you may want to dilute it with other vegetable juices. Dr. Lipski suggests V-8 or tomato juice—unless, of course, you've discovered that tomato triggers your heartburn. Another mix she likes is carrot-beet-celery juice. "It can really dampen the taste of the cabbage juice," she says. Cabbage juice is available at health-food stores and some grocery stores.

**Sip slippery elm.** Native-American and European cultures used slippery elm bark as a gentle, soothing natural remedy for heartburn and ulcers, says Dr. Lipski. It is safe in large quantities, whether you prefer to take it in lozenge form, chew on the bark, or brew it as a tea. For tea, simmer 1 teaspoon slippery elm bark in 2 cups boiling water for 20 minutes. Then strain and drink as much as you want; sweeten, if desired. Slippery elm bark is available at health-food stores and some drugstores and grocery stores.

## GIRDING YOURSELF AGAINST GERD

If you have heartburn two or more times a week or your heartburn persists to the point of causing inflammation or irritation of the esophagus, you may have a more serious form of heartburn called gastroesophageal reflux disease (GERD). With GERD, that stomach-closing LES muscle is either weak, overly relaxed, or too often relaxed. Bottom line: It doesn't stay shut the way it should to keep your stomach's acidic contents from backing up into your esophagus, explains Dr. Romero. This backup is known as reflux. GERD can cause regurgitation, excessive salivation, and difficulty swallowing.

While medicines can help relieve GERD symptoms, many people use them improperly, explains Dr. Romero, and doctors may give inadequate instructions. Try putting out your internal fire with these suggestions, as well as the recommendations to soothe ulcers (see page 82).

**Start with antacids.** "The good part about antacids is that they work immediately," says Dr. Romero. "The bad part is that they last only about an hour." That's because once they've soaked up acid, they get flushed away when the stomach empties. "If you get a lot of acid at night, you might want to take your antacids right before you turn off the lamp," she suggests. Make sure the antacids you take don't contain stomach-irritating aspirin or heartburn-triggering mint, warns Dr. Romero. If you have problems with constipation, use Rolaids or other magnesium-based antacids because they will help you move your bowels as they relieve acidity. If you have problems with diarrhea, Dr. Romero advises you to choose Tums or other calcium carbonate–based antacids. These have a constipating effect and work well to absorb acid.

*If you don't get relief from reflux by using over-the-counter antacids, try OTC acid blockers, such as Zantac or Tagamet HB.*—Yvonne Romero, M.D.

**Choose a stronger OTC, if necessary.** "If you find yourself requiring several antacids every day, consider choosing an over-the-counter (OTC) H2 receptor blocker medicine, also known as histamine receptor antagonists," says Dr. Romero. "These medicines don't neutralize acid, as antacids do. Instead, they decrease how much acid your stomach produces." H2 receptor blockers are available in such brands as Axid AR (nizatidine), Mylanta AR (famotidine), Pepcid AC (famotidine), Tagamet HB (cimetidine), and Zantac (ranitidine). These pills must be dissolved by the stomach and absorbed into the bloodstream, then travel back to the blood vessels of the stomach where the medication can turn off the pumps that make stomach acid, explains Dr. Romero. Because this process takes time, she recommends you take these medicines on a regular, scheduled basis for optimal benefit. "It's most effective to take H2 blockers at bedtime, so I leave those on the nightstand," she says.

Or consider a combination medicine, such as Pepcid Complete, which contains antacid *and* an H2 receptor blocker. Take it every day to get immediate symptom relief from the antacid, plus longer lasting acid inhibition from the H2 receptor blocker, says Dr. Romero. "If you take your medicine like clockwork, over time you will develop a nice blood level of the drugs that will cut down on acid production," she says.

**Get a prescription.** Talk to your doctor if you still have nighttime acid breakthrough heartburn or reflux, even though you take an OTC H2 receptor blocker faithfully every day. It may be more economical for you to switch to a higher prescription dose of an H2 receptor blocker at that point, says Dr. Romero. Another prescription option is a proton pump inhibitor (PPI), including Aciphex (rabeprazole), Nexium (esomeprazole), Prevacid (lansoprazole), Prilosec (omeprazole), and Protonix (pantoprazole). A PPI is even better than an H2 blocker at turning off the pumps that produce stomach acid. Dr. Romero suggests the best way to take them: "You wake up, pee, take your pill, wait 20 to 60 minutes, then eat breakfast." This helps ensure that the medicine will work when your breakfast stimulates acid production.

**Try BESS or Stretta.** For either of these outpatient procedures, no incision is required. The doctor uses an endoscope, a tube that is threaded down your throat to your stomach. The Bard's Endoscopic Suturing System (BESS) uses a tiny device like a sewing machine attached to the endoscope to put stitches in the LES to draw it tighter, like a drawstring bag, explains Dr. Romero. With Stretta, microwaves scar the area between the stomach and esophagus to tighten it. Both procedures make patients feel better, but they do not actually stop reflux, says Dr. Romero. You still get the acid damage to the esophagus; it just doesn't hurt as much.

**Consider fundoplication.** Perhaps you don't want to take pills every day for the rest of your life, or maybe your insurance won't pay for them. If either is the case, you may want to consider a surgical option. The most common is fundoplication, a procedure for severe GERD in which the top of the stomach is wrapped around the bottom of the esophagus to tighten the lower esophageal sphincter.

## ULCERS: HEALING THE HOLE IN YOUR STOMACH

An ulcer is a sore in the lining of either your stomach or duodenum, which is the first section of your small intestine that connects to your stomach. At least four million Americans know the burning pain of an ulcer. And although duodenal ulcers historically have been a predominantly male complaint, recent data indicates that women now share the pain equally. Women may still be more likely to develop stomach ulcers.

Doctors used to think that stress, lifestyle, and a digestive-fluid imbalance created ulcers. These factors may indeed play a role and aggravate an existing condition. But research shows that the cause behind a majority of cases is either infection with the *Helicobacter pylori* bacteria or continued use of nonsteroidal anti-inflammatory drugs (NSAIDs), such as aspirin and ibuprofen, explains **Yvonne Romero, M.D.**, an esophagologist and assistant professor at the Mayo Medical School in Rochester, Minnesota. Other factors include such irritants as coffee, alcohol, and cigarettes, but the jury's still out on whether they cause, aggravate, or contribute to the development of ulcers, says Dr. Romero.

An ulcer usually announces itself with a burning pain in the upper, center abdomen, between your navel and breastbone. The fire often begins a few hours after a meal or in the middle of the night.

> *If you have belly pain that gets better when you eat, then you have an ulcer. If you have pain that gets worse when you eat, then you have reflux (heartburn and* GERD).—*Yvonne Romero, M.D.*

If you think an ulcer sounds a lot like heartburn and gastroesophageal reflux disease (GERD), you're right. Even doctors have a difficult time differentiating between the three, says Dr. Romero. The medical rule of thumb says that if you have belly pain that gets better when you eat, then you have an ulcer. If you have pain that gets worse when you eat, then you probably have reflux (heartburn and GERD). But real life isn't always that simple, says Dr. Romero—truth is, "there's no way to say based on symptoms."

To be sure that what you have is really an ulcer, your doctor may perform an endoscopy. Your doctor threads a thin, flexible tubelike instrument called an endoscope through your mouth and into your esophagus, stomach, and duodenum. A tiny camera attached to the endoscope allows your doctor to view and photograph your gastrointestinal (GI) tract. Your doctor may also pass small instruments through the endoscope to take a tissue sample.

Your doctor may perform a blood test to check for the presence of antibodies to *H. pylori.* Or she may test a stool sample or your breath. If the bacteria are found there, she will prescribe antibiotics to kill them. Usually, she'll prescribe additional medicines to help heal injured tissue.

There are many conventional and alternative remedies you can try to soothe your battered stomach. Try the suggestions for soothing heartburn (see page 75) and GERD (see page 78), as well as this advice from *Elizabeth Lipski, Ph.D., C.N.N.*, a clinical nutritionist in Asheville, North Carolina.

**Nix NSAIDs.** About 10 percent of stomach and duodenal ulcers are caused by regular use of NSAIDs, such as aspirin, ibuprofen, and naproxen, says Dr. Lipski. Acetaminophen, such as Anacin-3 and Tylenol, is gentler on the stomach than other pain relievers. Talk with your doctor about pain relievers.

**Drink lots of water.** If you drink four to six 8-ounce glasses of water when the pain is bad, it may disappear. "Diluting the stomach acids really helps," says Dr. Lipski. "There's no exact science, but it seems to work."

**Fix some flax.** Flaxseed helps ulcers two ways: Duodenal ulcers are associated with low levels of linoleic acid, an essential fatty acid found in flaxseed and flaxseed oil. And ground flaxseeds buffer excess stomach acids and ease inflammation. Flaxseed and its oil are sold at health-food stores, as well as some grocery stores and drugstores. Dr. Lipski recommends 2 to 3 teaspoons ground flaxseed daily.

**Munch on fruits and veggies.** One study showed that the risk of developing ulcers fell 54 percent in men who ingested the most vitamin A. (They ate seven servings of fruits and vegetables a day.) To get vitamin A in your diet, eat carrots, pumpkin, spinach, and sweet potatoes. If you want to take a supplement, Dr. Lipski recommends 10,000 to 25,000 International Units (IUs) vitamin A daily, but notes that pregnant women should not exceed 10,000 IUs.

*For alternative remedies for ulcers, you can try* DGL *licorice, aloe-vera liquid, or ground flaxseed.*
—*Elizabeth Lipski, Ph.D., C.N.N.*

**Try licorice.** Chew two to four tablets deglycyrrhized (DGL) licorice three times a day, recommends Dr. Lipski. Licorice helps heal the stomach mucous lining, but pure licorice contains a substance that can lead to an increase in blood pressure. It's been removed in DGL licorice "so you get most of the medicinal benefits of licorice root without unwanted side effects," says Dr. Lipski. DGL licorice is available at health-food stores.

**Add aloe vera.** This plant soothes and heals such mucous membranes as the stomach lining. You can find liquid aloe vera in health-food stores. Follow package directions for drinking this remedy.

**Go for glutamine.** The digestive tract uses glutamine, an amino acid, to heal stomach and digestive tract problems. Dr. Lipski suggests starting with 8 grams a day. If you find it helpful, continue at that dosage until you no longer have symptoms for at least a week. If symptoms are improved but not eliminated, either remain on the same dosage or increase it to 15 to 16 grams glutamine daily. If you don't experience any benefit at that dosage, see a doctor or naturopath. Some people require up to 40 grams glutamine daily. The most common side effect is constipation. Glutamine is sold at health-food stores and some grocery stores.

## GALLBLADDER DISEASE: WOMEN ARE AT GREATER RISK

Gallbladder disease develops when something obstructs or slows down the flow of bile—a liquid that helps aid digestion—on its way from the liver through the gallbladder to the intestines. A common culprit is a high-fat diet, says *Elizabeth Lipski, Ph.D., C.N.N.,* a clinical nutritionist in Asheville, North Carolina. Too much dietary fat makes bile sluggish and allows cholesterol crystals to form, which eventually clump together and form gallstones.

Fortunately, the majority of gallstones are "silent," producing no symptoms. Silent stones can be as small as a grain of sand. Large gallstones may be as big as a Ping-Pong ball and can cause severe abdominal pain that increases rapidly and lasts 30 minutes to several hours. The pain often resembles that of a heart attack and can be in your back and shoulders. You may also have nausea, bloating, and belching. If you also have sweating and fever, see a doctor immediately.

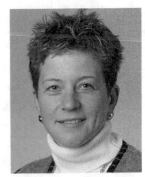

Every year, doctors perform about half a million surgeries to remove gallbladders when gallstones block the ducts, or outlets, through which bile flows or when the gallbladder is inflamed by bacterial infection or chemicals in bile.

Just being female puts you at higher risk of gallbladder disease, says *Lise Alschuler, N.D.,* clinical medical director at Bastyr University Center for

*Lose weight to reduce your risk of getting gallbladder disease, advises Lise Alschuler, N.D.*

Natural Health in Seattle. Being over age 40 further increases the risk. The following also put you at higher risk of developing gallstones.

- You are overweight.
- You have excess estrogen (such as from pregnancy, birth control pills, or hormone replacement therapy).
- You are of Native-American or Mexican-American heritage.
- You take fibrates, a class of cholesterol-lowering drug. (These medicines increase the amount of cholesterol in bile, which promotes gallstone development. The more commonly used statin class medications do not.)
- You have diabetes.

## PREVENTING GALLSTONES

Gallstones can be painful, so head them off before they become a problem.

**Skim off the fat.** Dr. Lipski recommends a diet low in fat, protein, and sugar, as well as high in fiber, to help prevent gallstones from developing. There's no one-size-fits-all rule for how much of these every woman should consume because "each person is individual," says Dr. Lipski. She recommends you gradually change your diet to learn what works best for you. Most women do well on a diet that emphasizes natural foods (rather than processed), with at least five to nine servings of fruits and vegetables per day. They'll also provide plenty of fiber. As for fats, the type matters more than the amount. "Avoid all hydrogenated or partially hydrogenated fats and shortenings," says Dr. Lipski. Those are typically found in processed foods, tub margarines, and many fried fast foods.

**Lose weight.** Being even moderately overweight raises your risk of developing gallstones, says Dr. Lipski. If your body mass index (BMI) is between 25 and 30, you're considered overweight. (To find your BMI, see page 479.)

**Don't crash-diet.** Shoot for a healthy weight-loss speed: no more than two pounds per week. "Don't decrease your caloric intake by more than 500 to 700 calories per day," says Dr. Lipski. Extremely low-fat, low-calorie diets actually increase your risk of developing gallstones, she notes, because sudden weight loss concentrates cholesterol in the bile. Fasting for more than 14 hours is also a no-no because it slows gallbladder movement. Moderate changes are healthier. Eat a bit less and move a lot more, advises Dr. Lipski.

**Exercise.** A scientific study found that 30 minutes of such vigorous aerobic exercise as running, jogging, and bicycling, five times a week, prevented gallstone problems in 34 percent of participants, reports Dr. Lipski. Couch potatoes were at greatest risk of developing the stones.

**Try alternative therapies.** The following may have some benefits.

- Lecithin: Lecithin makes cholesterol more soluble and, thus, less likely to form stones. Dr. Lipski recommends taking 500 milligrams a day of phosphatidyl choline, the most biologically active form of lecithin.
- Vitamin C: Researchers at the University of California at San Francisco found that women with low vitamin-C levels were at high risk for gallbladder disease. They suspect the reason is because ascorbic acid (vitamin C) helps convert cholesterol into bile acids. To correct the deficiency, experts recommend eating one large orange each day or taking 1 to 3 grams vitamin-C supplement. Reduce the dose if you experience diarrhea, says Dr. Lipski.

## TREATING GALLSTONES

The good news about gallstones is they don't always cause a crisis. Even if an ultrasound detects gallstones, you don't need treatment if you don't have symptoms, says *Lisa Forman, M.D.*, assistant professor of medicine in the department of gastro-enterology and hepatology at the University of Colorado Health Science Center in Denver.

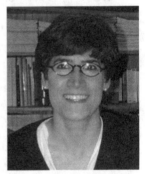

*Don't ignore your gallstone symptoms, advises Lisa Forman, M.D. Once the pain starts, it won't go away without treatment.*

Many people who have gallstones don't have any symptoms. But once you *do* start having symptoms, "it's likely your symptoms will continue," coming back again and again, says Dr. Forman. That's the signal that you'll eventually have to do something about them. And that's when you and your doctor will decide which treatment best suits you and your individual medical circumstances.

Before deciding to begin treatment, Dr. Forman looks for these classic gallstone symptoms of a condition known in doc-talk as biliary colic.

- Chronic, episodic pain, meaning you have bouts of pain that recur, sometimes within a few hours and sometimes not until years later
- Pain located in midabdomen (sometimes radiating to the right shoulder)
- Sudden onset, often immediately following a meal, especially if you've eaten foods high in fat
- Pain that increases to a peak and then declines gradually over several hours

"Often, people are referred for gallstones surgery because they had an abnormal liver function test," but that doesn't mean they have gallstones, explains Dr. Forman. She sees too many patients whose doctors inappropriately performed gallbladder operations when patients actually had liver disease. She cautions women not to rely solely on abnormal liver function tests to tell you that you need gallbladder treatment. If you're not having classic gallbladder symptoms, ask your doctor to check for other conditions that could cause abnormal test results.

*Don't agree to surgery just because you had one abnormal liver function test. If you're not having symptoms, ask your doctor to check for other conditions.—Lisa Forman, M.D.*

Almost everyone who gets gallbladder treatment eventually has surgery, says Dr. Forman. It may be an emergency if a gallstone perforates the gallbladder or there is infection, blocked bile ducts, or pancreatitis. You can't self-diagnose, she cautions, though usually you'll have a fever, feel rotten, and be in pain with nausea or vomiting, and your skin may turn yellow.

Before the 1990s, gallbladder removal meant surgery with a 5-inch incision. Today, many people can have laparoscopic surgery that requires only four tiny incisions in the abdomen and a short recovery time. If you opt for laparoscopic gallbladder removal, ask how many procedures your doctor has done—the more the better. "You don't want an untrained surgeon doing your laparoscopic gallbladder removal," advises Dr. Forman.

## DIVERTICULOSIS: MORE FIBER IS KEY

Diverticulosis is a condition that belongs to modern times: It was first noticed around 1900, about the time that processed foods were introduced into the American diet. Today, probably because our diets are so low in fiber, diverticulosis affects about half of all Americans by age 60, says *Jan Rakinic, M.D.*, a colorectal surgeon and associate professor of surgery at Southern Illinois University School of Medicine in Springfield.

Diverticula are small pouches that develop in the wall of the colon. These are weak spots that bulge out when the colon has to work too hard to push along small, hard stools. Once the pouches form, they never go away, notes *Elizabeth Lipski, Ph.D., C.N.N.*, a clinical nutritionist in Asheville, North Carolina, and author of *Digestive Wellness*.

Fortunately, most people don't experience pain with diverticulosis. But you may be constipated, have more gas than usual, and have a little discomfort in your lower left abdomen.

If the diverticula become inflamed or infected, trouble begins. Now you've moved into a condition known as diverticulitis, which can cause sudden and intense abdominal pain.

Luckily, fewer than 25 percent of those with diverticulosis ever develop diverticulitis, says Dr. Rakinic. Most first-time diverticulitis patients who have acute symptoms can recover with intravenous antibiotics and food restrictions. If these don't help, some people need surgery to remove an inflamed section of the colon.

When inflammation is mild, you may be able to prevent further attacks. The main treatments are increased fluid and fiber intake, says Dr. Rakinic. Combined, the two make stools bigger and softer so that it's easier for the colon to push them through.

To prevent diverticulosis and cope with diverticulitis, follow the tips for coping with constipation (see page 90), as well as this advice.

**Feed yourself with soft fiber.** When you're recovering from a diverticulitis flare-up, soft-fiber foods are easier to tolerate than raw foods and whole grains. Stick to cooked vegetables and fruits, vegetable soups, and such easy-to-digest grains as oatmeal, suggests Dr. Lipski. After the flare-up subsides, your everyday diet should contain lots of fruits, vegetables, whole grains, and legumes.

**Be prepared for surgery.** With proper management—fluid, fiber, and avoidance of problem foods—most people never require surgery, says Dr. Rakinic. But if you have repeated diverticulitis attacks, you'll probably need surgery at some point to remove the part of the colon where the inflamed diverticula are located, she explains. The surgeon cuts out the problematic part and reconnects the ends. It may sound drastic, but by the time you've had several attacks, your colon is so scarred that the next attack could cause a perforation in the colon wall and an abdominal infection known as peritonitis. If that happens, it's a surgical emergency.

## INFLAMMATORY BOWEL DISEASE: A CONSTELLATION OF PAIN

The two forms of inflammatory bowel disease (IBD) are ulcerative colitis and Crohn's disease. About two million Americans have IBD, women and men in equal numbers. With this autoimmune disease, the immune system attacks a part of the body as if it were a foreign invader. IBD usually starts between ages 15 and 40. Medical science doesn't know what triggers the problem.

Ulcerative colitis is a disease that causes inflammation and sores in the lining of the colon and rectum. It produces bloody diarrhea and stools containing mucus or pus. Flares vary in frequency and severity, and may be accompanied with a fever and abdominal pain. Treatment focuses on getting the disease under control, then controlling the flares, says *Ellen J. Scherl, M.D.,* assistant professor of medicine at Cornell University and director of the Inflammatory Bowel Disease Center at New York Presbyterian Hospital.

Crohn's disease is similar to ulcerative colitis but can show up in any part of the digestive tract from mouth to anus. It most commonly affects the end of the small intestine, resulting in pain in the lower right side of your abdomen. Symptoms vary widely, depending on what part of the digestive system Crohn's affects, but commonly include cramping, abdominal pain, diarrhea, fever, weight loss, bloating, rectal bleeding, and joint pain. As with ulcerative colitis, Crohn's attacks vary in frequency and severity.

*Talk with your doctor to make sure you are getting a strong enough dosage of medicine to keep your IBD symptoms at bay. Keep taking your medicine even when you aren't having symptoms.*—Ellen J. Scherl, M.D.

To control symptoms for ulcerative colitis and Crohn's disease, follow the tips for managing diarrhea (see page 93), as well as this advice.

**Educate yourself.** Don't count on your doctor to know the latest. Find out everything you can about your condition, says *Ritu Verma, M.D.,* section chief of clinical gastrointestinal services at Children's Hospital in Philadelphia. An excellent starting point is the Crohn's & Colitis Foundation of America (www.ccfa.org, 800-932-2423).

**Maximize medication.** "Talk to your doctor and make sure you're taking the maximum medication," says Dr. Scherl. Too often, patents reduce their doses on their own as soon as they feel better, she says. Medications are used to not only treat acute symptoms, but also to keep them away so that you have periods when you are symptom-free. Commonly used drugs are Azulfidine (sulfasalazine), Colazal (balsalazide), and Dipentum (olsalazine). Your doctor may also suggest using steroid and aminosalicylate enemas and suppositories to treat inflammation in the lower large intestine or rectum. For more severe cases or during a flare-up, stronger drugs are used to calm the immune system. These medications include Deltasone (prednisone), Entocort (budesonide), Folex (methotrexate), Imuran (azathioprine), Medrol (methylprednisolone), Orasone (prednisone), Prednisolone (prednisone), Purinethol (mercaptopurine), Rheumatrex (methotrexate), and Solu-Medrol (methylprednisolone).

*It's fine to take probiotic and omega-3 fatty acid supplements with your prescription medications for managing IBD.*
*—Elizabeth Lipski, Ph.D., C.N.N.*

**Avoid fiber during flares.** When you're feeling well, eat as much fiber as you can, but when you're having a flare or feel one coming on, fiber can make your symptoms worse, says Dr. Scherl. While you're in danger of a flare, avoid nuts, raw fruits and vegetables, corn hulls, and seeds. Stick to mild or steamed foods, such as bananas, potatoes, and rice.

**Try probiotics.** Beneficial bacteria—such as *Lactobacillus acidophilus, Bifidobacterium,* and *Saccharomyces boulardii*—can help ease IBD symptoms by restoring the balance of good and bad bacteria in the digestive system, says *Elizabeth Lipski, Ph.D., C.N.N.,* a clinical nutritionist in Asheville, North Carolina. Look for a probiotic supplement that contains both *L. acidophilus* and *Bifidobacterium* (it may contain others as well), she suggests. While you're having symptoms, Dr. Lipski suggests you take two capsules, three times per day (for a total of six per day); if you're using the powder, take a total of ½ to 1 teaspoon each day, divided into two or three doses per day. For general maintenance, Dr. Lipski recommends one to two capsules or ⅛ to ¼ teaspoon powdered probiotic supplement per day. It's fine to take probiotics with prescription medications and omega-3 fatty acid supplements, she says.

**Get enough omega-3.** Omega-3 fatty acids may help reduce the injuries IBD causes in the digestive system, says Dr. Verma. Eat salmon or mackerel three times a week to get your dose. Or take at least 1,000 milligrams omega-3 supplements daily. If you have IBD, you may increase that up to 3 to 4 grams daily, says Dr. Verma.

## CONSTIPATION: GETTING THINGS MOVING AGAIN

Even if you think you're as regular as clockwork, your personal plumbing may be more sluggish than you realize. For the average American, it typically takes 36 to 72 hours for food to complete its route through the digestive system. That doesn't sound bad until you learn that the optimal stool transit time is 12 to 18 hours—that's one-third to one-fourth less than the national average, says *Elizabeth Lipski, Ph.D., C.N.N.,* a clinical nutritionist in Asheville, North Carolina. A healthy transit time for food, she says, is 12 to 24 hours. Longer than 24 hours, and you're probably constipated.

Constipation is sometimes a symptom of a medical condition, such as an underactive thyroid gland, irritable bowel syndrome, diverticular disease, or colon cancer. But a lot of constipation stems from our habits, says *Jan Rakinic, M.D.,* a colorectal surgeon and associate professor of surgery at Southern Illinois University School of Medicine in Springfield. Correct those habits, and the problem goes away.

Take this advice to curtail your constipation.

**Don't rely on laxatives.** If you overuse laxatives to correct the problem, your digestive system can become dependent on them, leaving you worse off than before. Instead, focus on eating enough fiber, drinking enough water, and getting enough exercise.

**Drink plenty of water.** Make it least 48 ounces a day—extra, if you're drinking caffeinated beverages, because they can be dehydrating. Taking in lots of fluid makes stools softer and easier to pass, says *Ritu Verma, M.D.,* section chief of clinical gastrointestinal services at Children's Hospital in Philadelphia.

**Feast on fiber.** Eat lots of high-fiber foods, such as oatmeal, bran, and fresh fruits and vegetables. Fiber makes stools softer, bulkier, and easier to pass without straining, and increases bowel movement frequency. If you can consume 25 to 30 grams fiber a day, bowel movements should be a breeze. (For more information on high-fiber foods, see page 489). "Wheat germ is an excellent source of fiber," says Dr. Verma. "You can sprinkle it on yogurt, ice cream, salads, and other foods, or you can add it to baked foods." If you're already eating fruits, vegetables, and bran, then taking 2 to 4 tablespoons wheat germ daily is enough. If you're not getting other fiber, increase the amount of wheat germ you eat. You can't get too much, adds Dr. Verma.

**Go slow.** "It's important to add fiber to your diet slowly," notes Dr. Lipski. "Going too fast can cause gas and bloating." How slow? There's no set schedule to follow when you're adding fiber because each person's body is different. "Most people won't have any problems," she says, but if you experience any discomfort or negative changes in bowel habits, "just back off a bit and remember to drink plenty of water and exercise regularly."

*Psyllium is a natural laxative that you can't become dependent on. If you're a new user, avoid gas by starting with the minimum recommended dose and gradually increase to 1 teaspoon at each meal.—Elizabeth Lipski, Ph.D., C.N.N.*

**Try psyllium seeds.** Psyllium seeds and psyllium-seed husks add bulk and attract water to stools so that waste is easier to pass. Psyllium is available at health-food stores and as the main ingredient in such fiber supplements as Metamucil and Perdiem. "I tell my patients to use Metamucil or one of the other fiber supplements on the market, once a day, every day," says Dr. Rakinic. Follow the directions on the label.

Don't think of a fiber supplement as a laxative, but as a healthy way to add bulk to aid digestion. Since it is a natural product, the benefits come without causing a laxative dependency. Plus, psyllium doesn't irritate the digestive system, notes Dr. Lipski. Sudden increases in psyllium can cause gas and cramps, so she recommends building your tolerance gradually. Start with the minimal dose recommended on the package until you can handle 1 teaspoon psyllium with each meal. Fiber soaks up water, so you should drink 8 ounces water with psyllium.

**Exercise every day.** Make sure you get 30 minutes of exercise, whether you walk, do step aerobics, or ride a bike. Exercising helps move solid waste through the digestive tract, says Dr. Verma.

> *Keep your digestive tract moving with 30 minutes of exercise every day.*
>
> —*Ritu Verma, M.D.*

**Retrain your bowel.** If you rely on laxatives—even herbal laxatives and enemas—your bowels can become lazy and dependent on these aids, warns Dr. Lipski. You may wind up needing more and more laxative to get the needed results. Instead of taking laxatives, retrain your body to move your bowels regularly by sitting on the toilet and relaxing for up to 20 minutes each morning. Over time, your body will remember how to function without laxatives. Once you're retrained, take time for a bowel movement each morning.

**Heed the call.** Never ignore the urge to move your bowels. The longer a stool stays in the digestive tract, the more moisture it loses and the harder it is to pass, explains Dr. Rakinic. If you get in the habit of ignoring the urge, you may become constipated.

**Check medication package inserts.** Some medicines can cause constipation as a side effect. These include narcotic pain medicines, calcium and iron supplements, and some high blood pressure medications.

**Consider magnesium.** If none of the suggestions above work for you, try taking magnesium, suggests Dr. Lipski. First, talk to your health-care provider about trying magnesium, especially if you have any kidney problems. This mineral helps normalize intestinal contractions to move waste out quickly. Signs you might need more magnesium include insomnia, muscle weakness, sensitivity to noise, tendency to startle easily, and muscle twitches, especially in such small muscles as the eyelids. Start with 400 to 600 milligrams each day and increase gradually, if needed. Foods rich in magnesium include bulgur, spinach, yellow cornmeal, beans, and tomato paste.

# DIARRHEA: COPING WITH THE RUNS

It's no fun having diarrhea, but it may actually be good for you. The body uses diarrhea as a method of quickly removing whatever's making it sick—whether the offender is bacteria you picked up from a dirty diner, a virus, a food that disagreed with you, or something else.

Technically, diarrhea is defined as an abnormal looseness of the stool. It may include changes in stool frequency, consistency, urgency, and continence, says **Christina M. Surawicz, M.D.**, professor of medicine at the University of Washington Harborview Medical Center in Seattle and former president of the American College of Gastroenterology. "It can be fairly common," she says.

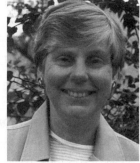

*Diarrhea isn't usually serious. But you should see your doctor if it lasts longer than a week or if you become dehydrated, says Christina M. Surawicz, M.D.*

In fact, worldwide, diarrheal diseases are among the leading causes of disease and death. In the United States, diarrhea is the second most commonly reported illness, after respiratory infections, says Dr. Surawicz.

The following are three main types of diarrhea.

- Bloody diarrhea: This may be a symptom of inflammatory bowel disease or other types of colitis, severe infection, or diverticulitis. See your doctor if you experience even one day of bloody diarrhea.

- Fatty diarrhea: This can be a symptom of celiac sprue (a bowel disease that prevents fat absorption from the intestinal walls) or malabsorption due to pancreatic disease. It's not always easy to tell if you have fatty diarrhea, known as steatorrhea, so your best bet is to have your doctor order special tests to measure stool fat, says Dr. Surawicz. In the meantime, these are clues that indicate you might have fatty diarrhea: if stools appear greasy, if you see oily droplets on the toilet bowl water, or if you have to flush the toilet more than once to remove the waste. See your doctor if you experience more than a week of fatty diarrhea.

- Watery diarrhea: This can be caused by many things, including a viral infection, food poisoning, intestinal infection, stomach flu, or medication or food or drink that didn't agree with you. See your doctor if you experience more than one week of watery diarrhea.

A brief bout of mild, uncomplicated diarrhea isn't usually serious. But if you have fever or severe abdominal pain, you become dehydrated, or symptoms last longer than a week, Dr. Surawicz recommends seeing your doctor.

Remember this advice when you have diarrhea.

**Check before you medicate.** "Diarrhea is the body's way of getting rid of something disagreeable: food, microbes, or toxins," says *Elizabeth Lipski, Ph.D., C.N.N.,* a clinical nutritionist in Asheville, North Carolina. The faster the bad stuff gets out, the sooner you'll get better. If you can't wait and plan to take an antidiarrhea medicine, check with your doctor first to be sure it's safe for your symptoms. Such medicines as Lomotil (diphenoxylate and atropine) and Imodium (loperamide) that slow gut motility (movement that pushes waste out) should not be used for diarrhea caused by invasive bacteria or toxins, says Dr. Surawicz. She cautions you to suspect dysentery caused by bacteria or toxin if you have bloody stools, fever, abdominal pain and cramps, or tenesmus (a symptom of rectal inflammation that makes you feel as if you have to go to the bathroom, but only small amounts come out when you do).

**Eat bland and binding foods.** The BRAT diet gets its name from bananas, rice, apples, and toast (dry). It settles indigestion and upset stomach, and also helps relieve diarrhea because these foods are "bland and binding," says Dr. Lipski. Other good choices: soda crackers, chicken (baked or roasted, without skin or fat), and eggs.

**Avoid dairy products.** When you have any type of diarrhea, it can be initially harder to digest products that contain lactose, which is the main sugar in milk. Stick to the BRAT diet and avoid dairy products until you feel better. Lactose intolerance can also be the cause of diarrhea. If your diarrhea goes away when you remove dairy products from your diet, talk to your health-care provider about whether you might be lactose-intolerant. (For more information, see "Lactose Intolerance: Mad-at-Cows Disease," page 97.)

**Avoid artificial sweeteners.** Mannitol, sorbitol, and xylitol are used to sweeten sugar-free soft drinks, candies, and gum. Even small amounts can cause diarrhea in people who are sensitive to these substances, says Dr. Lipski.

**Try probiotics.** There are more than 500 different types of bacteria in the gut. Some are neutral, some are beneficial, and others can cause disease. Good bacteria help digest food and even manufacture vitamins. Bad bacteria generate bloating, diarrhea, and other problems, including symptoms of irritable bowel syndrome (IBS) and inflammatory bowel disease (IBD). Probiotics are supplements that contain beneficial bacteria, such as *Lactobacillus acidophilus* or *Bifidobacteria.* They are available without prescription at health-food stores and drugstores. These beneficial bacteria treat diarrhea by combating the overgrowth of harmful bacteria in the gut that is typical of traveler's diarrhea and antibiotic-induced diarrhea, says **Cynthia Rudert, M.D.**, an Atlanta gastroenterologist. Look for a probiotic supplement that contains both *acidophilus* and *Bifidobacteria* (it may contain others as well), suggests Dr. Lipski. She recommends you take freeze-dried, refrigerated supplements for the best potency. While you're having symptoms, take two capsules, three times a day (for a total of six per day). If you're taking the powder, she advises you take a total of ½ to 1 teaspoon each day, divided into two or three doses. If you still have symptoms,

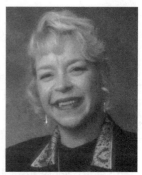

Taking an OTC probiotic supplement can help clear up a typical case of diarrhea, suggests Cynthia Rudert, M.D.

make sure you see your physician to rule out other disorders that involve gas and bloating.

**Check the label.** Taking an excess of vitamin C and magnesium—including antacids that contain magnesium salts—can cause diarrhea, notes Dr. Lipski. If you have diarrhea but no other symptoms of illness, try cutting back on these supplements. If that stops the problem, stick with the reduced dosage.

**Stay hydrated.** Drink plenty of fluids to avoid becoming dehydrated, a common side effect of diarrhea. Sip tepid water or any other liquid that you can tolerate, avoiding milk and caffeinated beverages.

## FLATULENCE: ABOUT THE GAS WE PASS

There must be dozens of euphemisms for—and hundreds, maybe thousands, of jokes about—this perfectly natural occurrence. Flatulence is simply air that has accumulated in the large intestine. When expelled, it is known as flatus. (Releasing air in the digestive tract upward through the mouth is called belching or, in doctor-speak, eructation.)

Causes of flatulence can include bacteria acting on undigested food, high-fiber foods, air swallowed while eating, foods our bodies can't digest (such as in lactose intolerance), pancreatic disease, irritable bowel syndrome, malabsorption, antibiotics, and diverticular disease.

Most people pass about 1 pint to a ½ gallon of gas a day—that's a little over a dozen flatus, whether you notice them or not. Drinking carbonated beverages and eating a high-fiber diet can increase flatulence. The majority of flatus is made up of odorless oxygen, carbon dioxide, nitrogen, and hydrogen. The stinky part comes from hydrogen sulfide, which smells like rotten eggs, as well as other trace gases given off by decomposing food in the colon, says *Elizabeth Lipski, Ph.D., C.N.N.,* a clinical nutritionist in Asheville, North Carolina, and author of *Digestive Wellness.*

Beans, legumes, broccoli, and cauliflower are prime gas producers. But they're also foods that are good for you, notes *Jan Rakinic, M.D.,* a colorectal surgeon and associate professor of surgery at Southern Illinois University School of Medicine in Springfield.

*If you tend to be gassy, don't drink with a straw. You swallow a column of air with each sip, which can cause gas.*—Ritu Verma, M.D.

Instead of giving up nutritious foods, see if these suggestions work for you.

**Chew slowly and chew well.** Undigested food produces gas. Since chewing is the first step in digestion, make the most of it. Give the enzymes in your saliva a chance to do their job and start breaking down food, suggests Dr. Lipski.

**Soak beans.** Soaking dried beans overnight before cooking them makes them easier to digest and, thus, cuts their gassiness, says Dr. Rakinic.

**Add enzymes.** If beans are on the menu, try taking Beano. This commercial product contains an enzyme that breaks down the sugars in beans that our bodies have trouble digesting, says Dr. Rakinic.

**Try Gas-X.** Such over-the-counter gas-reducing products as Gas-X are effective, says *Ritu Verma, M.D.,* section chief of clinical gastrointestinal services at Children's Hospital in Philadelphia. It's fine to take them every day, as long as you follow the manufacturer's directions.

**Go green.** Chlorophyll also reduces gas and odor, adds Dr. Rakinic. Try one to two capsules, two to three times daily as needed, or follow package directions. Chlorophyll capsules are available at health-food stores.

**Avoid bubbles.** Swallowing air—whether from carbonated drinks, chewing gum, talking while eating, or drinking through a straw (with each suck, you swallow a column of air inside the straw)—can cause gas. People who are prone to having a lot of gas should limit these gas-producers, notes Dr. Verma.

Avoid sorbitol-sweetened sugarless gums, which can cause gas if you're sorbitol-sensitive.

**Eat yogurt.** You'll be eating gut-friendly bacteria that help reduce gas. Dr. Rakinic suggests you try to eat a cup a day. Make sure the label says "with active cultures" or "live culture." This ensures the product contains such gas-reducing friendly bacteria as *Lactobacillus acidophilus*. If you can't stomach yogurt, take *acidophilus* capsules and follow dosage recommendations on the label.

**Exercise.** When you exercise, your muscle movements push gas out of your gastrointestinal tract, even if you don't notice, says Dr. Verma.

## LACTOSE INTOLERANCE: MAD-AT-COWS DISEASE

Do you find yourself having to leave the room after you eat a bowl of ice cream because of embarrassing gas? You might be lactose-intolerant.

Being lactose-intolerant means your body doesn't make enough of the lactase enzyme, which is necessary to break down milk sugar in order to digest dairy products. Eat a lactose-containing food, such as ice cream or milk, and you may experience nausea, cramps, gas, bloating, and diarrhea within 30 minutes to 2 hours.

In the United States, rates of lactose intolerance are highest among those of Asian, African-American, Native American, Mexican, and Jewish ancestry. Nearly 50 million Americans are lactose-intolerant, according to the American Gastroenterological Association. And that doesn't include "lactase deficient" people who notice that dairy foods cause problems that don't occur when they eat other foods.

What should you do if you suspect this is your problem? Consider these recommendations.

**Ask your doctor for a test.** The hydrogen breath test can determine if you are lactose-intolerant, explains *Charlene M. Prather, M.D.*, director of the Gastrointestinal Motility Center at St. Louis University School of Medicine. After drinking a lactose-containing liquid, your breath is measured every 15 minutes to detect hydrogen. Normally, we don't have measurable amounts of hydrogen in our breath. But undigested lactose causes bacteria in the colon to produce hydrogen, which gets picked up by the bloodstream and travels to the lungs, where it's exhaled.

**Keep a food-and-symptoms diary.** If you suspect you are lactose-intolerant, write down what you eat, when you eat, what symptoms you have, and when they occur, suggests *Susan L. Burke, M.S., R.D., C.D.E.,* director of nutrition services for eDiets.com.

**Try taking lactase.** Lactase-fortified products, such as milk and cottage cheese, are available in grocery stores, says Burke. These products contain lactase, the enzyme that your body lacks, so that you are able to digest dairy foods without having lactose-intolerance symptoms. Lactase supplements are available at health-food stores, advises Burke. How much the enzyme helps depends on how much enzyme you produce on your own. In other words, don't assume you can eat a whole bowl of ice cream after taking lactase. It may be fat content, rather than the lactose, that is causing your abdominal distress, says Dr. Prather. Go easy until you know how much the lactase helps.

**Try soy instead.** Soy may be a good substitute for dairy products, particularly soy products fortified with calcium and vitamin D, suggests Burke. Look for soy milk, cheeses, and yogurts.

**Read labels carefully.** Lactose may be hidden in such prepared foods as breads and baked goods, nonkosher lunchmeats, instant potatoes and soups, candies, processed breakfast cereals, mixes, and margarines.

## HEMORRHOIDS: TAKING AIM AT THE PAIN

Hemorrhoids are swollen or inflamed veins in the anus and lower rectum. Internal hemorrhoids develop beneath the lining of the anus and are painless, even when they bleed during a hard bowel movement. Sometimes, however, they become prolapsed, meaning they protrude outside the anus and can't be pushed back into place. External hemorrhoids are found under the sensitive skin near the anus and can cause pain when a blood clot forms, often after a hard stool. The clot usually gets reabsorbed over two to three weeks but occasionally will erode through the skin and cause some painless bleeding.

What creates a hemorrhoid? Internal abdominal pressure caused by constipation, diarrhea, pregnancy, chronic coughing, and weight lifting. They are somewhat like the varicose veins you may have in your legs, in that if blood pools in these veins, they swell. "What happens is these cushions of veins lose their attachments to the underlying tissue," explains *Jan Rakinic, M.D.,* a colorectal surgeon and associate professor of surgery at Southern

Illinois University School of Medicine in Springfield. "Then they slide up and down. When they slide toward the outside where they're not supposed to be, they bleed."

*Don't expect a drugstore cream to cure a chronic case of hemorrhoids. Changing your diet and exercise habits will do you more good.*
—*Jan Rakinic, M.D.*

If you experience bleeding during bowel movements and feel small, itchy lumps around your anus, you could have hemorrhoids. Luckily, preventing them is simple. Take action to prevent and correct constipation so you can pass stools without straining (see page 90) and follow this advice.

**Skip the creams.** Over-the-counter hemorrhoid preparations are generally not harmful, but Dr. Rakinic isn't convinced they're helpful either. One caution: Pay attention to the label and follow directions carefully. If you buy a product that contains steroids, such as hydrocortisone, and use it for more than the recommended two weeks, the steroids can cause thinning of skin around the anus and make it more vulnerable to trauma. Bottom line? She doesn't recommend these products. People expect creams to do what can only be accomplished with changes in diet and lifestyle, says Dr. Rakinic.

**Try sitz baths.** Soaking in a tub of warm water soothes hemorrhoids and helps relieve inflammation, says **Ritu Verma, M.D.,** section chief of clinical gastrointestinal services at Children's Hospital in Philadelphia. If you have a handheld showerhead, you can direct the spray toward your bottom for the same effect. Use normal bath temperature water, and soak or aim the spray at the hemorrhoids for at least five minutes. Do this at least two times a day.

If you're past the point of prevention, you'll be glad to know that there are new and effective treatments that don't involve scalpels. "Probably 95 percent of the people who come to me with complaints of hemorrhoids don't need surgery," says Dr. Rakinic. The goal of treatment is to shut off the blood supply to a hemorrhoid so that it goes away. Nonsurgical procedures include a rubber band ligation, in which a special rubber band is wrapped around the hemorrhoid (after a few days—typically 4 to 10—the hemorrhoid falls off), or sclerotherapy, in which a chemical is injected into the hemorrhoid and cuts off its blood supply. Both are pain-free outpatient procedures that can be repeated if you develop more hemorrhoids.

## CELIAC DISEASE: THE SECRET EPIDEMIC

Celiac disease is an autoimmune disorder that damages the small intestine and prevents absorption of nutrients. People who have it cannot tolerate gluten, a protein found in cereal grains, such as wheat, barley, and rye.

"Celiac disease is the most common missed diagnosis in medicine," says *Cynthia Rudert, M.D.,* an Atlanta gastroenterologist who is also medical advisor to the Celiac Disease Foundation and Gluten Intolerance Group of North America. "It may affect as many as 1 in every 179 individuals." Symptoms vary, but include fatigue, mental cloudiness, diarrhea, gas, bloating, constipation, and weight loss or gain.

Your risk for celiac disease is increased if you have another autoimmune disease, such as diabetes, thyroid disease, a vitamin $B_{12}$ deficiency, rheumatoid arthritis, and even chronic fatigue syndrome, fibromyalgia, and alopecia," says Dr. Rudert.

Previously, doctors thought celiac disease only affected the gastrointestinal tract, but now they've learned it can cause anemia, joint pain, and food sensitivities, including lactose intolerance. And, "most importantly for women, osteoporosis and infertility," says *Michelle Pietzak, M.D.,* a celiac disease specialist and pediatric gastroenterologist at the University of Southern California Keck School of Medicine and Childrens Hospital Los Angeles.

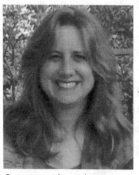

*Be your own best advocate, urges Michelle Pietzak, M.D. If you think you may have celiac disease, insist that your doctor test you for it.*

When people who are gluten-intolerant eat foods that contain gluten, the villi—tiny stalklike projections that line the small intestine and aid in nutrient absorption—are injured. Damaged or destroyed villi make your body unable to properly absorb nutrients from food.

The only real treatment is a gluten-free diet. "Fortunately, the damage to the villi is reversible," says Dr. Rudert. "On a gluten-free diet, those villi can heal within six weeks to six months and become normal again." But you do not need to initiate a gluten-free diet until you have a confirmed diagnosis of celiac disease, she says.

*A gluten-free diet is a must if you have celiac disease. Read food labels carefully to avoid eating anything that contains gluten.—Michelle Pietzak, M.D.*

If you think you have celiac disease, be sure to heed these recommendations.

**Get tested.** "People go from doctor to doctor to doctor, and because there is a lack of awareness of this disease, they're often not tested for it," says Dr. Pietzak. That's why she urges women to "be their own advocates" and keep looking until they find a doctor who will test them. Ask for a simple blood test called a celiac panel.

**Back up with biopsy.** Up to 20 percent of celiac patients may have "normal" blood tests, even though they have the disease, says Dr. Rudert. If you have the symptoms and your blood test doesn't show any abnormal findings, ask your doctor about having a small-bowel biopsy. Blood testing alone is not adequate to make a diagnosis of celiac disease, says Dr. Rudert, so your doctor is likely to confirm the findings by doing an intestinal biopsy, even if your blood test is positive. There is a subgroup of individuals that are screened appropriately for celiac disease and do not have it, yet are gluten-intolerant and respond to a gluten-free diet. In light of other associated diseases and symptoms associated with celiac disease, it is important to have the correct diagnosis.

**Have your family screened.** If you are diagnosed with celiac disease, other family members may need to be screened.

**Take charge of labels.** Become an avid label-reader, advises Dr. Pietzak. Read the ingredients of everything you eat to make sure that the food does not contain gluten. The gluten-free diet is difficult because some processed foods contain gluten that isn't indicated on the label, says Dr. Pietzak. If you aren't sure about a food's ingredients, contact it's manufacturer before you eat it.

**Seek support.** Join one of the major celiac support groups, such as the Celiac Disease Foundation (www.celiac.org). You'll get diet tips, information on food ingredients, and coping skills.

## COLORECTAL CANCER: PREVENTION AND DETECTION ARE POSSIBLE

This third most common cancer strikes almost 160,000 Americans each year, affecting women and men in nearly equal numbers and killing about 57,000. Yet it is a very curable disease if caught early. In fact, removing certain types of polyps is one way to prevent cancer.

"Know what your risk factors are," advises *Carol Ann Burke, M.D., F.A.C.G., F.A.C.P.,* director of the Center for Colon Polyps and Cancer in the Department of Gastroenterology and Hepatology at the Cleveland Clinic Foundation. Your colorectal cancer risk increases with age, increasing significantly after age 60. Additional risk factors include the following.

*Getting regular exams is your best defense against colorectal cancer, says Carol Ann Burke, M.D. The odds are in your favor if you get treatment early.*

- History of colon polyps: Polyps are mushroom-shaped growths on the lining of the colon. Most are benign, but the tendency to develop precancerous polyps, known as adenomas, raises your risk for colorectal cancer.
- Sibling, parent, or child with colorectal cancer or adenomatous polyps: Two inherited syndromes that particularly carry a high risk of colon cancer are hereditary nonpolyposis colorectal cancer and familial adenomatous polyposis. These families experience early onset (before age 50) and multiple generations with colorectal cancer.
- History of inflammatory bowel disease

Get regular exams to ensure that if you do get colon cancer, it will probably be caught when the tumor is curable. "Don't wait until you have symptoms," says Dr. Burke. "When cancer is caught early, your survival rate is as high as 90 percent."

Colon cancer guidelines recommend getting the following tests, starting at age 50—or sooner if you have any of the risk factors described above.

- Check out your entire colon: Every 10 years, get a colonoscopy to examine the entire colon. In this procedure, your doctor threads a thin, flexible tube through your anus and into your large intestine. The scope can be connected to a video camera to allow the doctor a better view of the inside of the colon. Your doctor may take biopsies at the same time, if needed. If you've had a hysterectomy, have scarring, or find the scope too uncomfortable for other reasons, ask the doctor to use a pediatric, or child-sized, colonoscope, suggests Dr. Burke. It does the job just as well with less discomfort. If your doctor says you have polyps, ask her to tell you exactly what kind of polyps were found. Most are benign, and only adenomatous polyps can develop into colon cancer, explains Dr. Burke.

There are two other procedures for viewing the entire colon without a colonoscopy. One is a double-contrast barium enema, in which your doctor inserts a thin tube through your anus to administer a chalky substance, as well as air, into your colon and then takes X-rays to view the colon for abnormalities. The other test is a virtual colonography. Your doctor inserts a thin tube through your anus to pump air into your colon, then uses a special CT scan test to look for abnormalities in the colon. Neither of these tests finds smaller polyps as effectively as a colonoscopy does. Plus, if your doctor sees a polyp or any other abnormality during one of these tests, you still need to have a colonoscopy for a biopsy.

*Don't wait until you have symptoms. Starting at age 50, get a colonoscopy to protect yourself from colorectal cancer.*—Carol Ann Burke, M.D., F.A.C.G., F.A.C.P.

- Test your stool for hidden blood annually: The fecal occult blood test (FOBT) detects the presence of hidden (or occult, meaning not visible to the eye) blood in stools. Hidden blood in the stool may indicate bleeding from a polyp or an early-stage cancer. The FOBT is a home test that is available in two forms.

One involves getting three fecal smears. You can get one of these tests, such as the Hemoccult, from your doctor or pharmacist. You collect very small stool samples from the toilet paper after you wipe and put the samples onto cards. When you complete this series of tests, you seal up the cards and immediately mail them to your doctor or lab.

To avoid false positives, read the instructions carefully about food or medications they recommend restricting in the days before you take the test. Some foods, such as rare red meat, horseradish, and some fruits or vegetables, can cause false positives. Some medications and vitamins, such as vitamin C, can cause false negative results.

The second type of FOBT involves dropping a test strip in the toilet water after you've had a bowel movement. While this may seem less messy and, therefore, a more appealing option, Dr. Burke warns that this method is not recommended by experts because it may not be as accurate as the smear type of test.

> *Ask your doctor for a fecal occult blood test that you can do at home. This annual test screens for early signs of colorectal cancer.*
> —*Carol Ann Burke, M.D., F.A.C.G., F.A.C.P.*

- Get checked for precancerous polyps in your lower intestines: Get a flexible sigmoidoscopy every five years. This test is similar to a colonoscopy, but the tube is not as long, so it examines only the lower part of the colon.

Dr. Burke says a colonoscopy is the preferred screening method. The annual FOBT and five-year sigmoidoscopy are better used together than either method alone, she says.

Meantime, it can't hurt to take these preventive measures.

**More fiber, less fat.** A high-fiber diet helps prevent colon cancer, says ***Ritu Verma, M.D.,*** section chief of clinical gastrointestinal services at Children's Hospital in Philadelphia. Adequate amounts of fiber and water help keep the colon healthy, while a diet low in fiber and high in fats and meat raises your risk of colorectal cancer. Although widely publicized research in 2001 found that high-fiber diets were not protective, experts still recommend them. The American Institute of Cancer Research noted that the findings "should not prompt people to abandon diets that have been consistently linked to reducing the risk of colon cancer."

**Get more calcium.** Studies show that routinely taking calcium carbonate supplements—the kind of calcium found in Tums—may lower your risk of colon cancer. Getting calcium in the diet from low-fat dairy or other calcium-rich foods may also be beneficial.

**Try folate supplements.** A large, long-term study found that a daily multi-vitamin containing 400 micrograms folate (folic acid) decreased the risk of colon cancer in women between ages 55 and 69, says Dr. Burke. Those who took the folate multivitamin for 15 years reduced their cancer risk by 75 percent; those who took it for 5 to 10 years reduced their risk by 20 percent. Doctors don't know why or how it works yet, but they suspect the vitamin helps protect against DNA mutations that could cause cancer.

**Take baby aspirin.** Another study found that a daily low-dose (80 milli-grams) adult aspirin or baby aspirin decreased the risk of recurrent colon polyps by 19 percent. However, even low-dose aspirin can cause side effects, so be sure to talk to your doctor first, cautions Dr. Burke.

# 5 Ears

chapter

## Now Hear This

*A man falls in love through his eyes,*
*a woman through her ears.*

—Woodrow Wyatt, British MP and journalist
"To the Point"; London *Sunday Times;* March 22, 1981

Woodrow Wyatt was arguably correct in his supposition, but he captured only part of the picture. Your ears are more than an arrow in Cupid's quiver. They help you to hear and, therefore, to communicate.

Ears also play a vital role in keeping your body balanced and your stomach settled. They're also the perfect places to hang jewelry. So many reasons exist to keep your ears in the best possible shape. Whether your ears ache, itch, make noise, or stop hearing, you'll find just what you need to know to maintain their health in the following pages.

### PREVENTING HEARING LOSS: WHAT DID YOU SAY?

We all want to feel a part of the conversation, and nothing takes us out of it faster than a hearing problem.

About 28 million Americans have some hearing loss. Sometimes, it's caused by disease, such as arteriosclerosis, diabetes, or meningitis. Other times, it's a result of noise exposure, chronic ear infections, a perforated eardrum, ototoxic drugs (medications, such as aspirin, that can hurt your inner ears' hair cells), or a condition called otosclerosis (in which one of the middle-ear bones hardens, interfering with sound transmission to the inner ear). It can even be caused by something as seemingly innocuous as earwax.

The most *preventable* cause of hearing loss is exposure to excessive sound. "The noise doesn't have to be as loud as a bomb going off," says *Jo Shapiro,* *M.D.,* chief of the division of otolaryngology at Brigham and Women's Hospital in Boston. "It can also be as low as an electric razor or a hair dryer but for a prolonged period of time."

# Even the noise of a hair dryer can harm your hearing if exposure is long enough.—Jo Shapiro, M.D.

If you notice some hearing loss, see your doctor. You will probably be referred to an audiologist, who will perform tests to help diagnose the cause and degree of your hearing loss. "There are some serious problems related to hearing loss, like tumors of the nerves of hearing or balance, or diseases of the middle ear," says **Stephanie Moody Antonio, M.D.,** an otolaryngology fellow with the House Ear Clinic in Los Angeles. Only your doctor can tell if you need a hearing aid or require surgery.

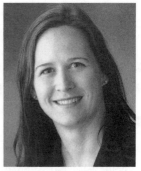

Hearing loss can indicate a related health problem, says Stephanie Moody Antonio, M.D. See your doctor to determine if you need a hearing aid or some other treatment.

Once you've lost some hearing, there's not much you can do, apart from wearing a hearing aid. But about 15 percent of adults with hearing loss can benefit from medical treatment.

Here is some sound advice for preventing hearing loss in the first place.

**Beware the volume.** "Noise is neglected as a public health hazard, and it can really damage your hearing," says Dr. Shapiro. You may have had the noise exposure in your 20s or 30s, but the effects often don't show up until your 50s. Sound intensity is measured in units called decibels. Sounds higher than 80 decibels can damage hearing, depending on the length of time you're exposed to them. These are some noises to watch out for.

- Lawn mower or truck traffic: 90 decibels; hearing damage can occur in eight hours.
- Vacuum cleaner: 94 decibels; damage can occur in five hours.
- Movies: Up to 112 decibels; damage can occur in 24 minutes.
- Walkmans: Between 85 and 110 decibels; damage can occur in 30 minutes.
- Rock concerts, clubs: 125 decibels; damage can occur in seven minutes.
- Exercise class music: Between 100 and 110 decibels; damage can occur in 30 minutes to two hours.
- Gunshots: Up to 140 decibels; damage can occur immediately.

**Cover your ears.** "For short-lived loud sounds—like when you're walking past a jackhammer—you can put your fingers in your ears," says Dr. Shapiro. "But if you're going to be around noise for an extended period—if you're using the jackhammer yourself—you need ear protection." Carry foam earplugs wherever you go. If a sound is too loud, pop the plugs in to protect your ears. "You can tell if noise is a threat—and requires plugs—if it makes your ears uncomfortable, you have to yell to be heard, or your ears ring when the sound quiets," she says.

**Improve your communication environment.** This is one of the best strategies you can employ if you have trouble hearing, says Dr. Antonio. "Use face-to-face conversation. Ask people to articulate and speak at a normal rate," she says. "If you don't understand, ask your friends to rephrase. Also, reduce background noise in the household." It can also be helpful to focus on the visual aspects of hearing, such as lip movements and facial expressions.

## HEARING AIDS: WHAT YOU NEED TO KNOW

*Hearing aid technology has come a long way. There are digital, programmable hearing aids so tiny that they can barely be seen. So don't automatically reject a hearing aid because you think it will be intrusive and ugly.*

There are four styles for sensorineural hearing loss (nerve deafness), which occurs when sensory cells in the cochlea are permanently damaged:

- In-the-ear (ITE) aids: An ITE aid fits in the outer ear of an adult with mild to severe hearing loss. These aids are made of hard plastic.
- Behind-the-ear (BTE) aids: Worn behind the ear, a BTE aid connects to a plastic mold that fits inside the outer ear. Sounds travel into the ear by way of the mold. BTE aids are used in people with mild to profound hearing loss.
- Canal aids: A canal aid is worn inside the ear canal. Such aids come in two sizes: The in-the-canal (ITC) aid fits the size and shape of the ear canal, and the completely-in-canal (CIC) hearing aid is largely concealed in the ear canal. Both types are used for mild to moderately severe hearing loss.

- Body aids: These aids are used only for people with profound hearing loss. A body aid is attached to a belt or wire and then connected to the ear by a wire. This type of hearing aid is quite large and, thus, is used only when no other kind of aid is a viable option.

For a person with sensorineural hearing loss who doesn't find a hearing aid helpful—or for someone who was born deaf—there is a small electrical device called a cochlear implant. The implant improves hearing by bypassing missing hair cells. It does not provide perfect hearing but helps a deaf person better understand speech and other sounds.

"Hearing aids can make a positive difference in a person's life," says *Deborah R. Price, Au.D.,* an audiologist in Dallas.

## TINNITUS: WHEN THE SOUNDS WON'T STOP

Having tinnitus is like housing a noisy little troll in your ear. Millions of Americans live with this troll, which makes one or more of the following sounds: whistling, ringing, clicking, roaring, or buzzing. For some people, the episodes are periodic; for others, the troll never shuts up. Two million people in the United States are disabled by the severity of their condition.

Tinnitus, the perception of sound in one or both ears or within your head, is more a symptom than a disease. It is usually the result of loud or prolonged noise exposure, hearing loss, or certain medications. Doctors haven't nailed down the physiological mechanism, but it's thought to result from the electrical discharge of tiny hearing receptors, called hair cells, in the inner ear, which then send ringing sound signals to the brain. "The area of the brain perceiving tinnitus is near the area where people perceive phantom limb pain—pain that feels like it is coming from an arm or leg that has been amputated," explains *Shelley Hill, M.D.,* an otolaryngologist at Southern California Permanente Medical Group in Panorama City, California.

Tinnitus has been linked with taking more than 12 aspirins a day, earwax, temporomandibular joint disorder (TMD), exposure to loud noise, a head or neck injury, high or low blood pressure, tumors, diabetes, salt, tobacco, and alcohol. Anti-inflammatory drugs, antibiotics, sedatives, and antidepressants can also cause tinnitus. To find out if a drug may be damaging to your ears—referred to as ototoxic—ask your physician or pharmacist.

Tinnitus may signal serious medical problems within the ear, including high-frequency hearing loss, so have it checked out by a hearing specialist.

*Taking a few aspirin a day is harmless. But a daily dose of 12 or more can cause tinnitus.—Shelley Hill, M.D.*

Nothing stops tinnitus, but you can reduce its irritating effects.

**Try white noise.** Tune a radio between stations to create static, turn on a fan, or get a fish tank, fountain, or white-noise machine that makes sounds resembling a rainstorm or waterfall. There is also an instrument called a tinnitus masker that can be worn like a hearing aid. "Any kind of low-level background noise will help mask the sound," says *Eileen Raynor, M.D.,* assistant professor of otolaryngology at the University of Florida in Jacksonville.

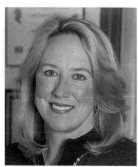

*Eating salty foods may make your tinnitus worse, warns Deborah R. Price, Au.D. Try to avoid processed foods and canned soups.*

**Cut out the sodium.** Too much salt can impair blood circulation, making tinnitus worse, says *Deborah R. Price, Au.D.*, a Dallas audiologist. Foods that harbor salt include processed foods, canned soups and vegetables, and soy sauce. Check nutrition labels and buy foods with low sodium levels.

**Avoid the din.** When a noise is too loud, the sound waves that enter your inner ear are too intense. This can damage nerve endings and send abnormal signals to the brain, which then causes buzzing or hissing. Tinnitus may occur after a single loud noise, such as a gunshot or firecracker, but it more commonly results from prolonged exposure to moderate sounds, such as industrial machines and loud music.

**Don't overdo aspirin.** The salicylic acid in aspirin can damage nerve cells in the ears, leading to tinnitus. One or two aspirin a day won't hurt, but a dozen or more might, says Dr. Hill.

## ONE WOMAN'S STORY: TINNITUS

*Maryann Eidemiller, 56, a freelance writer from Greensburg, Pennsylvania, was hit by a drunk driver in 1996. She isn't sure if it was the head injury or the pain medication she took while recovering from the accident that caused her tinnitus, but the noise has been in her head ever since.*

"It's extremely annoying," Maryann Eidemiller says. "I feel like I have cotton in my ear all the time, and when the room is quiet, the noise buzzes, clicks, or sounds like I have a seashell next to my ear." The only time Eidemiller doesn't hear the noise is when she's focused on *other* noise.

She tried a hearing aid, which worked to make outside sounds more clear. However, it also amplified the buzzing, so Eidemiller gave it back after the 30-day trial period.

Instead, she has found ways to ease the noise. "What really works for me is watching my diet, particularly my sodium intake," she says. She carefully reads food labels and has given up most processed foods, including frozen dinners and canned soup. She's also stopped eating out, because there's too much salt in restaurant food. She uses a lot of fresh cracked pepper to spice up a recipe. When people eat at Eidemiller's house, she puts a salt shaker out and announces, "You're going to have to add salt yourself." She drinks a lot of fluids to make sure her sodium ratio doesn't get so high that it causes fluid retention and the resulting clogged feeling in her ears.

"I've learned to accept my tinnitus," Eidemiller says. "I realize there is nothing I can do to make it go away entirely." This acceptance has also helped her to cope.

# EARACHES: QUIET THE PAIN

Your ears are vulnerable to attack in three places: the inner ear, middle ear, and outer ear.

## INNER-EAR INFECTIONS

An inner-ear infection can hit like a violent stomach virus. "There's no pain or fever, but you're extremely dizzy, whirling around, and throwing up," says *Shelley Hill, M.D.*, an otolaryngologist at Southern California Permanente Medical Group in Panorama City, California. Inner-ear infections result from bacteria or a virus that inflames the balance, or vestibular, system of the inner ear.

You should see a doctor to rule out other possible conditions. If you do have an inner-ear infection, your doctor will determine which type. Bacterial inner-ear infections require antibiotics. The viral form won't respond to antibiotics, but your doctor may be able to give you medication to ease your dizziness. Other than that, bed rest is your best bet. The recovery period for an inner-ear infection is usually about six weeks, over which time your dizziness will slowly improve.

These are some things our experts recommend that you can do to ease the pain of an inner-ear infection.

**Use a drugstore remedy.** "For the dizziness, try over-the-counter motion sickness remedies like Dramamine," suggests *Deborah R. Price, Au.D.* But don't use one for more than a week, or it will delay your recovery.

**Reduce salt.** Cutting back on sodium can also help, says Dr. Hill. Too much sodium may make your body retain water. That excess water can create pressure on the balance nerve.

**Stop exercising.** Overall, limiting strenuous activity is the best treatment for the first two to three weeks. "You should get up and walk around, but if you overdo it, you will continue to feel dizzy," says Dr. Hill. So give your balance nerve and body some time to recover and stick to activities that you feel comfortable performing.

## MIDDLE-EAR INFECTIONS

Middle-ear infections, also known as otitis media, occur most often in young children because their eustachian tubes—which connect the middle ear with the back of the nose—are narrower and more vulnerable to infection. Some adults, however, are just cursed with a higher-than-average susceptibility to ear infections.

## OUTER-EAR INFECTIONS

An outer-ear infection, also known as swimmer's ear, could more appropriately be called wet ear, because you're susceptible to it any time you get your head wet. Swimmer's ear is an infection of the skin in the ear canal. Water gets in the canal and brings bacterial or fungal particles with it. Normally, the water runs back out, and the bacteria and fungi don't wreak any havoc. But if there's a small break in the skin or the skin stays soggy, the bacteria and fungi can flourish and infect the outer ear.

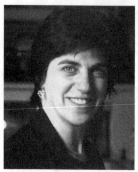

Like a middle-ear infection, swimmer's ear is extremely painful. "It hurts to touch the ear or chew," says Dr. Hill. You can differentiate between the two infections by pulling on your earlobe. If the tug worsens your pain, it's swimmer's ear. With swimmer's ear, your hearing may also become muffled as a result of the swollen skin blocking your ear canal, and there may be yellow-green pus coming from the ear opening.

If you think you have swimmer's ear, have your physician check it out. She'll probably prescribe antibiotic drops. "If you're diabetic and you get swimmer's ear, this infection can get very serious, so go to your doctor *immediately*," warns *Jo Shapiro, M.D.*, chief of the division of otolaryngology at Brigham and Women's Hospital in Boston.

*A swimmer's ear infection can be very dangerous if you're diabetic, so see your doctor as soon as you suspect trouble, warns Jo Shapiro, M.D.*

*If pulling on your earlobe increases your pain, then you have swimmer's ear, not a middle-ear infection.*

These are some things you can do on your own to prevent swimmer's ear or relieve its symptoms.

**Dry clean.** Water and swimmer's ear don't mix, so keep your ear dry when you have this infection. To prevent water from entering your ear while you shower, Dr. Shapiro recommends putting petroleum jelly on a piece of cotton and sticking it in your affected ear before you step under the spray. "Petroleum jelly prevents the water from soaking through the cotton," she explains. Take out the cotton as soon as you're done in the shower.

**Give your ear a shot of alcohol.** Alcohol helps evaporate water, and vinegar is a natural antibacterial. "If you tend to get swimmer's ear, put a mixture of half rubbing alcohol and half vinegar in a medicine dropper, and put a few drops in your ear," suggests *Eileen Raynor, M.D.*, assistant professor of otolaryngology at the University of Florida in Jacksonville.

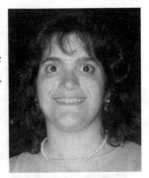

Homemade eardrops of rubbing alcohol and vinegar may help prevent recurring bouts of swimmer's ear, says Eileen Raynor, M.D.

Tilt your head sideways so that one ear faces up. Pull your earlobe up and backward, and insert the drops. Jiggle your earlobe to get the drops into the ear canal, then turn your head to let them drain out. Repeat with the opposite ear. Use this mixture to help prevent water from settling in the ear canals and avoid infections. The eardrops make your ear canals more acidic and, therefore, less appealing to bacteria, Dr. Raynor says.

**Say no to cotton swabs.** "If you look on a cotton swab package, it says, 'Don't use inside the ear,' " says Dr. Hill. Swabs push wax further inside the ears, irritate the sensitive skin of the ear canals, and can make the ears bleed, causing pain and infection.

## EARWAX: CLEARING OUT THE CLOGS

It may be a little gross, but earwax is normal and healthy. While the rest of your skin produces oil to use as a natural protectant, your ears make wax. It protects them from dirt, water, fungus, and bugs. It also prevents them from getting dried out and itchy.

Earwax is produced in the outer part of the ear canal. Normally, it falls out on its own as more is produced. "The ear is self-cleaning, so I wouldn't monkey with it if you don't have a wax-buildup problem," says *Jo Shapiro, M.D.*, chief of the division of otolaryngology at Brigham and Women's Hospital in Boston.

In some people, the wax doesn't fall out easily. Trouble arises when the ear keeps producing wax, and it builds up. "As women age, they tend to produce dryer, more obstructing wax, simply because of changes within the

## SHOULD I SEE A DOCTOR?

*Not all ear troubles require immediate medical attention, and different symptoms require different professionals.*

"Ear disease and problems with balance, ear pain, ear infections, and ear tumors are treated by an otologist or an ear, nose, and throat (ENT) doctor," says *Catherine Palmer, Ph.D.,* director of the Center for Audiology in Pittsburgh. "Hearing loss is evaluated and treated by an audiologist—a person with a master's degree or Ph.D. who specializes in hearing testing," she says.

### How to Assess Hearing Loss

If you think your hearing might not be up to par, *Deborah R. Price, Au.D.,* suggests asking yourself these questions:

* What kind of communication problems am I having?
* Do I ask for repetition?
* Do I misunderstand people?
* Am I embarrassed about my hearing loss?

If you answer yes to any of the questions, you may want to talk to your doctor about a hearing aid, says Dr. Price.

### Symptoms That Need Care

These are some warning signs that should send you to your health-care provider:

**Abrupt hearing loss:** If your hearing suddenly disappears in one ear, get to the doctor immediately. Generally, this kind of unexpected sensorineural hearing loss can be reversed with medication, says *Jo Shapiro, M.D.,* chief of the division of otolaryngology at Brigham and Women's Hospital in Boston. But treatment must be sought quickly. "We only have a two-week window to treat this," she says. After that, the loss may become permanent.

**Ear pain:** If the pain is severe—and especially if it is accompanied by drainage, a foul odor, or fever—you probably have a middle-ear infection and need antibiotics. See your physician.

**Sudden dizziness:** If dizziness comes on suddenly—and you also have congestion, ear pressure, or the symptoms of a cold—you may have an inner-ear infection. Most of the time, the infection is caused by a virus and doesn't require antibiotics. Err on the side of caution with any new symptoms of dizziness, though, and call or see your doctor. Dizziness can also be related to heart problems, blood loss, or a stroke, says *Eileen Raynor, M.D.,* assistant professor of otolaryngology at the University of Florida in Jacksonville.

**Ringing ears:** Also known as ringing in the ears, tinnitus can signal a number of medical problems, including damage to nerves in the inner ear, thyroid problems, or allergies. "In rare cases, tinnitus can signal a tumor on

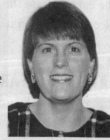

*Have tinnitus checked by a physician to be sure it's not a symptom of a tumor, recommends Catherine Palmer, Ph.D.*

the nerve that leads from the brain to the inner ear, so it's best to see a physician," says Dr. Palmer.

wax gland," says *Stephanie Moody Antonio, M.D.*, an otolaryngology fellow with the House Ear Clinic in Los Angeles. A hearing aid can also make wax worse, because it packs the wax down. If you have wax problems, you may need to visit your doctor a few times a year for a cleaning.

*Cotton swabs are not designed to be used inside the ear—it says so on the package. The ear is self-cleaning, so don't fool with it unless you have an unusual buildup of earwax.*

—*Jo Shapiro, M.D.*

Doctors recommend the following at-home treatments for earwax buildup.

**Put nothing smaller than your elbow in your ear.** This folk wisdom rings true. "If you just *have* to use a cotton swab, use it on your very outer ear only," says Dr. Shapiro. "If you put it in the ear canal, you might create a huge wax plug and then have to come in and see me."

**Soften the wax.** "There are different kinds of over-the-counter wax softener drops, like Debrox or Cerumenex," says Dr. Shapiro. "Put a few drops in once a month to soften your wax so it falls out on its own."

**Lubricate it.** Mineral oil loosens the wax so that it falls out more easily. "If your eardrum has been examined by your doctor and has no holes, put a few drops of mineral oil in your ear once a week or once a month as needed," says Dr. Antonio.

**Dissolve it.** If you have normal ears and are sure you don't have a perforation in your eardrum, try hydrogen peroxide to dissolve excess wax. "Using an eyedropper, put two to three drops in your ear and let it bubble out," says *Eileen Raynor, M.D.*, assistant professor of otolaryngology at the University of Florida in Jacksonville.

**Irrigate it.** "If you have earwax buildup, buy an ear-irrigation kit," says *Shelley Hill, M.D.*, an otolaryngologist at Southern California Permanente Medical Group in Panorama City, California. The kits are available at your audiologist's office or a drugstore. Each includes an oil that softens the wax, syringe to flush out your ear, and bowl. Follow package directions carefully.

# EARLOBE PROBLEMS: EARRINGS AND MORE

Earlobe problems go beyond heavy earrings that cause pain. Here are some common complaints, along with our experts' advice on preventing or resolving them.

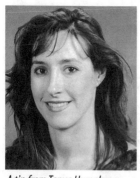

A tip from Tanya Humphreys, M.D.: If you're allergic to the metal in a pair of earrings, apply a coat of nail polish to the back of each earring.

**Try petroleum jelly.** Dry or scaly lobes are probably due to dry skin or dermatitis. "If a woman has a tendency for dry or sensitive skin, some petroleum jelly applied as needed should take care of the problem," says *Tanya Humphreys, M.D.*, director of cutaneous surgery at Thomas Jefferson University in Philadelphia.

**Watch out for nickel.** Red or crusty lobes are most likely caused by an allergic reaction to jewelry. Nickel is the most common allergen, and it's in a variety of jewelry metals. "Look for higher-grade metals, which are less likely to contain nickel, like sterling silver, stainless steel, or gold, 18-karat or higher," says Dr. Humphreys. If your ear is really inflamed, try a topical over-the-counter steroid. A 1-percent hydrocortisone cream or ointment works best. Anything stronger requires a prescription. Apply a thin coat of nail polish over the backs of the allergy-inducing earrings and let them dry before wearing to decrease symptoms, she advises.

**Select earrings carefully.** Hairbrushes, clothing, tangled long hair, and toddlers are all threats to pierced earlobes. This is especially true if you're sporting hoops or dangly earrings. So first and foremost, avoid big earrings whenever possible, especially heavy ones. If you do tear a lobe, apply direct pressure for at least 20 minutes to stop the bleeding, which can be profuse on an earlobe, says Dr. Humphreys. "Applying ice can also be helpful on the way to the doctor or emergency room," she adds. The good news is that pierced earring–hole tears can be repaired easily. "It's done under local anesthesia because we have to do a little plastic surgery, but the ear can usually be pierced again," says *Jo Shapiro, M.D.*, chief of the division of otolaryngology at Brigham and Women's Hospital in Boston.

# 6 Energy

## Stay-Well Secrets
## for Ultimate Vitality

*If the marathon that is your life has you on the run from dawn till long past dusk, you're probably worn out by the time you hit the sack. But what if you're so tired that you can barely function?*

The frenzy of everyday life devours our energy. We get so used to feeling frazzled that we forget what feeling good is like. "Being tired is *not* normal," says *Pamela Smith, R.D.,* author of *The Energy Edge.* "It's common, but not normal."

Why are we so exhausted? "Women have no boundaries. They're *always* on," says *Jesse Lynn Hanley, M.D.,* author of *Tired of Being Tired.* A typical woman expends her energies on others, juggling many roles and putting her needs last on the to-do list. No wonder she often finds herself dragging.

Poor diet, excess stress, and lack of exercise are just a few causes of low energy. Various conditions and illnesses can also give you that slogging-through-quicksand feeling. We describe several causes and conditions in this chapter and provide suggestions on how to cope and re-energize your life.

### FATIGUE: REVVING UP

When daily life is hectic, you might be inclined to neglect yourself. If there's not enough fuel in your tank to keep you going, you risk physical and mental burnout, says *Deborah Moskowitz, N.D.,* a naturopathic doctor and director of the Transitions for Health Women's Institute in Portland, Oregon. And, no, you can't rely on sugar and caffeine to get you through the day without eventually paying a penalty.

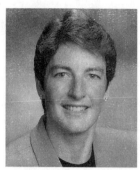

Cortisol and other hormones are secreted by the adrenal glands to help you deal with stress. Unfortunately, adrenal glands are not like that battery-driven bunny that just keeps going and going. The more these glands are required to respond to pressure-related demands, the sooner they'll give out—and they're not rechargeable.

If your adrenal glands are pushed beyond their capacity, you'll probably wind up with a collection of complaints, including fatigue, lethargy, and erratic blood-sugar levels, says Dr. Moskowitz. You're also likely to suffer from poor memory, mood swings, mild depression, and a reduced ability to manage stress.

If you need a tune-up, so to speak, consider these tips from Dr. Moskowitz.

**Get a grip.** Explore solutions to whatever is stressing you out. Get help with household chores, seek money-management advice, or change your work hours to avoid peak traffic. If necessary, start looking for another job.

**Tune in to tuning out.** Make time for mind-and-body relaxation therapies to relieve everyday pressures. (For techniques, see "Stress-Busters," page 283.)

**Boycott sugar and caffeine.** The charge they give you can also boost the release of stress hormones. Keeping your body high on these stimulants just wears you down.

> *Sugar increases the production of stress hormones, wearing you down. Take B-complex vitamins to promote energy and strengthen your nervous system.*—Deborah Moskowitz, N.D.

**Bump up your Bs.** Take a daily multivitamin containing B-complex vitamins to ensure you're getting the recommended amounts of vitamins and minerals—important nutrients you're probably not getting from meals. The extra B-complex vitamins in the supplement will promote energy, enhance your metabolism, and contribute to a healthy nervous system.

## ENDING CAFFEINE DEPENDENCY: JUST SAY NO TO JOE

*Trying to give up caffeine is a positive step, but cold turkey is not the way to go.*

Suddenly swearing off caffeine can leave you feeling weak, headachy, tired, and nauseated, says *Jesse Lynn Hanley, M.D.,* author of *Tired of Being Tired.* You need to ease off the stimulant slowly to avoid suffering withdrawal symptoms.

Start by giving up half a cup of coffee a day every few days. If you usually drink three cups a day, you'll be able to cut out caffeine altogether in two to three weeks. Mark your calendar each week to remind yourself how many cups of coffee (or caffeinated tea or soda) you can have each day.

Don't be fooled into thinking that decaf coffee is the solution to your java fix, since it actually contains *some* caffeine. And except for the Swiss Water Process variety, most coffees are decaffeinated with the chemical methylene chloride, a potential carcinogen.

To help your body adapt as it makes its way to a caffeine-free state, Dr. Hanley suggests taking supplements to increase your serotonin levels, which will help decrease your cravings. Thirty minutes before breakfast, lunch, dinner, and bedtime, take an herbal formula that contains 450 milligrams Saint-John's-wort and a preparation made up of equal parts sour jujube seed, California poppy whole plant, red sage root, hawthorn berry, and Saint-John's-wort. (Ask someone at your local health-food store for a recommendation.)

Do not use these supplements if you're already taking a selective serotonin reuptake inhibitor (SSRI), such as Prozac (fluoxetine) or Zoloft (sertraline); or an MAO inhibitor, such as Nardil (phenelzine) or Parnate (tranylcypromine).

---

**Exercise your right to exercise.** "I'm more resilient if I work out," says Dr. Moskowitz. She aims for getting physical activity at least three times a week to manage the stress of her busy life as doctor, wife, and mother of two small children—each a full-time position in itself. But even Dr. Moskowitz sometimes skips a session. When that happens, she makes sure to fit in a walk around the block. Dr. Moskowitz says exercise is important to her health because it provides the energy necessary to meet the needs of her family and patients.

A hectic schedule also demands a great deal of get-up-and-go from *Pamela Peeke, M.D., M.P.H.,* assistant clinical professor of medicine at the

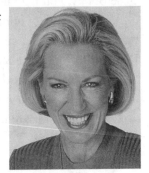

*If you need motivation to exercise, try this idea from Pamela Peeke, M.D., M.P.H.: Connect your workout with something that gives you joy.*

University of Maryland School of Medicine and author of *Fight Fat After Forty.* Dr. Peeke works out at least 30 to 45 minutes every day to keep her power levels up. That kind of commitment may seem daunting, but once you actually get moving, it becomes easier to keep going. "You can't wait for enough energy to move," she says. "You have to create it."

## You can't wait for energy. You have to create it.—*Pamela Peeke, M.D., M.P.H.*

Dr. Peeke seeks out physical challenges to help her stay motivated. One year, she ran the New York Marathon with a dozen of her patients; the next year, she scaled Mount Whitney. "When I'm working toward a goal, it's in the back of my mind every day," says Dr. Peeke. Whether she's walking on the treadmill, lifting weights, or running, she knows she's conditioning her body to do something more interesting later. "When you have a plan, then it's not just about exercise," she says. "If you connect exercise to something that gives you joy, you'll be that much more inclined to do it."

### SLEEPLESS NIGHTS: NOW I LAY ME DOWN...

Sleep is essential for good health. If you find your eyes wide open at the close of day, you may need to do more than count sheep.

What's ruining your slumber? Chances are, one of the sleep-thieves listed below is stealing the majority of your forty winks, says *Joyce A. Walsleben, Ph.D.*, director of the Sleep Disorders Center at the New York University School of Medicine and author of *A Woman's Guide to Sleep: Guaranteed Solutions for a Good Night's Rest*. She cites these as the top-10 culprits.

- Stress or anxiety
- Caffeine
- Light
- Illness
- Alcohol
- Fear
- Overcommitted schedule
- Depression or anger
- Noise
- Stimulants (diet pills, cold and allergy remedies, asthma medications)

To get the z's you need, Dr. Walsleben endorses "The Four Rs of Sleep," named by Joan Shaver, Ph.D., R.N., dean of the College of Nursing at the University of Illinois at Chicago. Check them out below.

**Regularize your sleep pattern.** Rise and shine at the same time every day. If you get up at 6 a.m. during the workweek, resist the temptation to sleep in on weekends. Avoid naps, unless you indulge in them regularly. Retire for the night at a set hour and try to snooze for the same length of time consistently. Some people require nine hours of slumber every night, while others do just fine with a mere seven or less. Discover your magic number—and stick with it.

> *You'll sleep better if you stick to a regular schedule. Go to bed and get up at about the same times every day.*—Joyce A. Walsleben, Ph.D.

**Ritualize your sleep behavior.** Reserve your bedroom for rest. Well, okay, and for sex, of course ... but that's another chapter. Turn in only when you're actually sleepy. Keep the room quiet, dark, and cool.

**Resolve stress before you retire.** Take up relaxation techniques, such as meditation or deep breathing. (See "Stress-Busters," page 283.) Dr. Walsleben also recommends keeping a kind of worry notebook as a means of venting your stress. On the left side of a piece of paper, jot down the issues that are troubling you. Then, on the right side, list possible courses of action that could resolve those issues. If you worry about money, for example, suggest things you can do to improve your fiscal future: postpone a vacation, pass up that new dress you've been eyeing, call a financial planner, or file a tax extension, to name a few options.

**Resist temptation.** Several hours before bedtime, avoid alcohol, caffeine, and tobacco, all of which can interfere with sleep.

When *Pamela Smith, R.D.,* finds herself short on shut-eye, she calls it a day at 8 p.m. So does *Pamela Peeke, M.D., M.P.H.,* assistant clinical professor of medicine at the University of Maryland School of Medicine—even if it means missing a favorite TV program. "That's what VCRs are for," she says.

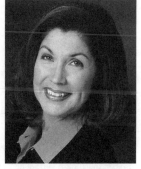

*Your brain won't let you sleep if you go to bed hungry, says Pamela Smith, R.D. Try eating a small late-night snack of cereal to keep your blood-sugar levels stable until morning.*

Smith provides this additional advice for your ticket to dreamland.

**Steady those hormones.** The symptoms of menopause can rob you of sleep. Hormone replacement therapy (HRT) helps regulate your hormones, which, in turn, eases night sweats and hot flashes. (For more information on HRT, see page 251.)

**Watch what you eat.** It's true that high-fat, high-sugar snacks may make you drowsy enough to sack out. But when your blood sugar drops a few

## MOTHER NATURE, M.D.:
## HERBS AND SUPPLEMENTS FOR SLEEPING PROBLEMS

*Many women prefer natural remedies that don't carry the risk of addiction or morning-after hangover, either of which can be a side effect of prescription medications.*

Herbs and supplements can help those plagued by sleeplessness, says *Shoshana Zimmerman, N.D.,* author of *My Doctor Says I'm Fine ... So Why Do I Feel So Bad?* Which one she advises depends on the reasons a patient isn't sleeping. Keep in mind that any supplement is safe to use only with the approval and supervision of your physician. All supplements discussed here should be available in your local health-food store or drugstore.

These are Dr. Zimmerman's herbal recommendations for arresting specific sleep-robbers.

**Stress and anxiety:** Either valerian or passion flower can be helpful.

Valerian has been shown to be more effective in liquid form rather than in powdered form. About 45 minutes before bedtime, take $1/2$ to 1 teaspoon valerian extract or 1 to $1^1/2$ teaspoons tincture. If you feel a little drowsy when you awaken, decrease your dosage.

If you prefer to take passion flower, combine 350 milligrams of the powdered form with

100 milligrams niacin, 50 milligrams vitamin $B_6$, 250 milligrams magnesium, and 100 to 300 milligrams 5-HTP. Take the passion-flower mixture about 45 to 60 minutes before you turn in for the night.

**Problems falling asleep or staying asleep:** Melatonin is a natural hormone produced by the pineal gland that is effective in inducing and maintaining sleep. If your body's melatonin levels are normal, taking a supplement won't help. "Supplements only produce sleepiness when you have a low level of melatonin," says Dr. Zimmerman. "If you take melatonin and it does not work, chances are you didn't have a deficiency." If you want to give melatonin a try, start slowly; taking too much can disrupt the body's natural wake-sleep cycle.

Many people respond well to dosages as low as 0.1 to 0.3 milligrams, taken about two hours before retiring for the evening. If you find that melatonin makes you too drowsy prior to going to bed, take it right before turning in. You may hours later, you'll wake up hungry and be unable to get back to sleep. Going to bed on an empty stomach is just as bad. If you haven't had enough to eat, your brain will stay alert until you satisfy your hunger. Good bedtime snacks combine protein and complex carbohydrates to keep blood-sugar levels stable throughout the night. Smith suggests a small bowl of whole-grain cereal with low-fat milk, half a turkey sandwich, or a banana with skim milk.

gradually increase the dosage, up to 3 milligrams, if necessary.

Dr. Zimmerman recommends the slow-release form of melatonin because it helps you stay asleep better than the rapid-release form.

Since melatonin secretes best in darkness, keep your drapes drawn, don't use a night-light, and shut off any lights that may shine into your bedroom.

**Middle-of-the-night wakening:** If you awake early and are unable to get back to sleep, Dr. Zimmerman suggests taking an Ayurvedic formula. Ayurveda is a holistic method of medicine that originated in India more than 3,000 years ago. The Tranquil Mind formula from Banyan Trading Company (www.banyantrading.com, 800-953-6424) is a mixture of herbs known to have a tranquil effect on the nervous system. Take one or two pills a half hour before bedtime.

When a racing mind occasionally keeps you from returning to dreamland, try a dropper of herbal kava extract to promote relaxation so that you can get back to sleep more easily. Although the U.S. Food and Drug Administration is investigating the link between kava and liver toxicity, Dr. Zimmerman says cases of adverse effects are extremely rare.

**Restless legs syndrome:** If you have this condition, you probably wake up repeatedly during the night due to often painful muscle contractions. Your sleep can be interrupted by twitching that you're not aware of, leaving you feeling drowsy the next day. If you have a family history of restless legs syndrome, you may have a deficiency of folic acid. Dr. Zimmerman treats this condition with 35 to 60 milligrams folic acid per day. Folic acid is available over the counter up to only 800 micrograms, so any higher dose requires a prescription. If you have no family history of restless legs syndrome, ask your doctor for a blood test to see if you have an iron deficiency.

**Midnight bathroom runs:** If sleep problems are caused by frequent trips to the toilet, reduce the volume of liquids you drink within a few hours of going to bed. That may prove helpful, but Dr. Zimmerman finds that many women must empty their bladders during the night, especially as they get older. If that sounds familiar, she recommends Banyan Trading Company's Kidney Formula, a mixture of herbs designed to improve what is known in Eastern medicine as weak kidney energy. Take one to two pills before bedtime. Be patient: It may take three to four months before you see results.

**Move your body.** If you walk, bike, or swim for 30 to 40 minutes a day, four times a week, you'll nod off faster and stay asleep longer than if you don't exercise at all. By boosting endorphins—your brain's feel-good chemicals—working out enhances your ability to deal with any stresses that may be keeping you awake. Just avoid strenuous exercise within three hours of bedtime, or you'll be too charged for slumber.

**Recline right.** Lying on your stomach for hours can cause back-and-neck muscle pain bad enough to chase away the sandman. Sleeping on your side can help you breathe more easily, thus reducing the likelihood of snoring, which can waken you during the night. To achieve the best sleep posture on your side, put a pillow between slightly bent knees to comfortably align your neck and spine. Prevent neck and shoulder aches by choosing a pillow that's thin enough to support your head without flexing your neck. Your back may get sore if you stay curled up all night to conserve heat, so make sure you're warm enough. Give yourself room to move. Remaining in one position for too long can make you feel stiff in the morning.

**Don't force the issue.** If you haven't fallen asleep within a half hour of retiring, get up and do something calming until you feel drowsy. (If you opt for reading, you might want to avoid a rousing murder mystery.) Try to stay awake until your eyes begin to close involuntarily. Don't look at the clock—the more you focus on the fact that you're not sleeping, the less likely you are to nod off.

If none of these tips are effective—and lack of slumber is interfering with your ability to function—ask your doctor about taking a prescription medication. (Always consult your health-care provider before self-medicating with an over-the-counter sleep remedy.) *Jesse Lynn Hanley, M.D.,* author of *Tired of Being Tired,* prescribes such short-acting drugs as Ambien (zolpidem), Ativan (lorazepam), or Sonata (zaleplon)—none of which should leave you groggy in the morning. Dr. Hanley recommends taking prescription medications no more than two out of every five nights so that you don't become dependent on them.

*To avoid becoming dependent on sleep medication, limit your use of these drugs to two or three nights a week, advises Jesse Lynn Hanley, M.D.*

## THE AFTERNOON SLUMP: TIPS FOR ALL-DAY ENERGY

Lunch is a thing of the past, dinner is still hours away, and you have many miles to go before you can legitimately wind down. You're hungry, tired, and cranky. If you regularly fall victim to this kind of dip, revamping your eating, drinking, and exercise habits may be needed to keep you going through the day.

Our experts suggest these lifestyle changes to beat the afternoon blahs.

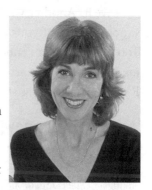

**Eat lightly, eat often.** Numerous minimeals spread throughout the day can help maintain energy levels, says *Susan L. Burke, M.S., R.D.*, director of nutrition services for eDiets.com. "Eating smaller meals, every two to three hours, keeps your engine revved," she says. Burke herself splits breakfast into two meals: At 7 a.m., she starts her day with a bowl of high-fiber cereal, a cup of nonfat milk, and a piece of fruit. Then she follows that up at 9 or 10 a.m. with a cup of nonfat yogurt (minus the fruit on the bottom, which is actually just energy-zapping preserves).

*Eat smart to maintain your pep throughout the day, advises Susan L. Burke, M.S., R.D. Build your diet on veggies, whole grains, fruits, and lean protein.*

**Bulk up.** If you crash an hour or two after lunch, revise your menus. The right foods help keep your blood sugar stable throughout the afternoon. Burke recommends a diet filled with whole-grain breads and cereals, whole fruit (fruit has fiber, juice has none), vegetables, salads, and such lean protein as fish, tofu, eggs, nuts, and legumes.

*Eat lightly every two to three hours to keep your energy high. For extra morning pep, split your breakfast into two meals.—Susan L. Burke, M.S., R.D.*

**Go for H₂0.** Boost your intake of water to boost your energy. Burke drinks three 20-ounce bottles during her work day, with a cup or two of herbal tea thrown in for good measure.

**Run stairs.** "It's guaranteed to get your heart and lungs working, and oxygen will flow to all your major muscle groups," says *Kelli Calabrese, M.S.,* author of *The Group Fitness Instructor Exam Preparation Manual* for the American Council on Exercise. As you build up your stamina, tackle more stairwells or take two steps at a time. For an added surge of power, swing your arms and breathe deeply.

**Move it.** Another way to avoid the midafternoon energy drain is to simply get out of your chair. Stretch at your desk or go for a short walk. Too busy for an extended exercise session? Three 10-minute intervals during the day are just as energizing as one 30-minute session, says Calabrese. Reduce pep-draining stress by sitting up tall, closing your eyes, and taking

## PAMELA SMITH'S POWER SNACKS

*When you need a nibble, pass up chips and candy bars in favor of something that will boost your energy.*

Nutritionist *Pamela Smith, R.D.,* says that a good snack contains at least 1 to 2 ounces of protein to stabilize your blood sugar for hours and a complex carbohydrate to give you a quick burst of energy. One key to eating right is having the right kinds of foods on hand. "The best intentions go out the window when you're not prepared," she says. Smith keeps some of these energizing snacks around at all times:

- Whole-grain crackers or cereal with a low-fat cheese, such as string cheese, part-skim mozzarella, or Laughing Cow Light cheese wedges
- Fresh fruit or a small box of raisins with low-fat cheese
- Half a lean turkey or chicken sandwich
- Plain, nonfat yogurt blended with fresh fruit or all-fruit jam
- Baked low-fat tortilla chips with fat-free bean dip and salsa
- Air-popped or low-fat microwave popcorn sprinkled with Parmesan cheese

- Whole-grain cereal with skim milk
- Health Valley graham crackers
- Rice cakes with natural peanut butter, which doesn't contain the sugar, vegetable oil, or preservatives found in processed varieties
- Homemade low-fat bran muffin with low-fat or skim milk
- Crisp bread (such as Ryvita, Kavli, or Wasa) with sliced turkey and Dijon mustard or light cream cheese and all-fruit jam
- Small can of water-packed tuna or chicken with whole-grain crackers
- Half a small whole wheat bagel or English muffin with 2 tablespoons light cream cheese
- Dill tortilla rolls: whole wheat tortilla spread with light cream cheese mixed with lemon juice, pepper, and dill
- Skim milk blended with frozen fruit and vanilla
- Trail mix: Combine 1 cup unsalted dry-roasted peanuts, 1 cup unsalted dry-roasted shelled sunflower seeds, and 2 cups raisins. Use 16 zip-lock plastic bags to store 1/4-cup portions.

deep breaths. With each breath, relax a different muscle group. Start with the muscles of the jaw, neck, shoulders, middle back, and abdominals, and move on down the body. Flex one set of muscles at a time, from head to toe, then repeat from toe to head.

**Slip in a stretch.** Elongating your muscles feels good. It also helps your posture and eases the aches and pains that come along with sitting at a desk all day, says Calabrese. Try this exercise: With both arms straight up overhead, reach toward the ceiling. Keeping both arms raised, stretch even higher with the right arm, holding the pose for a few seconds before switching to reaching with the left arm. Transition into a side stretch by bending to one side at the waist, extending the right hand toward the left wall. Hold for 10 to 30 seconds, while you take several deep cleansing breaths and try to relax the muscles a little more to enhance the stretch. Repeat on the opposite side. Need a good stretch for your neck? Drop one ear to your shoulder and repeat on the other side. Then let the weight of your head fall forward and relax.

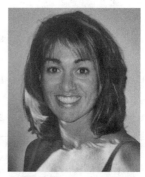

*Feeling dull at your desk? Get up and get moving, says fitness expert Kelli Calabrese, M.S. If you don't have time for a 10-minute walk, a few minutes of stretching and flexing will restore your pep.*

## CHRONIC FATIGUE SYNDROME: WHEN YOU'RE TIRED *ALL THE TIME*

Feeling draggy as you make your way through the day is difficult enough. But if you feel so worn out that you can't get through the day at all, you might have chronic fatigue syndrome (CFS). The name was coined in 1988 to describe a medical condition characterized by extreme fatigue, low energy, and at least four of the following symptoms.

- Impaired memory or concentration
- Sore throat
- Tender neck or armpit lymph nodes

- Headaches
- Nonrefreshing sleep
- Postexercise fatigue, lasting more than 24 hours
- Muscle and multijoint pain

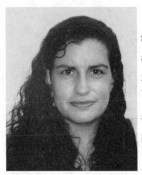

*There is no simple cure for chronic fatigue syndrome, says Nassim Assefi, M.D. With a prescription for exercise and physical therapy, most CFS patients can lead normal lives.*

Researchers don't know exactly what causes CFS, says **Nassim Assefi, M.D.,** the women's health attending physician in the departments of adult medicine and obstetrics and gynecology at the University of Washington at Seattle. Theories abound, but no study has been able to nail down a specific trigger. According to the Centers for Disease Control and Prevention, CFS affects adults of both genders and all racial groups. Few people recover from CFS completely, but just as few get continuously worse. The majority of people with CFS lead normal lives, with periodic recurrences of symptoms.

The difficulties of treating CFS and its many symptoms have led to no proven effective remedies, says Dr. Assefi. Rather, the most common approach is to address each symptom individually, such as prescribing physical therapy for muscle pain.

One treatment most physicians do recommend is regular exercise. Though Dr. Assefi advises patients to begin slowly, she strongly believes that the more they work out, the less tired they'll be in the long run.

*Regular exercise is key to living with chronic fatigue syndrome. In the long run, the more you work out, the less tired you'll be.*—Nassim Assefi, M.D.

Fitness expert **Kelli Calabrese, M.S.,** author of *The Group Fitness Instructor Exam Preparation Manual* for the American Council on Exercise, agrees. CFS patients usually have normal cardiovascular and metabolic responses to aerobic exercise. Their tolerance for activity may be limited at first, leaving them feeling even more fatigued and uncomfortable than usual. However, if patients start slowly and stick with a program, they usually see improvement in their energy levels and functional capacity. Calabrese warns CFS patients that they risk increased disability if they don't exercise regularly.

## ONE WOMAN'S STORY: CHRONIC FATIGUE SYNDROME

*Rebecca Kopf was diagnosed with chronic fatigue syndrome (CFS) at age 26. Previously, she had worked out five to six days a week, even as she pursued a career in marketing. Then CFS changed her life.*

"I had an abundance of energy," Rebecca Kopf recalls of the days before the diagnosis. But once CFS hit, Kopf simply couldn't get enough sleep. She dozed late on weekends, lay around all day, napped in the afternoon, and conked out by 8 p.m. She even had to take a nap at work. Fortunately, her employer was understanding, allowing Kopf an hour-long break every day in her office.

It wasn't just Kopf's sleeping patterns that suffered, though. Her plunging energy levels brought her workout regimen to an abrupt halt. Kopf's once healthful eating habits also deteriorated because she was too exhausted to care about what she ate. Lack of vitality made it too difficult to shop, make a meal plan, or even prepare food. Kopf remembers one trip to the grocery store when she became so overwhelmed by fatigue that she abandoned a full cart and went home. "It became easier to grab a sandwich from a fast-food restaurant or deli than to prepare something as simple as a salad or tuna sandwich," she says.

Seeking help, Kopf attended a seminar on CFS. She was impressed with the doctor leading the discussion and made an appointment to see him. That turned out to be the best thing she could do for herself.

"This sounds like a cliché, but he treated not only my symptoms, but also *me* as a person," she recalls. The physician recommended such dietary changes as eliminating alcohol and caffeine, including chocolate. He also helped her cope with the debilitating depression that frequently accompanies an illness such as CFS. "At the time, CFS was seen by many as an excuse, rather than as something real," says Kopf. "It was very difficult not to be heard or understood—and it was quite depressing."

Nearly a decade later, Kopf says that, overall, she feels great. She doesn't consider herself cured, but she has learned to live successfully with CFS. For example, she no longer tries to push through her fatigue but gives herself time to rest. That means taking an occasional day off from work or working out. "Those days are few and far between, though," she says. As a rule, she exercises five days a week and even recently ran a marathon.

Kopf is a self-confessed overachiever who once tried to fill her personal and profession schedules with nonstop activity. She now realizes—and would like other CFS sufferers to know—that it's okay to relax and limit the number of projects taken on. She believes in giving herself permission to sleep more and exercise less.

*Rebecca Kopf has learned to cope successfully with CFS. She recognizes her limits, keeps her work schedule realistic, and puts exercise and rest in perspective.*

Calabrese suggests this exercise program for CFS patients.

**Aim for aerobic.** A well-rounded workout regimen includes aerobics, stretching, and resistance training. Start by walking and, after several weeks, add stationary cycling and water aerobics in a heated pool. Alternate activities throughout the week. These low-impact exercises are particularly beneficial because they are not likely to aggravate any muscle or joint pain you may have. This routine is excellent for building your cardiovascular endurance and incorporates activities that you can continue throughout your life.

Here's an easy formula for determining the number of heartbeats per minute you should aim for while working out.

- 220 minus your age = your maximum heart rate (MHR)
- MHR x 60 percent = your lowest target heart rate
- MHR x 75 percent = your highest target heart rate

When you begin an exercise program, shoot for about 40 percent of your maximal heart rate. Gradually progress to 60 percent over 12 to 15

## A WOMAN'S RIGHT TO THE *RIGHT* TREATMENT: CHRONIC FATIGUE SYNDROME (CFS)

*Mainstream physicians used to treat the very idea of CFS with skepticism, if not downright hostility. Though that attitude has changed, getting proper treatment can still be problematic for many CFS sufferers.*

CFS is difficult to diagnose because its varied symptoms overlap with so many other conditions, including multiple sclerosis (MS), lupus, a thyroid disorder, and depression.

For that reason, "it's important to find a physician who is committed to the diagnostic process," says *Kim Kenney,* president and chief executive officer of the Chronic Fatigue and Immune Dysfunction Syndrome Association of America.

It's helpful to provide your doctor with a detailed account of your symptoms. Keep a written record of your observations and, if possible, note any connections with events or conditions in your daily life. For example, one important clue to CFS is fatigue that lasts more than 24 hours after exertion. Another indicator is whether symptoms are made worse by emotional or physical stress. "Any stressor can set someone with CFS back for two or three days," says Kenney. "That's one of the unique features of this illness."

Look for a physician you like who specializes in CFS. Then stick with him or her, even if your symptoms don't improve immediately. It will be to your benefit to have one doctor who knows you manage your condition. To find a physician who treats CFS, call your local hospital or state medical association and ask for a referral. Or check the CFIDS Web site (www.cfids.org) for a local support group, which should be able to provide you with a list of doctors in your area.

weeks. As your fitness level improves, you can build toward the high range but be careful not to exceed it and stress your heart unduly.

**Start slow and build.** When you have CFS, you need to exercise at a lower intensity than other people. If a workout is too intense, it's likely that you will tire rapidly and give up before experiencing any benefits. Your aerobic sessions should initially last 5 to 15 minutes, building bit by bit to 30 to 45 minutes. Exercise on alternate days, three or four times a week, for the first month. Then strive for working out most days. Once you can comfortably perform 30 minutes of continuous cardiovascular activity, gradually increase the intensity.

> *The best time to exercise? That's probably first thing in the morning if you have chronic fatigue syndrome.*
> —*Kelli Calabrese, M.S.*

**Pick the right hour.** The best time of the day to exercise is whenever your symptoms seem less severe. For most women with CFS, that's usually first thing in the morning, says Calabrese.

**Tone with weights.** Consult a personal trainer or physical therapist to develop a program for you. When you are proficient at the routine, add 1- to 2-pound weights to boost your strength. Increase the weight by degrees as you build up your stamina—you can buy half-pound magnets to attach to the dumbbells. Or stick with the same poundage and work up to performing another set (15 repetitions equal one set). Once you can handle two sets comfortably, then pump up the pounds. You may only be able to do about 10 repetitions at the heavier weight, but you can gradually boost that number as you get stronger. "The idea is to keep your workouts progressive and keep your body challenged," says Calabrese.

**Extend yourself.** Slow stretching exercises should focus on the hips, thighs, and shoulders, where CFS symptoms are frequently felt. Do one to three repetitions of each stretch, holding for 10 to 30 seconds. Sit with your legs bent and the soles of your feet together. Slowly tilt your torso forward. Maintain the stretch, then relax and repeat. (For a stretching exercise that focuses on the upper body, see page 127.)

## ANEMIA: WHEN EVEN YOUR BLOOD IS TIRED

You drag through each and every day. Maybe you feel dizzy, lightheaded, and short of breath. Perhaps you have heavy menstrual periods. You might include little or no meat in your diet. If any of these scenarios hit home, you might be anemic or have low blood levels of iron.

Anemia can be associated with an underlying disease, such as cancer, but most women who are anemic suffer from iron-deficient anemia, says **Nassim Assefi, M.D.,** women's health attending physician at the University of Washington at Seattle.

Dr. Assefi explains that your body needs iron to manufacture red blood cells. These cells contain hemoglobin, the protein that transports oxygen in the blood. Too little iron results in less hemoglobin, which translates into less oxygen and, subsequently, less energy.

The recommended dietary allowance (RDA) is 10 to 15 milligrams elemental iron, with premenopausal women and nursing mothers requiring the higher amount. Pregnant women need an increased dose of 30 milligrams.

Never take iron supplements without first checking with your doctor. Too much iron can be just as harmful as too little, interfering with the absorption of zinc and resulting in even more fatigue. Loading up on iron can also cause immune-system problems and may boost your chances of heart disease.

*Vitamin C aids absorption of iron, so take your supplement with a glass of orange juice. Don't swallow your pill with cola, coffee, or tea—all block iron.—Jesse Lynn Hanley, M.D.*

If you have iron-deficient anemia, ask your physician about taking one to three tablets of iron sulfate daily. Constipation is a common side effect of iron supplements, so be sure to increase your fiber intake, drink plenty of water, and exercise regularly, suggests Dr. Assefi. A slow-release iron supplement, such as SlowFe, may be less likely to make you constipated.

These supplements may require up to six months of use to restore your iron reserves, so it's advised that you include high-iron foods in your diet as well. Lean red meats supply the most absorbable form of iron, says *Pamela Smith, R.D.,* author of *The Energy Edge*. She also recommends these foods as excellent sources of iron.

• Dried apricots or raisins
• Prunes and prune juice
• Dried beans
• Dark green, leafy vegetables, such as spinach and kale
• Whole grains and cereals
• Well-cooked oysters and clams
• Poultry
• Tuna, shrimp, and sardines

Smith offers these additional tips to help your body absorb and use iron.

**Space supplements out.** The more iron you consume at once, the less the body actually takes in. Eating small iron-rich meals every two to three hours can help you absorb iron more effectively.

**Eat protein with every meal.** Protein facilitates iron absorption. In addition to such high-protein foods as lean meats and poultry, be sure to add low-fat cheeses and nuts to your daily menus.

**Get your Cs.** Vitamin C increases the absorption of iron. Enhance your diet with such fruits as oranges, grapefruits, strawberries, and pineapples; and such vegetables as broccoli, cabbage, and cauliflower. If you take an iron supplement, swallow it with orange juice or any other juice that's high in vitamin C.

**Flavor your water.** A spritz of C-laden lemon, lime, tangerine, or orange juice in your water not only makes a tasty drink, but also assists with iron absorption, suggests *Jesse Lynn Hanley, M.D.,* author of *Tired of Being Tired*.

# Check with your doctor before taking additional iron. Too much iron in your blood can lead to even more fatigue.

**Just say no.** Cola, coffee, and tea contain tannic acid, which interferes with your body's taking in of iron. Avoid downing supplements with any of these drinks. In fact, you should consider eliminating these beverages from your diet altogether, says Dr. Hanley. At the very least, limit your consumption to one cup a day at most.

## DIABETES: SUGAR HIGHS AND LOWS

Diabetes affects how your body makes or responds to insulin, the hormone that regulates delivery of blood glucose to organs and tissues, where it's converted into energy. Insulin resistance refers to a condition in which your body simply can't use the insulin available. This disorder can progress to full-blown diabetes, says *Elizabeth Lee Vliet, M.D.*, founder and medical director of HER Place: Health Enhancement and Renewal for Women in Tucson and Fort Worth, and author of *Women, Weight, and Hormones.* Diabetes is a serious metabolic disorder, she explains. The following are three types.

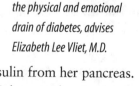

- Type I or insulin-dependent diabetes: This form occurs when the pancreas doesn't produce enough insulin. You must supply the insulin your body needs via injections or an insulin pump.
- Type II or noninsulin dependent diabetes: This is the most common form of the disease and results when your body doesn't respond to naturally produced insulin. It can often be controlled with exercise and changes in diet.

*Exercising will help you offset the physical and emotional drain of diabetes, advises Elizabeth Lee Vliet, M.D.*

- Gestational diabetes: This occurs when a pregnant woman's body is unable to use the insulin from her pancreas. It usually clears up after the birth of the baby. A bout with gestational diabetes increases the risk of developing Type II later in life.

This serious metabolic disorder is physically and emotionally stressful, says Dr. Vliet. If you don't control your blood sugar with exercise, diet, and medication, you can become overweight and dehydrated as you fluctuate between dangerously high and low sugar levels. At best, you're probably left feeling drained. At worst, you can damage your arteries, resulting in high blood pressure, kidney and nerve damage, vision and memory loss, cognitive impairment, heart attack, or death.

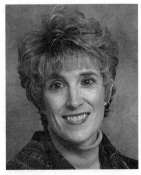

*Half of people with Type II diabetes don't realize they have it. Women over the age of 45 should be tested every three years, even if they do not have obvious symptoms, advises Anne Daly, R.D., C.D.E.*

About half of people with Type II diabetes don't realize they have it, warns *Anne Daly, R.D., C.D.E.,* president of Health Care and Education for the American Diabetes Association. See your doctor immediately if you notice any of its signature warning signs, which include unusual thirst, frequent urination, blurred vision, and unexplained fatigue. Even if you're not experiencing any symptoms, Daly says it's important to have your blood-glucose levels checked during routine physicals, especially after age 45. If test results are normal, continue to be screened every three years or at the interval recommended by your physician.

## CONTROLLING DIABETES WITH EXERCISE

Exercise plays an important role in any treatment regimen for diabetes, says fitness specialist *Kelli Calabrese, M.S.* It eases the depression that often accompanies chronic illness by releasing feel-good endorphins. Working out also helps you control or lose weight, which in turn helps regulate blood sugar. Exercise improves your body's cardiovascular function, as well as its ability to use glucose. It also assists in lowering blood pressure, reducing insulin resistance, and improving cholesterol levels.

Because exercise can affect blood-sugar levels, it's a good idea to work with your doctor to develop a safe and effective plan to help control your diabetes. Your physician can rule out such complications as diabetic retinopathy (damage to small blood vessels in the retina, which can lead to blindness), cardiac disease, and kidney or nerve problems. These difficulties won't necessarily keep you from exercising, but they may limit the type or intensity.

Daly recommends that you ask your doctor the following questions.

- How often do I need to exercise? What time of day is best for me?
- How long do I need to make my workouts?
- How intense do I need my exercise program to be?
- Should I do the same fitness program every day? Or can I vary it?
- How should I monitor my blood sugar before, during, and after exercise?
- Are there any types of exercise I should avoid?
- Which symptoms should I watch out for?
- What precautions should I take?
- Should I take less insulin or change my injection site before I exercise?
- How do I modify my meal plan?
- Will oral medications have the same effect if I exercise?

Once you get the go-ahead from your doctor, follow this advice from Daly to exercise safely.

**Start slow.** Work up to 30 minutes of physical activity a day. If you haven't exercised before, start out by walking around the block.

## SHOULD I SEE A DOCTOR?

*You can try sleeping more, working less, exercising more, and stressing less. But what if you still feel exhausted?*

If you can't identify the source of your fatigue, see your health-care provider as soon as possible. Unexplained tiredness and lethargy that lasts more than a few weeks can be symptomatic of many serious conditions and illnesses, says **Redonda Miller, M.D.,** assistant professor of medicine and director of Executive Women's Health Program at the Johns Hopkins University in Baltimore. Such causes run the gamut of the flu, mononucleosis, menopause, low thyroid function, medication side effects, depression, anxiety, stress, cancer, and heart disease to a vitamin-D deficiency.

When a woman complains of exhaustion, Dr. Miller conducts a physical examination that includes such routine lab tests as blood counts, thyroid function, blood-sugar level, and a urinalysis. The results can alert her to conditions such as hypothyroidism, diabetes, anemia, and a hormone imbalance.

If nothing shows up in the lab work, Dr. Miller looks for lifestyle factors that can sabotage energy. "The most common reason for fatigue in my patients is that they have no time for themselves and get little sleep," she says.

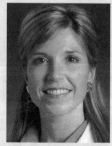

*A doctor can determine if your unexplained fatigue is a medical problem, says Redonda Miller, M.D. For busy women, the cause is often lack of sleep.*

**Listen to your body.** Stop *immediately* if you experience fatigue, pain, shortness of breath, or that slumping feeling that means your blood sugar is falling.

**Prepare your muscles.** A workout session should include 5 to 10 minutes of warm-up exercises and gentle stretching. Follow that up with at least 20 to 30 minutes of aerobic activity, such as walking or swimming, that gets your heart pumping and increases your circulation. Never exercise to the point that you feel weak or can't breathe.

**Know when to say when.** If you can't carry on a conversation while working out, then you're exercising too intensely. Slow down. Cap off the aerobic portion of your program with 5 to 10 minutes of cool-down exercises and more stretching.

## MANAGING THE STRESS OF DIABETES

Even if your diabetes is under control, the strain of supervising your condition day in and day out can be exhausting, says *Laurinda Poirier-Solomon, M.P.H., R.N.,* author of *Women & Diabetes.* Monitoring your glucose levels, keeping up your exercise, and paying attention to what you eat are must-dos. All require effort—and energy.

But women with diabetes are like most other women in that they often rank themselves last on the list of people to look after, says Poirier-Solomon.

Squeezing take-care-of-yourself time into your already-busy schedule can be overwhelming. Open yourself up to assistance, suggests Poirier-Solomon. Don't be afraid to ask for some help with doing household chores, chauffeuring the kids, or running errands. "Retire Superwoman—permanently," says Poirier-Solomon.

Stress-relieving techniques, such as meditation and yoga, are very helpful for women with diabetes—as they are for everyone else. (For more

*Nobody can do it all, especially when you add the stress of managing diabetes. Don't try to be Superwoman, says Laurinda Poirier-Solomon, M.P.H., R.N.*

information, see "Stress-Busters," page 283.) Also beneficial is sharing your feelings and fears about the disease. Your local hospital may have a diabetes support group or education program. If not, contact the American Diabetes Association (www.diabetes.org, 800-342-2383) to find out about resources available in your community.

# Eyes
## Seeing Your Way Clear

*Here's looking at you, kid.*
—Rick Blaine (Humphrey Bogart), *Casablanca*

Your eyes are your windows on the world. To give them the care they deserve, don't ignore any eye problems. Take the time to remedy relatively minor conditions, such as eyestrain and dry eyes, and don't delay seeing your doctor for any vision problems.

Here's expert advice on how to give your eyes a little TLC and how to spot some of the more common eye-related diseases and disorders, such as macular degeneration and cataracts, so that you can keep a clear view of the world around you.

### MACULAR DEGENERATION: LIVING WITH VISION LOSS

Even though *Lylas G. Mogk, M.D.,* is an ophthalmologist, her training and expertise couldn't prevent her father from developing macular degeneration at age 79. But his experience with the disease influenced her to help others. She opened the Henry Ford Health System Eye Care Services and co-authored, with her daughter, *Macular Degeneration: The Complete Guide to Saving and Maximizing Your Sight.*

Dr. Mogk describes macular degeneration as the breakdown of the macula. It is a small area responsible for detailed central vision in the center of the retina, the tissue at the back of the eye. People with macular degeneration retain peripheral (side) vision, but their distance and close central vision are both affected. This makes activities that require detail, such as reading, difficult or even impossible without the aid of extra lighting and magnifying devices. The ability to drive may also be compromised.

Macular degeneration is often referred to as age-related macular degeneration (ARMD, or just AMD). ARMD is one of the most common causes of vision problems in Americans ages 65 and older, says Dr. Mogk. Research suggests that ARMD may have a genetic factor: If a family member had the disease, you're more likely to develop it. And for reasons as yet unknown, ARMD affects Caucasians at a much higher rate than African-Americans or Hispanics, and women more than men.

ARMD has two forms: dry and wet. Most people have the dry form, which is characterized by a very slow breakdown of the macula. One early sign of the dry form that doctors can see during an exam is the formation of small yellow spots, called drusen, on the retina. The drusen gradually enlarge and cause areas of the macula to atrophy and eventually cause loss of central vision. ARMD often occurs in just one eye, but may later occur in the other eye. It may take several years before you notice any significant loss of vision with dry ARMD, says Dr. Mogk. Dry ARMD develops so slowly, many people are able to manage very well for an extended period with adaptations, such as reading large-print publications and using magnifying lenses for some daily activities.

ARMD almost always starts as the dry form. In approximately 10 percent of cases, it evolves into the wet form, which is more severe because it involves the growth of abnormal new blood vessels beneath the macula. These fragile blood vessels leak blood and fluid under the macula, causing damage, rapid vision loss, and eventual scarring.

If you get regular checkups, your eye doctor can identify ARMD before you ever notice any loss of central vision, says Dr. Mogk. She may take these steps to diagnose the condition.

- Dilate your pupils: To see as much of your retinas as possible, your doctor uses eyedrops that dilate your pupils. The doctor views each eye's macula using a handheld instrument called an ophthalmoscope.
- Test your vision with an Amsler grid: Your doctor may ask you to look at a grid that resembles a piece of graph paper with a dot in the center. You'll cover one eye and stare at the dot. People with ARMD are likely to see wavy lines or blind spots when looking at the dot, especially when new blood vessels are developing under the retina. If you have early signs of ARMD, your doctor may give you an Amsler grid so you can monitor your vision at home.
- Check your eye's blood flow with a fluorescein angiography test: Your doctor may perform this test if she thinks you might have wet ARMD. She'll inject a fluorescent dye into your arm, then photograph the blood

vessels in the retina as the dye passes through. If the photos show evidence of new, leaky blood vessels under the retina, your doctor can determine if and how they can be treated. ICG is a similar test that uses indocyanine green dye.

## TREATMENT OPTIONS FOR ARMD

If you have the wet form of ARMD, your doctor may treat you with a procedure called laser photocoagulation. She can perform this procedure right in her office, using a laser to seal off abnormal blood vessels under the macula to prevent further leakage. After the 30-minute procedure, you can usually resume your daily routine, says Dr. Mogk. Laser photocoagulation can delay additional vision loss in 70 percent of patients who undergo it. But the procedure comes with a trade-off: You may lose a little vision now to prevent greater loss later. This is because the heat of the laser beam can damage a tiny spot in the macula as it passes through to reach the vessels underneath.

Photodynamic therapy (PDT) is a recent variation on the laser procedure that combines laser treatment with the use of the drug Visudyne (verteporfin), says Dr. Mogk. PDT has less risk of vision loss than photocoagulation laser surgery. The doctor injects Visudyne into your arm, and it's carried in your bloodstream to the abnormal blood vessels behind the macula. The laser's light activates the drug, which seals the leaking vessel. Since it's light—not heat—that is important to this procedure, the doctor can use a cool laser, which doesn't damage the macula and impair vision, explains Dr. Mogk. While laser surgery cannot restore lost vision, it may slow down or delay further damage to your central vision.

There is no cure or treatment for the dry form of ARMD, but nutritional supplements may help delay its progress, says Dr. Mogk.

## WHAT YOU CAN DO TO AVOID ARMD

Although macular degeneration can't be cured, research suggests you may be able to prevent it—or at least minimize your risk of developing it to some degree. Dr. Mogk advises you to take these steps.

**Wear sunglasses.** Yellow, orange, brown, or amber lenses provide the best protection. They block the high-energy blue wavelengths that may contribute to ARMD.

## MOTHER NATURE, M.D.: MACULAR DEGENERATION

*If you want to reduce the risk of losing your sight due to macular degeneration as you age, look for help in your refrigerator.*

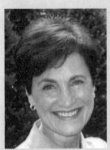

*Eat plenty of greens and fish, says Lylas G. Mogk, M.D. Their antioxidants and omega-3 fatty acids may help protect your eyes from age-related macular degeneration.*

Can the right foods preserve your sight? Maybe. That's the prescription suggested by *Lylas G. Mogk, M.D.,* co-author of *Macular Degeneration: The Complete Guide to Saving and Maximizing Your Sight.* She recommends a natural low-fat diet, with at least five servings a week of dark green, leafy vegetables to give you plenty of lutein and zeaxanthin, two antioxidants important for healthy maculae.

Antioxidants are chemicals that protect cells in the body from damage caused by excess free radicals. While our bodies produce free radicals simply by breathing oxygen, excess free radicals are produced by such external factors as the sun, pollution, and chemicals, explains Dr. Mogk. She recommends routinely eating such antioxidant-boosting vegetables as collard greens, kale, mustard greens, parsley, spinach, Swiss chard, and watercress. Red peppers and romaine lettuce contain smaller amounts of lutein and zeaxanthin but are also good options.

Research on the correlation between nutrition and age-related macular degeneration (ARMD) is new, and more studies are necessary, says Dr. Mogk.

In 2002, the Institute of Ophthalmology completed a study that found that taking supplements of antioxidants and zinc had a modest effect on slowing the progress of ARMD. To reap the benefits of these supplements, Dr. Mogk recommends taking four pills a day of Ocuvite PreserVision or ICaps AREDS Formula, available at drugstores. In addition to these, she says you should take 10 milligrams lutein and 250 micrograms selenium. Another recent study showed that omega-3 fatty acids may also protect the maculae, so you might add a daily dose of 2 teaspoons or two capsules of either flaxseed oil or cod liver oil.

"People with early ARMD should clearly be taking the whole amounts of the supplements, and others at high risk—such as older adults with family history of ARMD—are probably wise to take the whole amounts, although that's not absolutely proven," says Dr. Mogk. For those who have less risk, such as younger adults, taking a smaller dose of these supplements may be fine. "The whole topic is complicated, so I tend to offer the possibilities as they seem appropriate for each patient," she says.

No supplement is a proper substitute for a good diet, warns Dr. Mogk. And since some of the doses in these supplements are higher than the accepted daily recommendations, you should discuss their use with your primary-care doctor, especially if you have other medical problems or take prescription medications.

**Avoid smoke.** Smoking damages the retina, not to mention just about every other part of your body. Even secondhand smoke is potentially harmful.

**Consider nutritional supplements.** A recent trial sponsored by the National Eye Institute found that antioxidant supplements may help protect the macula in people who are at high risk for developing advanced ARMD. A smaller study at Harvard University suggested that omega-3 fatty acids, found in fish and flaxseed oils, may also help lower your risk for getting ARMD. (For more information, see "Mother Nature, M.D.," page 141.)

**Eat greens.** Make sure your diet includes plenty of antioxidant-rich dark green, leafy vegetables.

## GLAUCOMA: THE SNEAKY VISION THIEF

The greatest danger of glaucoma is its stealth: It can steal your eyesight without warning, says *Ruth Williams, M.D.,* a glaucoma and cataracts specialist from Wheaton, Illinois, who chairs the ophthalmology section of the American Medical Association. Early diagnosis and treatment provide the best chances to save your sight.

Glaucoma is a disease affecting the optic nerve, which carries images to the brain. Normally, a fluid called the aqueous humor flows throughout the eye and continuously drains through various channels. If the drainage is interrupted, as it is in glaucoma, pressure builds up within the eye. Left untreated, the increasing pressure pushes against and damages the optic nerve, eventually resulting in blindness.

Acute and chronic types of glaucoma are defined by where the fluid blockage occurs. Secondary glaucoma can result from an injury or inflammation of the eye, such as a cataract, eye tumor, advanced diabetes, or any condition that interferes with fluid drainage. This form of glaucoma may also develop in people who take corticosteroid medications.

Anyone can get glaucoma, but genetics clearly plays a role. People with a family history of glaucoma are at greater risk; so are African-Americans. Other risk factors include being older than age 50, being nearsighted, or having experienced past eye injuries. If any of these apply to you, Dr. Williams recommends you have your eyes checked by an ophthalmologist or optometrist at least once a year. It's during routine eye exams that most people learn they have chronic glaucoma, since they usually have no symptoms. You *can* have symptoms with acute glaucoma. Dr. Williams advises you to see your doctor immediately if you experience nausea, vomiting, decreased vision, blurry vision, halos around lights at night, pain and redness of the eye, haziness, or a dilated pupil. "Nausea, vomiting, and eye pain indicate an immediate emergency," she says. Blindness can occur in just two to five days, depending on the level of eye pressure.

During your annual eye examination, your doctor will perform a simple test, known as tonometry, that measures the pressure in your eye. An instrument called a tonometer directs a puff of air against each eye and then measures the time it takes to flatten the cornea, explains Dr. Williams. She says this is a good screening device, but the Goldmann tonometry test is a more accurate measure and is now used by ophthalmologists and many optometrists. In this test, the doctor numbs your eyes with anesthetic drops so that she can lightly press the instrument against each cornea to cause a slight indentation. The tonometer registers each eye's resistance.

Normal eye pressure can range from 12 to 22 millimeters of mercury. Women typically have higher normal pressures than men, and Asians have lower normal pressures than either Caucasians or African-Americans. Some people develop glaucoma at so-called normal pressures, while others with high pressures don't necessarily develop the condition. "That's why it's so important to be examined by a doctor who knows how to look at the optic nerve carefully," says Dr. Williams.

## WHO'S WHO IN EYE CARE

*There are three types of eye-care professionals.*

Both ophthalmologists and optometrists provide good primary eye care, says *Yvonne Johnson, O.D.,* director of medical affairs for Novartis Ophthalmics in Atlanta.

**Optometrists:** They provide most primary care. They are not physicians but have completed college, as well as four years of optometry school. Known as O.D.s, optometrists diagnose various eye disorders and can prescribe corrective lenses. In most states, they can also prescribe medications to treat eye diseases. Should you have a condition that requires surgery or medical care that an optometrist cannot provide, she will refer you to an ophthalmologist who specializes in your particular condition.

**Ophthalmologists:** These medical doctors receive specialized training in the diagnoses and treatment of eye diseases. They are the only eye-care professionals who can perform surgery.

**Opticians:** These professionals cannot examine eyes or prescribe corrective lenses. They follow the prescription written by an ophthalmologist or optometrist to make and fit eyeglasses or contact lenses.

Since a pressure reading alone does not necessarily refute or confirm glaucoma, the following tests may also be performed.

- Ophthalmoscopy: The doctor uses a lighted instrument to magnify the back of your eyes to view any damage to your optic nerves.
- Perimetry: Also known as a visual field test, this procedure requires you to look straight ahead while covering one eye. Intermittent dots of light are projected on a bowl-shaped screen, and you press a button whenever you see a light. The machine creates a printout, or map, that shows the range of your peripheral vision. A new test known as nerve-fiber analysis does not replace the perimetry test but can add to the information available to your doctor. An optic-nerve photograph is a similar test that can document the appearance of your optic nerves, explains Dr. Williams. Your doctor may repeat these tests every few years to check for areas of change.
- Gonioscopy: The doctor uses drops to numb your eyes, then inserts special contact lenses. Each lens has a mirror in it that allows the doctor to look sideways into your eye to check the angle between the iris and cornea, an area where blockage tends to occur.

*Consider it an emergency if you have nausea, vomiting, and eye pain. These could be symptoms of acute glaucoma that can lead to blindness in just days.*

—*Ruth Williams, M.D.*

## TREATING GLAUCOMA: PREVENTING BLINDNESS

Chronic glaucoma, the most common form, usually affects both eyes, says Dr. Williams. If the disease is caught early, it rarely leads to blindness. Medication is usually all that's required to lower the pressure in the eyes and prevent damage to the optic nerves.

Medications are available as pills, eyedrops, ointments, or inserts (thin strips of medication you put in your eye). A class of drugs called beta-blockers is used to decrease production of fluid in the eyes. Medicated eyedrops in this category include Betagan (levobunolol), Betimol (timolol), Betoptic-S (betaxolol), Ocupress (carteolol), OptiPranolol (metipranolol), and Timoptic-XE (timolol). Your doctor will decide if eyedrops or another form of medication is most appropriate for you, says Dr. Williams. If medication does not successfully control the pressure, your doctor may recommend you have laser surgery.

Laser surgery will likely be the initial treatment if you have acute or secondary glaucoma. Your doctor can often perform laser surgery right in her office, and you usually don't require much recovery time.

For more serious forms of glaucoma, your doctor may recommend microsurgery, which is more invasive and must be performed in a hospital or clinic. The doctor places a microscope several inches above your eye so that she can make a tiny cut in the white of the eye, known as the sclera. This opening becomes an artificial channel that allows fluid to bypass the blocked drainage canals, thus reducing pressure in the eye. The surgeon may also remove a small piece of the iris (the colored portion of the eye) to prevent future problems. While this surgery doesn't usually require that you go under anesthesia, you will likely have to protect your eye for about a week afterwards. You may not be able to drive, read, exercise strenuously, or get water in your eye.

## CATARACTS: SEEING THROUGH A CLOUD

"Having a cataract is like looking through a window that is fogged up," says *Ruth Williams, M.D.*, a glaucoma and cataracts specialist from Wheaton, Illinois, who chairs the ophthalmology section of the American Medical Association. A cataract is a cloudy spot on the normally clear lens of an eye that can occur at any time but is more likely as you age.

Like many eye diseases, cataracts can sneak up on you, says Dr. Williams. If the cloudiness is not located near the center of your lens, you may not even be aware of it. If you do have symptoms, you may notice the following.

- Painless blurred vision
- Sensitivity to light
- Frequent changes in prescription for eyeglasses
- Distorted or ghost images in either eye
- Poor night vision
- Seeing halos around lights
- Fading or yellowing of colors

Though cataracts are most often related to aging of the eyes, other risk factors include family history, such medical conditions as diabetes, previous eye injury or surgery, use of certain medications (steroids, for example, which may be prescribed for such illnesses as lupus or lung diseases), and long-term, unprotected exposure to sunlight.

Having a cataract doesn't necessarily mean that you'll have vision problems or need treatment. "Just because a cataract's there, doesn't mean it needs to come out," explains Dr. Williams. "It's really a vision decision." Most doctors would opt to remove a cataract only if it bothers you or vision loss interferes with your life.

If a cataract affects your vision, it must be removed surgically and replaced with a clear man-made lens. Cataract surgery is usually an outpatient procedure. Your eye should heal completely within a few days to a few weeks.

*Most doctors remove a cataract only if vision loss interferes with day-to-day life.—Ruth Williams, M.D.*

You may not be able to prevent cataracts, but research suggests you can delay their occurrence, says **Mandi D. Conway, M.D.,** professor of ophthalmology at Tulane University. These are her suggestions for preserving clear sight.

**Cover up.** Wear a broad-brimmed hat or sunglasses with UVA/UVB protection to protect your eyes when you're outside.

**Stop smoking.** Smoking has been linked to the development of cataracts, with some damage perhaps being irreversible. But a recent study found that people who were smoke-free for 25 years or longer lowered their risk of cataracts later in life by 20 percent, compared with those who continued to smoke. However, the risk of former smokers did not decline to the level of those who had never smoked.

**Cut back on salt.** An Australian study indicates that people who consume high-sodium diets have twice the risk of developing subcapsular cataracts, which is the most serious form.

**Eat your veggies.** Recent studies suggest that you may reduce the risk of cataracts with a steady diet of vitamins C and E, certain B vitamins, and the carotenoids lutein and zeaxanthin, found in such dark green, leafy vegetables as spinach, collard greens, kale, mustard greens, and turnip greens.

# PRESBYOPIA: FOCUSING AT ARM'S LENGTH

Can't see to read a menu anymore? Given up trying to read phone book listings? Does holding a book at arm's length only partially help you to focus? You could have presbyopia, commonly known as farsightedness. It's annoying. But it's also a fact of life, says *Eve Higginbotham, M.D.,* professor and chair of the department of ophthalmology at the University of Maryland in Baltimore.

As you age, the lenses of your eyes slowly lose their elasticity. By the time you're in your 40s, the lenses may be so rigid that they can't alter their shape enough to bring close objects into sharp focus, explains Dr. Higginbotham. Changes in the lenses cause most of the problem, but there may also be a decrease in strength of the muscles inside the eyes that squeeze the lenses, she adds.

Unfortunately, there's no way to prevent farsightedness. These are things you can do to enhance your vision.

**Identify the problem.** If you've never worn glasses and now find close objects blurry, see an eye doctor for an exam. She can determine if your condition is age-related or a symptom of a more serious problem. Most adults should have an eye exam at least once every two years.

**Try reading glasses.** Your doctor will be able to tell you if you need custom-made eyeglasses or if a pair of over-the-counter (OTC) reading glasses can do the trick. "People often buy glasses that are more expensive than

---

## SHOULD I SEE A DOCTOR?

*Regular exams are just as important for your eyes as any other part of your body.*

You should have a regular eye exam, even if you're not aware of any vision problems. That's often the only way to learn if anything is amiss with your eyes, says *Ruth Williams, M.D.,* chair of the ophthalmology section of the American Medical Association.

Vision care should also start early: Dr. Williams recommends that children have their first eye exam at 6 months and their second at age 3. They should be examined again before entering first grade and then every two years thereafter.

If you experience no vision problems, Dr. Williams recommends being examined every two to three years between ages 19 and 40, every two years between ages 41 and 60, and every year thereafter. If you need vision correction or have other eye conditions that need monitoring, your doctor will recommend an exam schedule for you.

See your eye doctor immediately if you notice decreasing or blurred vision, pain, or discharge, says Dr. Williams.

they really need," says Dr. Higginbotham. She suggests you start off with a +1.25 magnification, which may work for a few years. When you need stronger lenses, increase the magnification by 0.25 degrees (or diopters). Since OTC glasses are not expensive, you can buy several pairs and keep them where you're most likely to need them, perhaps by the computer and your nightstand.

**Alter your prescription.** If you require one prescription for seeing up close and another for seeing far away, bifocal lenses may be a good choice. Recent options for bifocals don't have visible lines in the lenses. Trifocals are also available, which allow you to look comfortably at a computer screen. Bifocal contact lenses are also available.

## CONTACT LENSES: HANDLE WITH CARE

*Some people don't like to wear eyeglasses, and laser vision surgery may not appeal to them either. Wearing contact lenses could be an excellent alternative.*

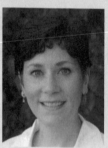

*Keeping your contacts clean helps keep them comfortable and effective, says Louise Sclafani, O.D. Choose and apply your makeup with care to avoid damaging a lens.*

Contact lenses offer practical benefits, says *Louise Sclafani, O.D.,* associate professor of clinical ophthalmology at the University of Chicago. She says they may offer better sight than eyeglasses do, and they move with your eye, allowing a natural field of vision.

Contact lenses have a few drawbacks, too. They tend to make everyone's eyes dry, but women who wear contacts may be especially prone to dry eyes because hormonal fluctuations can alter tear production, says Dr. Sclafani. Taking birth control pills, being pregnant, and experiencing menopause can also contribute to drying out your eyes. A contact lens can stick in place if your eye is too dry, which increases your risk of infection. If dry eyes become a problem, Dr. Sclafani says your doctor may ask you to switch to rigid gas-permeable lenses, such as Hydro2, which are made of a so-called wettable material that moves more easily on your eyes or to soft lenses specially designed for dry eyes.

Once you have the correct type of lenses, most people can wear contacts successfully if they follow their doctor's advice, says Dr. Sclafani. She suggests these dos and don'ts for getting the most from them.

**Follow the prescribed care routine.** Care varies depending upon the type of lenses you wear and how often you wear them. Special cleaning solutions are sometimes required. Don't use homemade saline solutions, since they can cause an infection that may result in blindness among soft-lens wearers.

**Go mono.** Ask your eye doctor about monovision, which is most commonly prescribed for contact-lens wearers. The prescription for one eye is for near vision, and the one for the other eye is for far vision.

## EYESTRAIN: TAKE A BREAK

Too many hours staring at a computer can leave you with tired eyes and an achy head. If that's the case, you could be experiencing eyestrain, says *Gerri Goodman, M.D.*, clinical instructor of ophthalmology at the Johns Hopkins Hospital in Baltimore. Other symptoms include redness, burning, blurred vision, sensitivity to glare and light, and difficulty concentrating.

**Stay on schedule.** If you're wearing disposable or planned replacement lenses, carefully follow the schedule for discarding used lenses.

**Don't use waterproof mascara.** Avoid lash-extending mascara, which contains fibers that can irritate eyes. Also avoid waterproof mascara, which is not easily removed with water and may stain soft contact lenses.

**Be careful with cosmetics.** Choose an oil-free moisturizer and a water-based, hypoallergenic liquid foundation, since cream makeup may leave a film on your lenses. Keep false-eyelash cement, nail polish and remover, perfume, and cologne away from the lenses, since they can damage the plastic. Wash your hands thoroughly before handling your lenses but avoid cream soaps and hand lotions, which leave a film on your hands that can be transferred to the lenses.

**Make up with lenses.** Put your lenses in before you put on makeup to avoid getting cosmetic particles on your lenses. But take your contact lenses out before you remove your makeup.

**Spray with care.** Avoid using hair spray while wearing your contacts. If you must spray your hair with your lenses in, close your eyes while spraying and keep them closed for a few seconds afterwards.

**Stay moist.** While using a hair dryer, blink frequently to keep your eyes from getting too dry.

**Get checked.** Keep regular appointments with your eye doctor during and after your adaptation period to make sure that the prescription works and the lenses don't need to be replaced. (For more information, see "Should I See a Doctor?" page 147.) Dr. Sclafani recommends you get a checkup as soon as possible if you experience any of the following problems:

- Blurred or fuzzy vision, especially if it comes on suddenly
- Red, irritated eyes
- Uncomfortable lenses
- Pain in and around the eyes

**For your eyes only.** Don't put a lens in your mouth or moisten it with saliva, which is full of bacteria and, thus, a potential source of infection. And never share lenses with someone else. Remember that all contact lenses are medical devices—even if you wear cosmetic tinted lenses without vision correction, you're still susceptible to the same hazards as other lens wearers.

Eyestrain can be caused by several conditions, such as the inability of one or both eyes to focus well, inability of both eyes to work together, or prolonged close work without a break. But prolonged computer use seems to be the culprit in a significant number of eyestrain cases these days. Dr. Goodman explains that most people tend to stare at a computer screen without blinking, which dries out your eyes and overworks the eye muscles.

Dr. Goodman has these suggestions to help you avoid so-called computer fatigue syndrome.

**Check the layout.** The distance between your eyes and the computer screen should be 17 to 26 inches.

**Keep materials close.** Keep any papers or books you're working with next to the screen at about the same distance from your eyes so that you don't have to constantly refocus.

**Adjust the brightness.** You want enough contrast so that you can comfortably view the screen without straining. Reduce glare by turning off overhead lights, if necessary. A desk lamp may be better than an overhead light for you. Go with whatever is most comfortable.

**Cut the glare.** Reduce glare from such sources as curtainless windows. Use an antiglare screen on your computer or move it away from windows.

**Blink.** Every 15 to 20 minutes, close your eyes. Then look away from the screen and blink.

**Fake it.** Keep a bottle of artificial tears on your desk and use them throughout the day. (For more information, see "Dry Eyes," page 152.)

**Consider computer glasses.** These are glasses specifically designed for use at midrange and close distances. They allow you to comfortably see the computer screen, as well as your paperwork, without having to refocus. They are not designed for distance vision.

## CONJUNCTIVITIS: SEEING RED

Conjunctivitis is a catchall for basic red eye (also known as pink eye), says *Yvonne Johnson, O.D.,* director of medical affairs for Novartis Ophthalmics in Atlanta. Though these conditions are not usually painful, they can be mighty unpleasant. There are three common types of conjunctivitis.

- Bacterial conjunctivitis: Especially prevalent in children, this condition is characterized by rapid onset of redness, grittiness, and a thick discharge that can make the eyelids stick together.
- Allergic conjunctivitis: This is one of the most common forms, also known as seasonal allergic conjunctivitis. The red, watery, itchy eyes usually occur in the spring and fall when the pollen count is high. However, if you have allergies to dust mites and animal dander, you may be in for red, itchy eyes year-round.
- Viral conjunctivitis: This form of red eye may accompany an upper respiratory virus and is marked by hot, watery eyes.

A bacterial infection can be treated with antibiotic drops or ointment, such as Ciloxan (ciprofloxacin), Ilotycin (erythromycin), or Tobrex (tobramycin). Apply a warm compress to the eye to loosen and wash away crustiness, suggests Dr. Johnson. If the condition is in one eye only, be careful not to let the same compress touch the other eye because you can spread the infection.

Allergic conjunctivitis can be treated with over-the-counter antihistamines that contain naphazoline. Or your doctor may prescribe such medications as Patanol (olopatadine) or Zaditor (ketotifen), which prevent the itchy eyes associated with allergies. Cool compresses can also take away the heat and discomfort caused by allergies.

Usually, no treatment is necessary for viral conjunctivitis—it simply has to run its course. But you can soothe the discomfort with artificial tears. (For more information, see "Dry Eyes," page 152.) Some viruses, such as the herpes virus, may require an antiviral eyedrop, says Dr. Johnson.

Dr. Johnson has this advice to help you cope with conjunctivitis discomfort.

**Don't rub.** Rubbing an itchy eye only irritates it further. It also increases the risk of transferring the infection to an unaffected eye.

**Switch to glasses.** Don't wear contact lenses until the condition clears up. Besides feeling uncomfortable, contacts will trap bacteria behind the lenses.

**Wear sunglasses.** This protection minimizes irritation from the sun's glare.

**Skip eye makeup.** Contaminated makeup applicators can transfer the infection from eye to eye.

**See your eye doctor.** Get a diagnosis to be sure you really have conjunctivitis. Some serious, sight-threatening eye conditions initially can appear to be red eye.

## DRY EYES: DON'T FORGET TO MOISTURIZE

Having dry eyes is manageable, but it's a regular condition for many people, says **Yvonne Johnson, O.D.**, director of medical affairs for Novartis Ophthalmics in Atlanta. Look out for these causes of dry eyes.

- Decongestants, diuretics, antidepressants, and antihistamines can reduce moisture in the eyes.
- A dry, dusty environment dries mucous membranes of the eyes.
- Contact lenses can hinder the lubrication action of tears in the eyes.
- Extended computer use can lead to insufficient blinking, meaning fewer tears to bathe the eyes.
- Lower levels of estrogen after menopause lead to changes in mucous membranes throughout the body, including the eyes.

Dry-eye symptoms include a stinging or burning sensation, tearing, sensitivity to light, and the feeling that there's a foreign body in the eye, says Dr. Johnson. When eyes become excessively dry, they can also develop a discharge. If the condition worsens or is left untreated, damage to the cornea can lead to reduced or blurred vision, says Dr. Johnson.

Dry eyes are treatable, says Dr. Johnson. You can soothe your eyes with an over-the-counter tear substitute, such as GenTeal. Be sure to choose a product that is labeled as unpreserved, since preservatives in products designed to "get the red out" will make the condition worse. You can use artificial tears as often as necessary. "Listen to your eyes," says Dr. Johnson. Some patients get relief from having their drainage holes (puncta) closed with special plugs so that tears are retained in the eyes, adds Dr. Johnson.

In addition to using artificial tears, Dr. Johnson has these suggestions to help soothe your dry eyes.

**Moisturize the air.** Use portable humidifiers in your home and office to combat overly dry air.

**Shun smoke.** Cigarette smoke is very drying to the eyes. Don't be around cigarettes—your own or anyone else's.

**Nix alcohol.** Alcohol dehydrates your body, which includes drying out your mouth and eyes. If you drink, keep it to a minimum.

**Take a break from contacts.** Contact lenses can dry out your eyes. They change the composition of tears, so give your eyes a rest whenever you can.

# VISION PROBLEMS: ASSESS LASER VISION SURGERY

If you're tired of squinting at the clock in the middle of the night or seeing yet another contact lens swirl down the drain, you might be interested in laser vision correction, also known as refractive surgery. This increasingly popular procedure can improve or correct nearsightedness, farsightedness, and astigmatism (a condition in which either near or far vision is blurred).

If you'd like to live free of spectacles and lenses, for the most part, consult a laser vision specialist to discuss your individual needs, advises *Gerri Goodman, M.D.*, clinical instructor of ophthalmology at the Johns Hopkins Hospital in Baltimore and one of the first ophthalmologists to perform laser eye surgery in the United States.

Laser in-situ keratomileusis (LASIK) is a vision correction procedure performed by an ophthalmologist or a refractive surgeon who uses a microsurgical instrument to create a flap in the cornea. (The cornea is the clear, front part of the eye that helps you focus.) A cool laser beam reshapes the cornea, then the flap is closed. Because the surface of the cornea is preserved, the correction is almost instantaneous.

Laser vision correction has been performed in the United States since 1995, says Dr. Goodman. Earlier procedures of this type were known as automated lamellar keratectomy (ALK) and photorefractive keratectomy (PRK). Dr. Goodman says LASIK is now the preferred treatment because patients recover more quickly, require fewer post-surgery visits, and experience less discomfort, risk of infection or scarring, and need for anti-inflammatory drops after this procedure.

LASIK is a relatively painless outpatient procedure that is effective even for patients with strong eyeglass or contact prescriptions. The worse your eyesight, the longer the procedure takes, says Dr. Goodman, but even the worst cases need only about a minute of laser time. Eyedrops are the only anesthetic required, but your doctor can give you a mild tranquilizer to help you relax, if necessary.

After the procedure, your eyes may feel irritated for a few hours, and you may experience some dryness for several days. You should be able to see well by the day after the surgery. If you had extremely poor vision, though, complete recovery can take up to eight weeks. Either way, you should notice significant improvement in your vision in a few days following the procedure, says Dr. Goodman.

You'll need to stay indoors for the rest of the day after your surgery, advises Dr. Goodman. Within a week, you should be able to follow your usual routine, including light exercise. For about a month after the surgery, you should wear eye protection, such as wraparound sunglasses, when outdoors. If your eyes are especially light-sensitive, you may even have to wear them indoors. For at least two months, it's a good idea to wear safety glasses if you're physically active or engaged in contact sports, says Dr. Goodman. She suggests avoiding gardening and water-related activities for two weeks to avoid the risk of infection from plant fungi and bacteria.

LASIK is relatively new. There are no long-term study results on it yet, but there appear to be no lasting negative effects on the eyes.

The cost of LASIK varies and depends on whether you have surgery on one or both eyes. Expect to pay about $1,800 to $2,000 per eye. The fee covers presurgery consultation and evaluation, the surgical procedure, medications and eyedrops, and postsurgical care, including eye exams for a year afterward. LASIK is usually not covered by insurance, but many vision centers offer flexible payment options.

As enthusiastic as Dr. Goodman is about laser surgery—she had the procedure more than 10 years ago—she says that LASIK is not necessarily a cure-all for every vision problem and warns that not everyone will achieve perfect eyesight. The weaker your prescription, the better chance you have to get positive results. You should also have a stable prescription, meaning that you are not a good candidate for LASIK if your prescription changes almost every year or has changed in the past 12 months. Surgery may be riskier for people who have unusually thin corneas or certain medical conditions, such as lupus, diabetes, glaucoma, cataracts, or rheumatoid arthritis. Some medications can also make surgery risky. Discuss your particular risks with the surgeon.

Dr. Goodman conducts an intense medical history and visual exam to determine whether laser correction is an appropriate choice for a patient. She notes whether the individual removes her eyeglasses during the conversation and, if so, how frequently. "By spending time with each person, I get a feel for what he or she needs," says Dr. Goodman. Sometimes, she talks patients out of having surgery. "If I can't give good results or the results they're hoping for, then I won't do the surgery," she says.

Anyone who opts to have LASIK surgery should have realistic and appropriate expectations: Know your probable outcome before you go in so that you're less likely to be surprised or disappointed with the results, advises Dr. Goodman. Only an estimated 5 to 15 percent of patients need follow-up surgery to help correct such side effects as blurring, difficulties with night vision, or, in few cases, eyesight that's worse than it was before the surgery.

If you get near-perfect or perfect vision from LASIK, you will no longer have to rely on contacts or eyeglasses to drive, play sports, or watch TV and movies. If you start out with a strong prescription, however, you might still need glasses for reading and close work.

To find a qualified LASIK surgeon, your eye doctor can refer you to an ophthalmologist who performs LASIK. Or visit the American Academy of Ophthalmology at www.aao.org and click on "Find an Eye M.D." for a list of academy members who perform LASIK. Ask any prospective surgeon the following questions.

- How long have you performed LASIK surgery?
- How many procedures have you performed?
- What is your success rate? How do you define success?
- How many of your patients have achieved 20/20 or 20/40 vision? How many have needed follow-up surgery?
- What is the chance for me, with my vision correction, to achieve 20/20 vision?
- What type of laser do you use? (Your surgeon should use one of the lasers approved by the U.S. Food and Drug Administration, listed at www.fda.gov/cdrh/lasik/lasers.htm.)
- What is involved in postoperative care?
- Who handles postoperative care?
- What are the risks and possible complications of LASIK?

Even if laser vision surgery is not an option for you now, that doesn't mean a new procedure down the road won't be the answer for you, says Dr. Goodman. New vision-correction techniques being developed include intraocular lenses, implantable contact lenses, and wavefront technology (the next type of laser technology). Most of these applications should be available within a few years.

# 8 Feet
........................................................................

## Caring For (and Repairing) Your Faithful Carriers

*They did not look at my face, they did not look at my hands ... what I did for the country ... they looked down at my feet.*

—Imelda Marcos, former first lady of the Philippines and shoe connoisseur

Ah, our feet. What woman doesn't adore adorning them with the latest in leather and suede? Or get a psychological boost from finding the perfect black boots? (Never mind that you already have three pairs in the closet.) Yet our footwear, the very things we adore, can be the source of our aching feet.

The reason is simple: Our shoes don't fit properly. In fact, most of us wear shoes one to two width sizes too small, causing nearly 90 percent of foot problems. No wonder that 9 out of 10 foot surgeries are performed on women, at an annual cost of $3.5 billion, with 15 million lost workdays. The problems are almost as numerous as Mrs. Marcos' footwear.

### BUNIONS: AVOIDING THE KNIFE

Think *bunion* and what comes to mind? Something gross, deformed, ugly? A bunion is actually a bony protrusion on the outside of a big toe. It's not a growth on the foot but a deformity at the toe joint that causes the bone to stick out. The bump you see is the joint bulging to the side. An emerging bunion may be mildly painful but not even noticeable without X-rays.

Over time, however, the protrusion causes the big toe to press against the next toe, and so on down the line. This forces the toes to overlap, resulting in calluses on the big toe and the next two toes, as well as hammer toes. (See "Hammer Toes," page 166.)

The bursa is a sac of fluid that protects the joint and overlays the bunion. It may become swollen, inflamed, and extremely painful. This visible deformity can also be accompanied with internal changes in the joint that are associated with degenerative arthritis. Then there are bunionettes, which are smaller versions of bunions that appear on the outsides of little toes.

If your grandmother or mother had bunions, it's likely you'll have them, too, since the tendency to develop bunions—rather than the bunions themselves—is hereditary. Therefore, what many women (and men) inherit is faulty foot development. What triggers the formation of bunions is probably shoes.

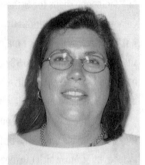

Look down. Are you wearing shoes that squeeze or pinch your feet? Is your closet full of high-heeled, pointy-toed shoes? If so, you've likely got bunion triggers wrapped around your toes right now.

*There's an easy alternative to painful bunion surgery: Wear sensible shoes that fit properly, says orthopaedic surgeon Gail Dalton, M.D.*

Surgery is an alternative treatment of bunions, but it should only be viewed as a last resort, says **Gail Dalton, M.D.,** a foot and ankle specialist and orthopaedic surgeon in Atlanta, who chairs the Orthoses and Footwear Committee for the American Orthopaedic Foot & Ankle Society (AOFAS). A better option is a two-pronged approach: controlling symptoms and preventing the deformity from getting worse.

With that in mind, here's how to avoid surgery.

**Shop for sensible shoes.** Try soft shoes made of leather or canvas. Opt for a large toe box, the area in the front of each shoe for the toes. (See "The Women Podiatrists' Guide to Choosing Healthy Shoes," page 162.)

**Stuff your shoes.** Nonprescription inserts found in drugstores may be helpful if you place excess pressure on the inside of a foot while walking, which is called overpronating. To discover if this is a problem for you, check the inside of the sole on each shoe for excessive wear. If you're not sure, bring your shoes to a podiatrist for a professional opinion.

If these inserts don't help, your doctor may prescribe special inserts called orthotics. An orthotic insert is tailor-made for your foot. It's like a custom-made dress, as opposed to an off-the-rack nonprescription insert that may fit okay, but not perfectly.

## DECIDING ON SURGERY

*A surgical procedure is not the answer to most foot problems. You might have better, easier choices.*

"Bunion surgery is not fly-by-night surgery," warns *Gail Dalton, M.D.*, an orthopaedic surgeon in Atlanta who chairs the Orthoses and Footwear Committee for the American Orthopaedic Foot & Ankle Society (AOFS). "It's a major operation." The success rate is high—85 to 90 percent of patients have good to excellent results—but that doesn't mean you should jump into it with both feet.

"When things go wrong in bunion surgery, they go wrong big time," says Dr. Dalton. That includes infection, which can mean multiple surgeries and even amputation. Nerve problems, a rarity, may result in a lifetime of pain.

That's why Dr. Dalton won't operate on anyone who hasn't first tried to wear shoes that fit right.

"There really are choices out there that give proper fit and are still fashionable. Surgery should be viewed as the last resort," she says.

Some women seek cosmetic surgery for non- or mildly painful bunions, hammer toes, or other foot problems solely for reasons of vanity—so that their feet will look nice in sandals, for example. *Cherise Dyal, M.D.*, an orthopaedic surgeon in Wayne, New Jersey, who chairs the Public Education Committee for AOFAS, argues against such procedures and stresses the risks of surgery to her patients. She strongly suggests that women try a sensible route—choosing wider shoes and lower heels, and paying attention to seams and linings—instead of surgery.

**Try moleskin.** Over-the-counter moleskin pads or foam may also help with small bunions. Place the pad directly on the top of a bunion to relieve pressure from your shoe.

**See an expert.** Start with your primary-care physician. If symptoms persist despite recommendations, ask for a referral to a podiatrist or orthopaedic surgeon who specializes in feet. If you have diabetes, you should *always* consult a health-care professional about your feet. Diabetes can cause a loss of sensation and higher risk of infection in your feet. To be safe, you may need to see a podiatrist for even such minor procedures as clipping toenails.

## HEEL PAIN: SOLVING THE NUMBER-ONE FOOT PROBLEM

Heel pain is usually associated with one of two areas of soft tissue: Pain can be in the Achilles tendon, which runs from the heel bone to the calf muscle. Or it can occur from the plantar fascia, a band of ligaments that starts at the heel and spreads across the bottom of the foot to the ball. Heel pain may be the primary reason people see a podiatrist, says *Suzanne M. Levine, D.P.M.*, a podiatric surgeon in New York City and author of *Your Feet Don't Have to Hurt: A Woman's Guide to Lifelong Foot Care.*

If the back of the heel is tender, you probably have Achilles tendinitis, especially if the pain gets worse with use. The pain generally improves with rest and medication, such as acetaminophen, aspirin, or ibuprofen (also known as nonsteroidal anti-inflammatory drugs, or NSAIDs). Chronic Achilles tendinitis that persists despite home treatments can lead to a rupture of the tendon and require a cast. So see your doctor if the pain hasn't improved after a week of resting and taking NSAIDs.

If the pain is in the plantar fascia at the bottom of your heel, you have plantar fasciitis. You feel the most pain when your heel hits the floor in the morning and less after stretching it or as you use your foot during the day.

Pain can also occur from problems in the bone, such as a heel spur. These bony protrusions composed of calcium that irritate the plantar fascia are so common that they're usually downplayed as a cause of heel pain. Even if your doctor sees one on an X-ray, that doesn't mean the spur is the cause of your pain. A spur may develop after weight gain (including pregnancy) or a sudden increase in exercise level (we can't win!). Some women get heel pain simply because the heel loses fat reserves as we age, which is why this complaint is more common among mature women (translation: over age 40).

*Losing weight may be the most effective way to eliminate arch and heel pain.*—Suzanne M. Levine, D.P.M.

Take these steps to combat heel pain.

**Don't be flat.** Instead, wear shoes with a 1-inch heel or athletic shoes with a padded inner arch. Avoid flats and uncushioned tennis shoes.

**Safeguard your feet.** Wear well-constructed athletic shoes when you exercise. Choose a shoe that has plenty of cushioning, good traction (the tread on the bottom of the shoe), and a stiff cup around the back and lower part of the heel that stabilizes your ankle. Replace the shoes when you see noticeable, uneven wear on the sole. Such wear depends on many factors, including how often you use the shoes and the severity of any foot abnormalities.

**Get soles with give.** Hold a shoe with the toe in one palm and the heel in the other hand. Flex the shoe between your palms. If it bends a little, it has give. Rigid soles can torture your heels.

**Lose weight.** "It's the most important thing many of us can do to banish arch and heel pain," notes Dr. Levine.

**Flex and stretch.** Before you get out of bed, flex and stretch each foot for 60 to 90 seconds. Rotating your ankle, flex your foot toward you and then stretch it away from you. This helps relieve the pain of plantar fasciitis.

## CALLUSES: IF THE SHOE DOESN'T FIT, DON'T WEAR IT

Normal calluses are good. The layers of dead, thickened skin protect body parts exposed to constant pressure. Guitar players, carpenters, and runners all develop calluses. Good calluses don't hurt, which means something is amiss if you have a painful one.

Calluses on your feet usually form when you wear shoes that aren't shaped like your feet (e.g., pointy-toed shoes) or aren't the correct size. In some women, calluses form when the body compensates for a physical irregularity in the foot's structure, which affects the way they walk. In all cases, calluses can be thought of as shields your body creates to protect against the pressure caused by ill-fitting shoes or foot irregularities. If you don't change to better fitting shoes or correct the foot problem, a callus will grow in diameter and thickness, eventually coming in contact with the shoe and causing pain from the pressure.

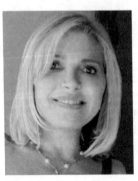

Wear inserts in your shoes to take the pressure off calluses, says Suzanne M. Levine, D.P.M. If a drugstore product doesn't do the trick, see a podiatrist for custom-made orthotics.

To conquer your calluses, follow the advice of *Suzanne M. Levine, D.P.M.*, a podiatric surgeon in New York City and author of *Your Feet Don't Have to Hurt: A Woman's Guide to Lifelong Foot Care.*

**Soften the pain.** An over-the-counter moleskin pad helps with occasional discomfort. Most brands are comparable in quality.

**Switch shoes.** If you wear the same shoes—or shoes with the same heel height—for eight or more hours a day, start varying your footwear. Wear 2-inch heels to the office, for example, but then slip on lower heeled or athletic shoes in the afternoon.

**Pick a pad.** An insert, heel pad, or metatarsal pad may relieve the pressure on a callus. Use inserts or pads in all your shoes (except open sandals) until you get relief. These products are available in most drugstores. If they don't help, talk with your doctor about the next tip: a prescription for orthotics.

**Get a prescription.** Calluses are often caused by a bone deformity or very high or low arches. If you have these problems or you've tried over-the-counter (OTC) inserts without relief, see a podiatrist about getting custom-made orthotics.

**Try some tea.** To soften calluses, steep a chamomile tea bag in 2 quarts warm water and soak your feet in the tea for 15 minutes. Using a pumice stone, gently rub the calluses to remove the dead skin. Follow up by applying a moisturizer. The best kind? Petroleum jelly, because it helps seal in natural oils and doesn't evaporate.

**Make a paste.** Mix 8 tablespoons mineral oil, ½ cup Epsom salts, 1 cup kosher salt, and 1 tablespoon baking soda. Apply to all callused areas on your foot. Put your foot into a plastic bag and wrap a warm towel around it. Remove your foot from the bag after 10 minutes. Gently rub a pumice stone in a circular motion over the callused areas until the dead skin is gone.

Be careful to avoid OTC products that contain salicylic acid, which can damage the skin. Do *not* attempt self-surgery: Taking a sharp instrument to your calluses can result in a serious infection.

## CORNS: COMFORT FOR THE LITTLEST PIGGY

Corns are the common colds of foot pain, notes *Suzanne M. Levine, D.P.M.*, a podiatric surgeon in New York City. Some tender loving at-home foot care can alleviate them.

Like calluses, corns are thickened areas of skin that form in response to friction from ill-fitting shoes. They usually develop on top of, between, or at the tips of toes and on the outside of the little toes. The core of a corn is live skin—complete with nerve endings—making corns more painful than calluses. They're usually yellowish but can turn red when inflamed.

Most over-the-counter corn remedies and pads contain salicylic acid, which can cause blisters.

Dr. Levine suggests you try these self-care remedies.

**Soak your foot.** Treat the affected foot to a soak in warm water and Epsom salts for 15 to 20 minutes. If the corn is inflamed, soak your foot for at least an hour and skip the next three steps.

**Be a softie.** Apply moisturizer to the corn. Petroleum jelly is the best choice.

**Wrap it up.** Use plastic wrap to cover the affected area for at least 15 minutes to continue softening it.

**Stone it.** Remove the wrap. Gently use a pumice stone on the corn until the dead skin is removed.

To ensure that a corn doesn't return, stop wearing shoes that irritate the area. If you don't, be sure to stock up on Epsom salts and plastic wrap.

## THE WOMEN PODIATRISTS' GUIDE TO CHOOSING HEALTHY SHOES

*If the shoe fits, you can wear it in good health. But how can you tell if a shoe is really right for your foot? Here are some tips and tools you can use to assess the shoes in your closet and help decide if the fashionable footwear in the store is a perfect fit.*

*Gail Dalton, M.D.,* is passionate about footwear. The chair of the Orthoses and Footwear Committee for the American Orthopaedic Foot & Ankle Society (AOFAS) and an orthopaedic surgeon in Atlanta, Dr. Dalton confesses to visiting shoe factories and stores while on vacation, all in a quest for sensible, comfortable—yet still attractive—shoes.

A healthy shoe should be no more than a half-inch narrower, wider, or longer than your foot.

Dr. Dalton recommends that you make your tracings late in the day, when your feet are at their largest. She says that if women used this method to test all their footwear, they would eliminate a lot of shoes. And that, of course, provides the perfect opportunity to buy more!

### MEASURE YOUR FEET

The key to comfort, she says, is making sure your shoes fit. All too often they don't. So Dr. Dalton recommends making foot tracings, which you can make in minutes.

- Put two pieces of sturdy white paper on the floor. Stand with one bare foot on each sheet. Trace each foot.
- Place a pair of shoes over the tracings. If you can still see the outline of the tracings, then you know your shoes are too small. Healthful shoes will cover the tracings.

"You'll see when a shoe simply doesn't fit," says Dr. Dalton. In most cases, shoes are too narrow. Less often, they're too long or too short.

### SHOE-SHOPPING SAVVY

Dr. Dalton suggests these footwear tips sanctioned by the National Shoe Retailers Association, the Pedorthic Footwear Association, and the AOFAS.

**Judge by fit, not by size.** "Shoe-measuring devices are standardized, but shoe sizes are not," says Dr. Dalton. A 7B from one manufacturer may not be the same as a 7B from another. In fact, even the same manufacturer's 7Bs are not all the same, because different styles and models are built on different lasts (a mold over which the material is stretched). The bottom line? "It's absolutely meaningless what size you measure out at. It's more important how the shoe fits your foot," says Dr. Dalton.

# PLANTAR WARTS: HIGHLY CONTAGIOUS, HARD TO CURE

They're painful, ugly, itchy, and develop on the bottoms of the feet. Plantar warts can appear as one large wart with smaller ones around it or as an assortment of many. They can resemble calluses but are more painful.

Caused by the human papillomavirus (HPV), plantar warts are highly contagious, especially in such moist settings as bathrooms and locker rooms. They can spread to your hands if you touch a wart on your foot.

**Measure often.** Have your feet measured regularly to provide a reference point. Feet grow longer and wider as we mature. Yet according to a 2000 survey by the American Academy of Orthopaedic Surgeons and the AOFAS, 78 percent of women don't have their feet measured when they buy shoes; 57 percent couldn't remember the last time they'd measured their feet.

**Think big.** Measure your feet late in the day when they are at their largest. Feet swell as the day wears on.

**It takes two.** Most people have one foot larger than the other, so be sure to measure both feet. Always fit to the larger foot.

**All rise.** Stand when measuring your feet. There should be about ½-inch leeway for your longest toe at the end of each shoe.

**Shape matters.** Always choose a shoe that conforms to the shape of your foot. If you have a narrow heel and a wide forefoot, ask for shoes that were made with combination lasts. This means the last for the heel was a different width (usually narrower) than the last used for the width of the ball of the foot.

**Go for comfort.** To ensure the best fit, make sure that the ball of each foot is comfortable in the widest part of the shoe and that your heel fits comfortably in the shoe with a minimum of slippage.

**Never be tight.** How many times have you said, "They're tight, but I'll break them in"? Forget about it! Shoes are like men: You can't change them once you get them home.

**Walk in both shoes.** That's the only way to make sure each feels right.

**Wear hose or socks.** Try on new shoes while wearing the type of stockings or socks you plan to wear with the shoes.

## SIGNS OF A GOOD SHOE

Here are a few extra tips to consider:

- Good shoes have rigid material under the arches for support. Midsoles should be flexible.
- The ideal heel is ¾ to 1-inch high. If you feel you must wear higher heels, switch between different heights during the day. "Treat high heels like a dessert," says *Cherise Dyal, M.D.,* an orthopaedic surgeon in Wayne, New Jersey, who chairs the Public Education Committee for the AOFAS. Like any indulgence, only splurge on them once in a while.
- Check the shoe's back and side for a counter, the stiff material that supports the heel. Shoes with counters are a healthy choice.
- Check the lining for irritants, such as wrinkles, loose lining, and ridges. If the shoes have any of these, be strong and leave them in the store—regardless of the price or color!

If you have been exposed to plantar warts, take these precautions.

**Scrub-a-dub-dub.** Scrub the bathroom floor with bleach after every bath or shower, even if you live alone (to avoid reinfection). HPV is a hearty virus.

**Change towels.** Use separate towels to dry your feet and then to dry the rest of your body.

*Scrub the tub with bleach after every shower to keep from reinfecting yourself with plantar warts.*

**Take aspirin.** This homemade treatment is recommended by New York City podiatrist *Suzanne M. Levine, D.P.M.,* author of *Your Feet Don't Have to Hurt: A Woman's Guide to Lifelong Foot Care:* Mix five crushed aspirins in 4 tablespoons bottled water with the oil from one vitamin-E capsule and 1 teaspoon liquid vitamin A. Using a cotton swab, apply the paste to the wart. Put your foot into a plastic bag for 15 minutes. Then use a pumice stone to gently remove the dead skin. Apply daily until the wart disappears.

**Try preparations and pads.** Over-the-counter preparations containing salicylic acid can help to slowly remove a wart. DuoFilm is a good brand because it allows you to control the amount of liquid you put on the pad. Put petroleum jelly on the skin around the wart to protect it from the acid on the pad. Cut the pad small enough to cover the wart only. Gently pumice the wart after you bathe each day, then apply a new pad.

**See your doctor.** If the pain continues or the condition doesn't improve with home remedies, see your physician to make sure you really have a plantar wart and not something else. Your doctor may treat warts with liquid nitrogen, which helps kill the virus-infected cells. You may require a few office visits, since warts can be deep and recur easily.

## ATHLETE'S FOOT: DRY, DRY AGAIN

Athlete's foot is a misnomer because you don't need to be an athlete to get this most common of fungal infections.

"A major cause of athlete's foot is too much moisture inside your shoes or socks," says *Gail Dalton, M.D.,* a foot and ankle specialist and orthopaedic surgeon in Atlanta, who chairs the Orthoses and Footwear

Committee for the American Orthopaedic Foot & Ankle Society (AOFAS). The result? Scaly, white patches between your toes and on your feet. The skin may not itch initially, but as athlete's foot progresses, the itching starts and gets worse. Soon, the skin may crack, redden, and smell.

To avoid this scenario, Dr. Dalton suggests the following.

**Wear clean, dry socks.** Damp socks are a prime breeding ground for fungus. Change socks as often as necessary to keep your feet dry.

**Lose your nylon socks.** Most doctors and the American Academy of Dermatology recommend wearing all-cotton socks to prevent athlete's foot. "Pure cotton breathes better, minimizing sweat and moisture," says Dr. Dalton.

**Let your feet breathe.** If you're wearing shoes made of synthetic materials, switch to sandals or leather shoes, or go barefoot whenever possible. Slip off your shoes under your desk at the office. Expose your toes to the sun.

**Don't share.** Wear flip-flops or shower shoes in locker rooms and pool areas to protect your feet in those damp environments.

If you get athlete's foot despite your best efforts, try such over-the-counter products as Desenex and Micatin. Make sure you use them as directed, otherwise the fungus may return. If you have diabetes, always see your doctor or podiatrist about any fungal infection on your feet.

---

## SHOULD I SEE A DOCTOR?

*If your feet hurt—and do-it-yourself remedies like those described throughout this chapter don't work—see a doctor, says* **Cherise Dyal, M.D.,** *an orthopaedic surgeon practicing in Wayne, New Jersey, and chair of the Public Education Committee for the American Orthopaedic Foot & Ankle Society.*

Go to your primary-care doctor or consult with either of the following foot doctors:

**Podiatrists:** These medical professionals are not M.D.s or O.D.s. Each typically receives a bachelor's degree before entering the four-year program at one of the seven colleges of podiatric medicine in the United States. Those completing the program receive their Doctor of Podiatric Medicine (D.P.M.). When they pass a state licensing exam, these doctors are eligible to practice in about one-third of states. Two-thirds require additional postdoctoral work, which can be completed in primary podiatric care, podiatric orthopaedics, or podiatric surgery. Each advanced program lasts one to three years.

**Orthopaedic surgeons:** These physicians attend undergraduate school and four years of medical school. Then they complete a five-year residency, during which they learn the fundamentals of orthopaedic surgery. This can be followed by one to two years of subspecialty training in the foot and ankle.

# HAMMER TOES: RELIEF FOR TENDER TOOTSIES

This condition gets its name from the toes involved looking like the hammers inside a piano. The name could also refer to the pain of hammer toes, which feels as if a hammer has been dropped on your foot.

A hammer toe is a deformity of the middle joint, usually in the toe next to the big toe, explains **Gail Dalton, M.D.**, a foot and ankle specialist and orthopaedic surgeon in Atlanta, who chairs the Orthoses and Footwear Committee for the American Orthopaedic Foot & Ankle Society (AOFAS). The pressure from wearing tight, pointy shoes forces the joint to bend and twist. This makes the tip of the toe point down and a bump, or corn, form on top. Over time, the tendon in the toe stiffens along with the joint and fuses the toe into a permanent deformity. Hammer toes and bunions often appear together. "Toes are like hair," Dr. Dalton tells patients who want to wear pointy-toed shoes. "If you part your hair one way long enough, it just stays that way. A foot with hammer toes is simply a foot that's molding to the shape of a pointy-toed shoe." Remember how Chinese women once bound their feet to make them dainty? "What women do today is simply foot binding in a milder form," she says.

Follow this advice to prevent and relieve hammer toes.

**Free your toes.** Get your feet out of the vise and into healthy, sensible shoes. (See "The Women Podiatrists' Guide to Choosing Healthy Shoes," page 162.) If you change footwear before the deformity progresses too far, you may avoid much pain. Open- and square-toed pumps are preferable to round-toed shoes.

**Pad it.** Use over-the-counter pads with straps to protect bumps and keep the toes flat, rather than pointed down. Wear them with shoes that have roomy toe boxes.

**Cool it.** Apply an ice pack to the area three to four times a day or take nonsteroidal anti-inflammatory drugs (or NSAIDs, such as ibuprofen) to relieve pain. If you're depending on drugs all or most of the time to relieve pain, see your doctor.

If your hammer-toe condition is extremely painful and advanced, you may need surgery. There are two options, both performed under local anesthesia: One involves stretching the tendon in the toe, which enables the toe to lie flat. The other requires removing the toe joint. Painful, advanced hammer toes usually necessitate the more aggressive option.

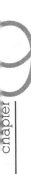

# Hair
## Tips for Top-level Problem Solving

*From fairy tales to advertising, our culture glamorizes shiny, vibrant locks. It's no wonder that a female's self-esteem seems to stem in part from whether she's having a good hair day.*

Experts agree that a woman's hair is a key component to her identity. Fortunately, methods and products are now available to address virtually any coiffure concern.

### OILY HAIR AND DANDRUFF: DON'T BE A FLAKE

Though it's certainly not a pretty thought, fungus lives on everyone's scalp. However, only about half of us end up with dandruff as a result. Your chances of being in that unlucky 50 percent depends on whether you've inherited an oily scalp.

"Dandruff is quite greasy," explains *Hilary Baldwin, M.D.*, a dermatologist in private practice and associate professor of dermatology at the State University of New York at Brooklyn. "The fungus feeds off the grease, making the skin itchy and scaly."

Consider these tips to reduce oil and flaking.

**Select the right shampoo.** Antidandruff shampoos are your best defense against current and future dandruff. Products that include salicylic acid reduce flaking but don't actually kill fungus. Coal-tar shampoos usually smell like asphalt, a scent most women prefer not to exude. Opt for a shampoo that contains ketoconazole, such as Nizoral A-D, or pyrithione zinc, such as Head & Shoulders. These kill the fungus that feeds off your scalp and reduce oil.

*Don't be in a hurry to rinse out an antidandruff shampoo. The longer the shampoo is on your scalp, the more effective it will be.*—Hilary Baldwin, M.D.

Whichever shampoo you use, it must reach your skin to work its magic, so massage it thoroughly into your scalp. Leave it on your hair for one minute before rinsing. The longer the shampoo interacts with your scalp, the more effectively it will kill fungus, so try not to wash the product off your scalp completely. You don't need to leave suds in your hair to do the job, but standing under a stream of water for another 10 minutes as you shave your legs will definitely counteract the shampoo's effects. "Make shampooing the last thing you do when in the shower," says Dr. Baldwin. If you use a conditioner, select one labeled as an antidandruff product.

**Style correctly.** Many women put too much mousse or gel in their hair. Scalp oil promotes dandruff, so the less greasy your hair the better. Rub a little styling product on your palms and then gently run your hands through your hair from front to back, recommends *Kornelia Jones,* a stylist at Mélange Salon at The Peninsula New York. Use your fingers or a comb to distribute the product throughout your hair, then style as usual.

## DRY HAIR AND SPLIT ENDS: PUT BACK THE MOISTURE

Blow-dryers, chlorinated water, sunlight, air pollution, and wind all conspire to damage the outermost layer of your hair, known as the cuticle, which is responsible for your hair's smooth, shiny appearance. If the cuticle peels off, the layers underneath are exposed, and you're left with dry, flyaway hair.

If your hair is dry, take these steps to restore luster.

**Choose a good conditioner.** Conditioners benefit your hair by repairing the shaft, increasing shine and strength, decreasing static electricity, and protecting from damaging ultraviolet radiation, says *Zoe Diana Draelos, M.D.,* clinical associate professor of dermatology at Wake Forest University in Winston-Salem, North Carolina. Look for products that include collagen

## SHOULD I SEE A DOCTOR?

*Few hair problems require a physician's care. But hair loss, dandruff, and unwanted fuzz are exceptions.*

Always consult your health-care provider if you're losing your hair, rather than try any self-care methods. Your physician will investigate possible causes, such as an iron deficiency, thyroid disease, or a hormonal imbalance. For example, a small percentage of women experience hair loss because their bodies produce too much of the hormone testosterone. In those cases, testosterone-blocking prescription medications may help. Excessive unwanted hair may also signal any number of other medical conditions, so have your doctor check out the source.

If your scalp is scaly and your antidandruff shampoo flakes out even after four to six weeks of use, see a doctor. You may have psoriasis, a condition that resembles dandruff. If that's your diagnosis, your physician will prescribe a topical steroid or mineral oil—or both—to reduce inflammation.

At-home hair-removal methods can sometimes cause an ingrown hair that raises a painful red bump. If it doesn't straighten itself out within a week, get a prescription for antibiotics. Wash ingrown hairs daily with antibacterial soap or dab on an antibacterial cream or benzoyl peroxide.

and silicone (sometimes listed as dimethicone). These ingredients penetrate the cuticle to replenish nutrients, says Dr. Draelos.

**Get a haircut.** Frequent trims—as often as every four weeks—snip away split ends and help your hair look smooth.

**Shun the sun.** Your hair shaft gets much of its strength from substances called sulfur molecules. When exposed to the sun, these molecules oxidize, which involves the same chemical activity that produces rust. As the molecules break down, hair becomes weak, dry, and rough. Resist rays by wearing an opaque hat, advises Dr. Draelos. Or condition your hair with a hot-oil treatment or leave-in conditioner that contains zinc oxide before heading outdoors.

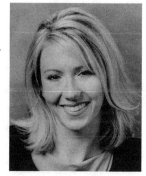

**Blow off the dryer.** After shampooing, let your hair air-dry until it's just damp. Then take this styling tip from *Corinne Wiedemann,* a training and service representative for Great Clips salons: Rub mousse or styling product into your moist hair, then blow-dry on the warm—not hot—setting to add volume.

*Dry heat can damage your hair, warns Corinne Wiedemann of Great Clips salons. Use mousse on damp hair, she advises. Then blow-dry on a warm setting.*

## GRAY HAIR: BRING BACK THE LUSTER

For many women, the appearance of gray hair is the first hint that their youth is fading. If it were just a color consideration, perhaps it wouldn't be as much of a problem. But gray hair also tends to feel like straw. Moisture in your hair drops as you age, causing even oily scalps to become dry.

Luckily, there are ways to bring color and vitality back to your locks.

**Condition longer.** Many conditioning products instruct you to leave them on your hair from three to five minutes per application. Once you start to go gray—and especially if your hair is already dry—go for the full five minutes to let your hair fully absorb the conditioner, says *Cathy Bateman,* director of education for haircolorxpress International, a chain of coloring salons based in Fort Lauderdale, Florida. If you color your hair, choose a product that contains chamomile, which helps condition without stripping. If you're opting for the natural look but desire the silky, smooth hair of your youth, Bateman recommends using a conditioner with keratin protein, which adds to the existing protein in your hair and strengthens the shaft.

*If you decide to stay with gray, use a conditioner with keratin protein to retain the silky, smooth look of your youth.—Cathy Bateman*

**Nod to nature.** For your first dye job, don't venture from within one to two shades of your natural color, suggests Bateman. This conservative approach allows you to blend away the gray without attracting the attention of friends, co-workers, and family. "Most women like to have a change without people saying, 'Oh, you colored your hair.' A lot of women like it when someone says, 'You look so good. Have you lost weight?' They didn't lose weight; they just enhanced their skin tones and brought out their natural beauty." If you're already completely gray, try a subtle light brown or dirty blond shade.

**Go deep.** If your hair thins as it grays, give it a thicker appearance by choosing a shade or two darker than your natural color—particularly if you're blond, says Bateman.

# HAIR LOSS: WHEN THIN ISN'T IN

Let's uncover the bald facts about the two common causes of lost locks.

Shedding, medically known as telogen effluvium, is linked to hormonal shifts, such as during puberty or pregnancy. An iron deficiency and such medical conditions as thyroid disease may also cause shedding, as can chemotherapy and other medications. Though shedding can alter looks dramatically, the hair usually grows back within 6 to 12 weeks after the affliction is resolved or the drugs are discontinued.

The genetic form of hair loss is called alopecia. With this condition, new hairs do not grow in to replace the ones that fall out. This results in thin hair all over your head, as well as a typical bald spot at the crown.

Whether you suffer from shedding or genetic hair loss, there are options that offer assistance in correcting the problem.

**Try minoxidil.** Despite the hype, Rogaine is not a guaranteed solution for a hair-loss problem. "Rogaine seems to help about half of women with hair loss," says *Mary Lynn Moran, M.D.,* a clinical faculty member at Stanford University in Palo Alto, California. This product is available over-the-counter at most drugstores. Start with the 2-percent solution and apply twice a day.

## A WOMAN'S RIGHT TO THE *RIGHT* TREATMENT: HAIR LOSS

*When losing your hair causes you to seek professional help, be prepared for a barrage of questions and tests that will assist in pinpointing the cause and best remedy.*

To find out if you have a genetic predisposition to hair loss, a doctor should ask about both male and female relatives who have experienced the same problem. She may also look into your dietary and supplement habits to learn if you're consuming too much or too little of key nutrients. A blood test is required to check your iron level, as well as to determine any hormonal imbalances.

Some physicians may not be as conscientious as they could be when it comes to the subject of thinning hair, says *Diane Hoss, M.D.,* associate professor of dermatology and director of the Hair Loss and Scalp Disorders Clinic at the University of Connecticut at Farmington. "A lot of doctors don't deal well with hair loss, and that's why a lot of women get upset," she says. "They feel that their doctors don't give their condition the attention it deserves." If your physician doesn't ask the appropriate questions or perform the necessary tests, consider making an appointment with another doctor.

Your best route may be straight to a dermatologist who specializes in hair loss and regrowth. Consult a phone book or search online at the American Academy of Dermatology's site, www.aad.org.

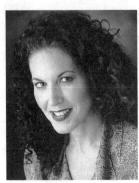

If you don't notice improved growth within six months, move on to the 5-percent solution. Hair lost to shedding usually grows back without the use of Rogaine, as long as you take steps to eliminate the cause of the problem. (See "Should I See a Doctor?" page 169.) However, there's no harm in trying Rogaine to help hair regrowth along.

**Take a hormone check.** Going on or off birth control pills can temporarily cause hair to fall out due to fluctuating hormone levels, says Dr. Moran. Also, some birth control pills contain a type of progesterone that can aggravate hair loss. If the change in your hair coincided with a change in your birth control prescription, discuss your symptoms with your gynecologist. In many cases, hair will grow back within six months. Otherwise, you may need to switch to a pill with a different form of progesterone.

*Talk with your gynecologist if going on or off your birth control pills coincides with your hair loss, advises Mary Lynn Moran, M.D. The fluctuation in your hormone levels may be the cause of your condition.*

**Consider a faux finish.** More women experience thinning hair than will ever be known because weaves and wigs effectively cover up baldness. A weave, also known as a partial hair replacement, is attached at a hair salon. A stylist braids, glues, or pins real or synthetic hair to existing hair, close to the scalp. The good news: When complete, the weave blends in imperceptibly with real hair. The bad news: A weave lifts up as your hair grows, so you'll need a touch-up about every four weeks. Weaves are expensive, running several hundred dollars for the initial application, plus $60 to $100 per alteration. If you'd rather not hassle with so many trips to the salon, consider wearing a wig. Shop for one before too much of your hair falls out so that you can closely match the wig to your natural color.

**Be wary of surgery.** Transplants are less than ideal for women because females tend to have thin hair all over their heads, rather than in one concentrated bald spot. To perform a transplant, a surgeon removes hair from where it is plentiful and will regrow on the scalp, then inserts grafts of one to six hairs each into small holes in the parts of the scalp where hair is thin or nonexistent. "There's a chance surgery can shock the surrounding follicles, causing them to go into hibernation," warns Dr. Moran. In other words, a transplant may replace some hairs but may cause even more to fall out—and not grow back. Get a second opinion before seeking surgery.

**Examine your diet.** Vegans—people who steer clear of eating *any* animal products—sometimes lose hair because they don't get enough protein or iron, says **Diane Hoss, M.D.**, associate professor of dermatology and director of the Hair Loss and Scalp Disorders Clinic at the University of Connecticut at Farmington. Some studies show that women who get at least 18 milligrams of iron—either through diet or supplements—reap the most benefits from Rogaine. This doesn't mean that you have to chow down on meat, the most easily absorbed source of iron. Instead, fill up on green leafy vegetables, whole grains, legumes, and iron-fortified breakfast cereals, advises Dr. Moran.

## PARTING WAYS WITH UNWANTED HAIR

*The hair on your head may not be your only concern. A woman is always on the lookout for methods and products to manage the hair on the rest of her body.*

There are five options for removing undesired hair from your underarms, legs, and bikini line, as well as elsewhere on your body. Below are the pros and cons of each:

• **Plucking:** This time-consuming method is best reserved for areas requiring little hair removal, such as the eyebrows or nipples.

• **Waxing:** This procedure can keep you smooth for several weeks, says **Holly Vance, Pharm.D.**, manager of pharmacy services for Drugstore.com in Bellevue, Washington. But it also stings and may leave your skin red for a day or so. Waxing rips hairs out at an angle, making ingrown hairs more likely to develop. Curly-haired women are especially prone to this side effect, so they should opt for another hair-removal method.

• **Bleaching:** This is one of the best options for hiding facial hair, since it doesn't leave stubble or an overly shiny appearance.

• **Depilatories:** These creams and lotions contain chemicals that dissolve hair and keep it from growing back for a few weeks. Be aware that a

depilatory will remove *all* hair it comes in contact with, including the fine, downy fuzz on your face. The result is an undesirable waxy look, says Dr. Vance. Because the chemicals in depilatories can cause skin reactions, always do a small test patch on your wrist before moving on to a larger area, particularly on your face. If any irritation develops, take a different route to removal.

• **Shaving:** This oldie but goodie is perhaps the easiest method for ridding yourself of hair. On the downside, stubble appears within about a day. For that reason, says Dr. Vance, you may prefer not to shave your facial or arm hair.

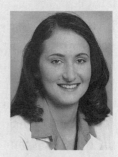

*A depilatory removes all your facial hair, including normal fuzzy down. The result can be a waxy and unnatural look, warns Holly Vance, Pharm.D.*

# 10 Heart, Blood, and Circulation
## The Flow Must Go On

*Almost twice as many women die from heart disease as from all forms of cancer combined, making it the number-one health threat for women.*

If you place a yearly breast exam higher than your routine cholesterol check on your priority list, you're not alone. Although women are eight times more likely to die from heart disease than from breast cancer, an American Heart Association survey found that only 8 percent of women ranked heart disease as their primary health concern.

Why are women so misinformed? Researchers have only recently studied the signs and symptoms of heart disease in women. Discoveries include the fact that women experience heart attacks differently than men. In addition to traditional pain in the chest, women are more likely than men to feel nauseated, tired, or dizzy.

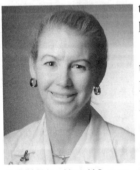

C. Noel Bairey Merz, M.D., says that standard treatment of heart conditions is based on men's symptoms. Doctors now realize that women experience heart attacks differently.

Lack of previous research means that some doctors are still ignorant of the signs and prevalence of heart disease in women. "Just as many women have heart attacks as men, but we continue to see that diagnosis can be delayed and treatment slower or not given at all," says *C. Noel Bairey Merz, M.D.,* medical director of Women's Health at Cedars-Sinai Medical Center in Los Angeles. That's why knowledge is your best defense against deadly heart disease. The more you learn about your heart, blood, and circulatory system, the better informed you'll be to stay healthy and get the proper tests and treatments.

# HEART DISEASE: A PRIMER FOR BETTER HEALTH

Each day, your heart pumps 2,000 gallons of blood through a web of blood vessels. This blood carries oxygen from the lungs and nutrients from the intestines to cells throughout your body. It picks up waste products along the way, dropping them off in the liver, kidneys, and lungs.

Your four-chamber, four-valve heart is the motor that keeps this stream moving. Overall, it works amazingly well, but—as with everything—it's susceptible to wear and tear.

Heart disease develops as fat, cholesterol, calcium, and other arterial discards get stuck on the inner lining of your arteries. This buildup can turn into what's referred to as plaque, which is similar to the gunk the dentist scrapes off your teeth every six months. In your heart, plaque doesn't get scraped away regularly and so can grow large enough to block blood flow.

Clogged arteries to your heart may eventually trigger a heart attack, but blockages occur in other parts of your body, too. If they're in your arms or legs, you'll experience pain and numbness, symptoms of peripheral artery disease. Obstructed arteries to your brain can trigger a stroke. Add high cholesterol or high blood pressure to the mix, and your risk of heart disease shoots higher than a bull stock market.

## CHOLESTEROL TRAFFIC JAMS

Despite its negative reputation, we actually need cholesterol for various bodily functions. Cholesterol is used to form cell membranes, tissues, and some hormones. But too much of the wrong type of cholesterol can end up damaging your arteries.

## SIZING UP YOUR GENES

*Heart disease and stroke tend to run in families and within particular minority groups.*

If you have a close relative who suffered a major heart attack in his or her 30s or 40s, that automatically puts you at higher risk for heart disease. Each additional relative who suffers from heart disease at a young age increases your risk.

African-Americans are prone to high blood pressure, heart disease, and stroke. Native

Americans run a high risk of diabetes. Talk to your doctor about both your family history and ethnic predisposition to disease. If your doctor knows you have a strong family history of a particular condition, she may be more likely to place you on medication sooner and test you more often.

Cholesterol is a soft, waxy type of bloodborne fat. Your body produces some, but the bulk comes from what you eat. Because dietary cholesterol can't dissolve in your blood, it needs an escort to get around in your body. The two types of these escorts are low-density lipoprotein (LDL), or so-called bad cholesterol, and high-density lipoprotein (HDL), or so-called good cholesterol.

Think of LDL and HDL as taxi drivers, with cholesterol as their passengers. LDL cabs tend to get stuck in traffic, sometimes wrecking or breaking down along the side of the road (aka your arteries). As more LDL and other substances get stuck, plaque piles up and can eventually grow large enough to clog an artery. If this happens, blood flow to the heart is reduced, which can trigger angina, the chest pain commonly associated with heart disease.

Not all plaque pileups get large enough to cause symptoms, but even small ones can be lethal. The most dangerous heart attacks occur when minimal deposits of plaque rupture. These younger, more unstable formations are too small to block blood flow when safely pasted to the side of an artery, but the "paste" doesn't always hold too well. If a small clump of plaque breaks free, its hard outer covering bursts and releases the softer, waxy inner substances into the blood. Other blood components quickly stick to this "wax," forming a large clot that can completely block an artery and quickly cause a heart attack.

HDL, on the other hand, is a skillful driver. It carries cholesterol out of your arteries and to your liver for disposal, with no accidents or tie-ups. HDL may even stop along the way at various LDL pileups, towing away some of the debris.

## PRESSURE BUILDING

Your heart creates pressure in your arteries every time it pumps, or contracts. Healthy, smooth arteries stretch to accommodate the flow of blood. Unhealthy, ridged arteries require the heart to pump more strenuously, just as a car must work harder to travel a rutted dirt road than to drive on smooth blacktop. This extra effort damages arteries and weakens your heart's pumping ability. Various factors, including high blood pressure, can cause your arteries to become ridged. Numerous minerals, including salt and potassium, interact to affect the health of your arteries, your blood pressure, and how well the muscles lining your arteries function.

Over time, elevated blood pressure can further damage blood vessels' linings, attracting plaque like sludge in sewer pipes and slowing blood flow. These conditions combine to require your heart to work even harder to pump blood through those clogged pipes.

## THE HORMONE CONNECTION

To some degree, estrogen protects women against heart disease. This female sex hormone lowers levels of bad LDL cholesterol, raises levels of good HDL cholesterol, and keeps arteries supple. But as you approach menopause and your supply of estrogen drops, so, too, do its protective effects. That was one reason doctors regularly recommended prescription hormone replacement therapy (HRT) after menopause. They figured that replacing lost estrogen would help maintain its protective effects on the cardiovascular system and, thus, reduce heart disease risk. New research finds this theory flawed.

> *If you have heart disease, don't start taking hormone replacement therapy.*
> —C. Noel Bairey Merz, M.D.

The Heart and Estrogen-Progestin Replacement Study (HERS), for instance, examined postmenopausal women who already had heart disease and found that HRT did not reduce their heart-attack risk. Instead, it slightly *increased* it, especially in the first year of therapy. Enough subsequent

### ARRHYTHMIA: NOT ALWAYS A PROBLEM

*Many people occasionally experience what feels like their heart is fluttering. Is it a heart attack?*

Probably not. The fluttery feeling is known as arrhythmia. It occurs when the heart's natural source of electricity in the sinus node (called the natural pacemaker) is not in charge of directing the normal pattern or rhythm. Other parts of the heart temporarily override the natural pacemaker, changing the beating pattern.

A heart normally beats 60 to 100 times a minute, but during an arrhythmia, it pumps less effectively, beating slower or faster than usual. The resulting fluttering sensation in your chest may be accompanied by other uncomfortable symptoms, such as lightheadedness, dizziness, or fainting.

Arrhythmias are common: One in five people experience an erratic heartbeat at some point in life. A fluttering or palpitation often turns out to be premature or early beats, which are not dangerous. Most people have early beats but often don't feel them. "Many of them are nothing, but you need to get it checked out and be told that it's nothing," says *Deborah L. Wolbrette, M.D.*, a cardiologist with Pennsylvania State University's Milton S. Hershey Medical Center in Hershey. If your fluttering occurs without other symptoms, you're probably fine. But if it's accompanied by dizziness, fainting, or nausea, you may have a serious problem. See a doctor to be on the safe side.

studies echoed these findings that in 2001 the American Heart Association stopped recommending HRT for treatment—or prevention—of heart disease.

In 2002, findings from the Women's Health Initiative (WHI) led the American Heart Association to take the position that HRT should not be prescribed as a means of preventing heart disease even in healthy women. The WHI was not set up to study HRT use for treatment of menopause symptoms or to test all forms of estrogen. More research is needed in these areas.

If you have heart disease and are not currently taking HRT, don't start, advises **C. Noel Bairey Merz, M.D.,** medical director of Women's Health at Cedars-Sinai Medical Center. If you're already on HRT and have been diagnosed with heart disease, talk to your doctor, she says, and ask about statins. Statins are a class of drugs that doctors often prescribe to treat heart disease. Some commonly prescribed brand names of these drugs are Lipitor (atorvastatin), Mevacor (lovastatin), Pravachol (pravastatin), and Zocor (simvastatin). Statins block a cholesterol-producing enzyme, thus lowering the risk for heart attack, stroke, arrhythmia, and angina. They also may possess positive side benefits, including strengthening bones and preventing dementia.

## PREVENTING HEART DISEASE: A FORMULA FOR LIFELONG HEALTH

Keeping your heart and circulatory system healthy is a simple formula:

*A healthy diet + moderate, consistent exercise + a healthy*
*weight − smoking = greatly reduced risk for heart disease and stroke*

All the elements work synergistically: Healthy diet and consistent exercise help keep your weight in check, while exercise also aids in quitting smoking.

### FOOD AS MEDICINE

Researchers now know that fruits, vegetables, and whole grains contain powerful nutrients that help keep the lining of your arteries healthy. They realize that high-fiber foods block fat and cholesterol from the blood, preventing them from turning into blood cholesterol.

They also understand that there is bad fat and good fat. Bad types of fat tend to increase cholesterol levels. These include saturated fats from animal products, like red meat and dairy, and trans fats from processed foods, like cakes, doughnuts, and chips. Good types of fat keep cholesterol levels low.

Examples are monounsaturated fats found in certain oils and nuts, and polyunsaturated fats also found in certain oils and in fatty fish like salmon. But eating healthfully for your heart doesn't mean eating only apples, carrots, and whole wheat bread. "You don't need to put a superbig emphasis on fiber, fruits, vegetables, and whole grains to see a huge difference in your health," says *Liz Applegate, Ph.D.,* lecturer in the department of nutrition at the University of California at Davis and author of *Eat Your Way to a Healthy Heart.* "Simply switching from a diet that is high in

## STROKE: A HEART ATTACK IN YOUR BRAIN

*The same lifestyle changes that lower your risk for heart disease can also lower your risk for stroke, the number-three cause of death and the leading cause of long-term disability.*

A stroke occurs when a blood vessel that carries blood to your brain becomes blocked or bursts, cutting off the oxygen and nutrient supply to part of your brain. If starved of oxygen and nutrients long enough, that region of the brain starts to die, affecting the part of the body it controls. Strokes can cause paralysis, hamper language, and diminish vision, as well as other problems.

It is important to recognize these early signs of a stroke—any of which can come on suddenly—so that you can get treatment and restore normal brain function as soon as possible:

- Numbness or weakness, especially on one side of the body
- Confusion, difficulty talking, or problems understanding conversation
- Loss of coordination and balance
- Vision loss
- Severe headache with no obvious cause

In addition to a following a heart-healthy diet, exercising, not smoking, and maintaining a healthy weight, you should make a special effort to reduce your exposure to stressful situations—and calm your reactions to them.

A Swedish study found that people with high blood pressure (a risk factor for stroke) who managed stress poorly nearly doubled their risk of stroke, probably because the body reacts to stress by increasing blood pressure and heart rate. Though it's difficult to change from a driven, high-stress person into a calm, easygoing one, study author Lena André-Petersson, M.S., says that knowing the dangers associated with your personality type can go a long way toward helping you decrease your stress levels.

Pay attention to how you respond to stressful situations in your life—a sudden change in work assignments, a confrontational teenager, or a long line at the grocery store. Do you blow up? Or do you take a deep breath and calmly work through it?

If you tend toward the volcanic approach, make a conscious effort to take a step back. Breathe deeply from your abdomen. Every time you exhale, blow out the air forcefully as if you were expelling the anger and tension. Practice this relaxation technique and others to stay calm in an explosive situation.

saturated fat to a diet that's higher in unrefined carbohydrates and lower in fat will help you lose weight and lower your cholesterol levels."

Follow Dr. Applegate's tips if you want to prevent heart disease—rather than treat an existing condition—or are embarking on your first healthy diet.

**Limit yourself.** Although meat contains important nutrients, such as zinc and iron, it also tends to provide the bulk of artery-clogging saturated fat in your diet. Ration daily red meat, poultry, pork, and lamb consumption to about 6 ounces, a portion size no larger than two decks of cards. Choose such lean cuts as sirloin and remove any visible fat.

*Which is worse on the cholesterol scale, eggs or red meat? If you guessed eggs, you'd be wrong. It's okay to eat eggs daily if you limit red meat and other saturated fats.*—Liz Applegate, M.D.

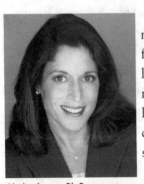

*Liz Applegate, Ph.D. suggests a diet based on fruits, vegetables, whole grains, and unsaturated fats found in nuts and fish to keep arteries healthy.*

**Substitute whenever possible.** Eat fish instead of meat at least once or twice a week. Fish contains a fat called omega-3 fatty acids. This type of fat helps lower blood cholesterol and triglyceride levels. It may even boost healthy HDL, as well as make blood less sticky and, thus, less prone to artery-blocking clots. Choose such cold-water fish as mackerel and salmon, which contain the most omega-3s.

**Bring back eggs.** Because one egg contains more than 200 milligrams dietary cholesterol, eggs have earned a bad reputation. But researchers now know that dietary cholesterol doesn't boost levels of blood cholesterol for 80 percent of people, assuming consumption of saturated fat is low. Dr. Applegate says it's safe to eat one to two eggs a day, as long as you keep red meat and other sources of saturated fat and cholesterol in check.

## ONE WOMAN'S STORY: STROKE

*While at work one day, Ohio state representative Joyce Beatty, then 50, started to feel uncomfortable. "I realized I had little control of my throat muscles. It was like I was choking," she says.*

"All of a sudden, this sensation riddled through the right side of my body," Joyce Beatty remembers. "My staff at first thought I was choking, and someone tried to do the Heimlich maneuver. Finally, someone called 911 and said that she thought I was having a heart attack. Neither I nor the people around me thought I was having a stroke."

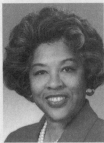

*Ohio legislator Joyce Beatty suffered a stroke that changed her life. Today, she manages her health with better diet and exercise choices.*

Fortunately, Beatty got to the hospital quickly, where doctors immediately recognized that she was indeed having a stroke.

She spent a month in the hospital and then more months getting physical therapy and electric-shock treatments to restore speech and control over the right side of her body. It was six months before Beatty felt normal again.

"Like many working women, I wasn't in touch with my personal health. I should have been more aware," she said. "I had high blood pressure. My maternal grandmother had had a stroke, but I didn't think it would happen to me. When we think about cardiovascular disease, we think it only affects people who are more into their senior years, rather than those in their 40s or 50s."

To reduce the chance of a recurrence, Beatty met with a registered dietitian who helped her shy away from artery-clogging fats and increase her intake of artery-friendly fats. Beatty completely gave up red meat.

In addition to blood pressure-lowering medication, she began taking the prescription drug Lipitor (atorvastatin) to lower her blood cholesterol, which was above 300 mg/dL. She started walking, jogging, or cycling for a half hour three times a week, actually putting exercise appointments in her date book.

Beatty reduced stress by calling it quits whenever she felt drained. "I balance my days better by listening to my body," she says. "When my body tells me that enough is enough, I stop. Instead of 12- to 15-hour days, if my body shuts down in seven or eight hours, I shut down, too."

The most important change was how Beatty deals with her doctor. Before the stroke, she got regular checkups but rarely asked questions. She'd say she felt fine, so her doctor didn't worry about her high blood pressure and high cholesterol.

Now she asks questions about every test: What do those numbers mean? Do my family history and other risk factors affect what the test results mean? What else can I do to improve? "The patient has to take the ownership," says Beatty. "You have to remind your doctor if you're in a minority ethnic group that is predisposed to stroke or heart disease. It is a dual responsibility."

**Load up on fruits and vegetables.** The American Heart Association recommends five or more servings a day, but go higher if you can. Dr. Applegate suggests that you eat as many as 6 to 12 servings. Both fruits and vegetables supply needed fiber, as well as an array of nutrients that work in concert to keep your arteries healthy. A serving equals one medium-sized piece of fruit, ½ cup fruit or vegetable juice, or ½ to 1 cup cooked of raw vegetables.

**Get milk.** Aim for at least two servings of low-fat dairy or other calcium-rich foods per day. Besides keeping bones strong, calcium helps regulate blood pressure. A serving equals 1 cup milk or yogurt, 1 ounce cheese, or ½ cup cottage cheese. If you can't handle dairy, take calcium supplements.

**Stick with whole grains.** Such whole grains as whole wheat bread and pasta supply a wealth of important nutrients, including vitamin E and various B vitamins, that help maintain the health of your arteries. Processed grains, such as white bread and white pasta, usually lack these nutrients. Aim to include four to eight whole-grain servings a day. A serving equals one slice of bread, 1 cup cold cereal, ½ cup hot cereal, or 1 cup cooked rice or pasta.

**Watch your saturated fats.** You can have five to eight servings a day. But be sure to measure carefully, particularly if you're trying to lose weight, because fat contains more calories per gram than protein or carbohydrates. One

## SHOULD I SEE A DOCTOR?

Many heart disease risk factors, such as high blood pressure and high blood cholesterol, have silent symptoms. That's why seeing your doctor for testing is so important.

Only tests for blood pressure, cholesterol, and blood sugar will let you and your doctor know whether anything is wrong:

- **Blood pressure:** When you see your gynecologist or family physician for a yearly exam, ask the nurse whether your blood pressure reading has changed from the year before.
- **Cholesterol:** Ask your gynecologist or family physician to test your blood cholesterol once every five years if you have no risk factors of heart disease, more often if you have risks. Get what is called a full cholesterol panel, which tests HDL, LDL, and triglyceride levels.

Usually, to get the full panel, you need to have a fasting test performed in the morning. Be sure to make note of your HDL and LDL results.

- **Blood sugar:** Ask your family doctor for a fasting blood-glucose test at age 45 and every three years after.

Keep your doctor informed about changes to your health. Tell your doctor about any of the following symptoms, even if they seem benign: shortness of breath, fainting, dizziness, fatigue, nausea, confusion, headache, thirst, blurry vision, sudden weight loss, or frequent urination.

serving equals 1 teaspoon vegetable oil, 2 teaspoons margarine, 1 tablespoon salad dressing, 2 teaspoons mayonnaise or peanut butter, 3 teaspoons seeds or nuts, an eighth of a medium avocado, or 10 small olives.

**Gravitate toward healthier, liquid fats.** Favor olive and canola oils over butter and margarine. If you're watching your weight, stick to the lowest number of recommended servings. For example, take in no more than six servings of starches and five servings of fats per day.

## ENERGIZING EXERCISE

Many physicians joke that if the benefits of exercise could be compacted into a pill, heart disease and other age-related illnesses would be history.

Lack of exercise increases your risk of high blood pressure—which damages the lining of your arteries and weakens your heart—by 30 to 50 percent. Physical inactivity also makes you more likely to gain weight and have abnormally low HDL cholesterol levels. Yet fewer than one in four women get enough activity to be considered heart fit.

*Lack of exercise increases your risk of high blood pressure by 30 to 50 percent. Make your goal 30 minutes, at least four days a week.*

Here are some things that will do your heart good.

**Aim for 30.** The American Heart Association recommends a half hour of intentional exercise three to four times a week, as well as increased activity on the other days. That means making a concerted effort to walk, jog, swim, or do some other form of aerobic exercise that you enjoy. The good news is that any chosen exercise doesn't have to be performed for 30 minutes in a row. It can be broken down, for example, to 20 minutes at lunch and 10 minutes after dinner. On off days, increase your daily activity by parking far from your destination, taking the stairs rather than the elevator, and playing with your dog or kids in the yard.

**Get a checkup.** If you've never exercised, check with your doctor before starting any activity or program. Certain conditions, such as angina or high blood pressure, can make some forms of exercise dangerous. Running and weight lifting are examples. Otherwise, get out there! Start walking regularly with your dog, kids, or spouse. Sign up for an interesting exercise class, such as yoga, tai chi, or African dance. Get caught up on those household tasks you've been putting off. Call some old friends and meet in the park for a stroll. Lack of exercise makes you lethargic, so even if you feel you haven't the energy, make yourself get moving—if only for 10 minutes at first. You may be surprised how quickly exercise increases your energy levels.

## THE IMPORTANCE OF WEIGHT CONTROL

The more pounds you carry, the harder your heart must work. This increases your risk for heart disease, high blood pressure, and stroke. It's like buying a huge car with a small engine. A small engine will last a lot longer powering a small car than it would a larger one. Losing weight helps lower levels of unhealthy LDL cholesterol, boost levels of healthy HDL cholesterol, reduce blood pressure, and improve blood-sugar control. Fortunately, an exercise regimen can help you burn off excess calories and better regulate your appetite.

To lose weight safely, you need to cut about 500 calories from your daily diet. If you're beginning an exercise program, remember that you'll burn an extra 200 or more calories each day, so take that into consideration. The easiest way to reduce calories is to cut back on foods that contain no nutritional calories, such as sugary snacks, soft drinks, and chips. For example, you could save 300 calories a day just by forgoing two 12-ounce regular soft drinks.

## TIME TO QUIT

You're probably aware that breathing smoke, tar, and nicotine into your lungs puts you at risk for more than just lung cancer. It also accelerates the artery-clogging process by damaging the lining of your blood vessels. In addition, smoking causes your blood vessels to constrict, making the blood stickier and increasing your risk of clots.

Studies have found that smokers experience a variety of health problems as a result of artery damage—from back pain caused by diseased arteries in the back to leg pain from diseased arteries in the legs to sexual dysfunction.

# TREATING HEART DISEASE: STOP AND REVERSE THE DAMAGE

You are at high risk for heart attack and stroke if you have been diagnosed with heart disease, dangerously high blood pressure or cholesterol, or diabetes or insulin resistance, or if you occasionally suffer from chest pain. You'll need to follow a strict diet, make a few strategic lifestyle changes, and engage in the proper form of physical activity for your health concern. Here's advice for health problems that increase your risk for heart attack and stroke.

## A WOMAN'S RIGHT TO THE *RIGHT* TREATMENT: HEART DISEASE

*Women notoriously play down their symptoms when they see a doctor—a tendency that can be dangerous.*

"When asked about their symptoms, women often almost apologize for being there," says **Deborah L. Wolbrette, M.D.**, a cardiologist with Pennsylvania State University's Milton S. Hershey Medical Center in Hershey. "They say, 'Oh, I know this is nothing,' 'I'm sorry that I'm here,' or 'This is silly. I know there is nothing wrong with me.' When you say that you don't think anything is wrong, you're saying exactly what your doctor wants to hear. So your doctor will respond with, 'You're right, there's nothing going on.'"

On the other hand, when a man sees a doctor, he says he knows something is wrong and tells the doctor to examine him. "Guess who gets the stress test? The man will get it, and the woman won't," says Dr. Wolbrette.

To complicate matters, many women have different heart-disease symptoms than men. So when a doctor asks a woman if she's feeling squeezing chest pain (a typical male symptom) and she honestly answers no, the doctor figures she doesn't have heart disease.

To turn this dangerous miscommunication around, Dr. Wolbrette suggests these tactics:

**Complain, don't apologize.** Shortness of breath, fatigue, dizziness, and fainting spells are all cause for a checkup. If you suspect something is wrong, you must see a doctor and explain how you are feeling. "It's not that the doctors are denying the women. It's how you present yourself. You need to be your own advocate," says Dr. Wolbrette.

**Learn the language.** Because symptoms, such as nausea or dizziness, can seem unrelated to heart disease, tell your doctor you've never felt quite this way before. You might say, "There's something going on, or I wouldn't be here." You might have to insist, adding, "There's something wrong. I know it doesn't sound like a heart problem, but there's something different. This doesn't feel normal." If appropriate, tell the doctor, "I can't do what I used to do." When your doctor realizes your symptoms are out of the ordinary, she usually takes notice.

**Get your questions answered.** If the doctor doesn't ask the right questions, tell her what's on your mind anyway. Don't let her rush out of the room before you have explained your symptoms and had all your questions answered. "If you are unclear about why your doctor isn't putting you on a medication for this problem or requesting a test for this problem, *ask*," says Dr. Wolbrette. "Believe me, your male counterparts do."

## HIGH BLOOD CHOLESTEROL: KEEPING LEVELS IN CHECK

You want a low LDL count and a high HDL count. And that's how the numbers generally run until you hit menopause, since estrogen tends to nudge HDL levels upward.

Blood also contains a fat called triglycerides. This dangerous blood fat has a tendency to get stuck along artery walls. Women with high triglycerides usually also have high LDL and low HDL levels. For an accurate picture of your heart health, you need to know your LDL, HDL, triglyceride, and total cholesterol counts, as well as your cholesterol ratio (HDL to total cholesterol).

*Some doctors feel that* HDL *standards are not high enough for women, which may mean women don't get early treatment.*—C. Noel Bairey Merz, M.D.

Because women naturally tend to have higher HDL cholesterol levels than men, some doctors fear women are still at risk in the generally accepted safety zone of 50 to 60 mg/dL. "There are those of us who think that women are less likely to get treated despite having similar risks as men," says *C. Noel Bairey Merz, M.D.,* medical director of Women's Health at Cedars-Sinai Medical Center. "The sad reality is that the current guidelines translate into fewer women being treated. Yet just as many women as men get heart disease, so we're obviously missing some of them."

Dr. Merz says more research will determine a better HDL number for women to shoot for, but she feels that 70 mg/dL may be a good goal. "It doesn't give you immunity from disease. It just counts as one negative risk factor," she says.

To raise HDL and lower your LDL and triglyceride levels, reduce your intake of saturated and trans fats, and eat more fish. You should also try the following heart-healthy diet tips.

**Bring on the beans.** Eating more soluble fiber is your best defense against high cholesterol, says *Liz Applegate, Ph.D.,* lecturer in the department of nutrition at the University of California at Davis. Soluble fiber traps fat and cholesterol in your intestines, preventing them from making their way into your bloodstream. Soluble fiber also slows cholesterol production in the liver. Ideally, aim for 25 to 30 grams of soluble fiber a day from food, not supplements. This shouldn't be a hardship—even baked beans count. "Most people think baked beans are junk food because of the sugar and bacon. But just one serving gives you 15 grams of soluble fiber," says Dr. Applegate. In fact, studies show that adding just 1 to 1½ cups of beans a day to your diet drops cholesterol levels. Other good sources of soluble fiber include fruits, whole grains (particularly oat bran), and vegetables.

**Switch your margarine.** Sold under the brand names Take Control and Benecol, this special margarine contains plant substances that act like fiber to suck fat and cholesterol from your intestines, says Dr. Merz. To get the right dosage, follow the manufacturers' suggestions.

**Back off the booze.** Alcohol seems to nudge good HDL cholesterol upward, particularly in postmenopausal women, says Dr. Applegate. Red wine and dark beer also contain phytochemicals (biologically active substances in plants) that may protect the heart by making the blood less sticky and relaxing the blood vessels. Studies show that different types of alcohol—wine, beer, and hard liquor—are associated with the same reduction in risk for heart disease. But too much alcohol can also raise blood pressure and increase your risk of breast cancer. If you don't currently drink, Dr. Applegate suggests discussing the pros and cons of alcohol consumption with your doctor. If you do drink, serve your alcohol with meals, which may increase the HDL-boosting effects.

And stick to just one drink daily. That's 12 ounces of beer, 4 ounces of wine, or 1.5 ounces of 80-proof distilled spirits.

**Experiment with soy.** Numerous studies suggest that a diet with upwards of 25 grams soy protein per day dramatically reduces LDL and total blood cholesterol levels and boosts HDL levels. Soy may work by interfering with cholesterol production in the liver, reducing the amount of fat the intestines absorb, or preventing LDL from getting stuck in your arteries.

The numerous soy products on the market—from breakfast cereals to burgers to flavored tofu—make meeting your 25-gram goal easier than ever. If a product claims to be a source of soy protein, it contains 6.2 grams or more per serving, says Dr. Applegate. The key to getting more soy in your diet is experimentation. Try soy ground round (a hamburger substitute) in soups, soy cheese on sandwiches, soy milk in cereal, and soy nuts on salad.

## ANGINA: A WARNING YOU MUST HEED

Once plaque builds up in your arteries, you officially have heart disease. Narrowed arteries may cause discomfort—called angina—during exertion or stress, when the heart can't get enough blood.

Angina is a warning that part of your heart isn't getting all the blood it needs, putting you at high risk of a heart attack. If you think you are having angina or have experienced it before, talk to your doctor. Be aware, though, that many women don't get that warning in the same straightforward way men do.

"The definition of angina as a squeezing, clenched-fist feeling in the chest was based on what men described," says *Deborah L. Wolbrette, M.D.,* a cardiologist with Pennsylvania State University's Milton S. Hershey Medical Center in Hershey. "It was presumed that women would feel it the same way, but we're learning they don't."

Instead of chest discomfort, women may feel nausea or fatigue, as well as heartburn, neck or arm pain, sweating, or other nebulous symptoms. So how do you know whether that nausea or fatigue is actually angina or just a reaction to something you ate? Don't try to diagnose the problem yourself, recommends *Alice Chang, M.D.,* an instructor at the Harvard Medical School. If you know you have gastroesophageal reflux disease (GERD) and your symptoms are familiar, try the usual treatments but call your doctor if the symptoms don't go away in a reasonable time. Women with diabetes have an increased risk for heart disease even before menopause, Dr. Chang says, and they are more likely to have atypical symptoms rather than classic chest pain. If you have diabetes, Dr. Chang advises that you be particularly concerned about nausea, heartburn, sweats, and neck or arm pain. She says women with diabetes should call their doctor whenever they have any unusual symptoms, especially if they last longer than 15 minutes.

If you have any warning symptoms, ask yourself the following questions.

- *Is what I'm feeling unusual?* If you've never felt quite this way before, you could be experiencing angina and should tell your doctor about it immediately. Symptoms can seem like heartburn but are more intense than usual or get worse despite your usual treatment.
- *What was I doing when I started feeling like this?* If you were raising your arms over your head (a common angina trigger in women), exercising, or doing something stressful—such as arguing with your teenager or balancing your checkbook—it could be angina. Extreme cold or heat, a heavy meal, alcohol, and cigarette smoking can also trigger an episode.
- *How long did it last?* Angina is often relieved by rest, when blood flow returns to normal or does not have to meet the demands of exercise. During a heart attack, however, blood flow is blocked long enough to cause permanent damage to heart muscle. Therefore, pain or symptoms that last longer than 15 to 30 minutes suggest possible heart damage. If you have symptoms for longer than 30 minutes but your electrocardiogram (EKG) and blood tests show no evidence of heart damage, you probably are not having a heart attack. Getting medical attention when suffering unusual symptoms and chest pain is extremely important in making a diagnosis. If you suspect you are experiencing angina, call your doctor for an evaluation as soon as possible.

The longer you have symptoms and delay treatment, the more heart muscle is damaged if you're having a heart attack and the higher your risk for heart complications later on. In studies looking at heart-attack treatment, women take longer than men to go to the hospital after the start of heart-attack symptoms. Partly, this is due to how long it takes to recognize atypical symptoms. But it also probably relates to a woman's role as a caregiver. A woman often takes time to prepare a meal or make sure that children or grandchildren are picked up from school before getting herself to the doctor's office or a hospital.

If your doctor says your symptoms are angina-related, keep a journal to help spot any patterns, including situations that cause and relieve symptoms. Then if you have pain that falls out of the pattern, you'll know to seek immediate medical care.

If your doctor has diagnosed you with heart disease, follow this advice.

**Minimize saturated fat.** For average women without established heart disease, the recommended dietary limit for saturated fat (a known artery-clogger found in animal products, such as dairy products and red meat) is 20 grams a day. But you'll want to cut back to 10 to 12 grams, says Dr. Applegate. You can do that by eating healthy, low-saturated fat sources of protein, such as soy and fish, instead of higher saturated fat animal protein foods, such as hamburger and pork.

*If you have heart disease, walking and yoga are the safest forms of beneficial exercise.—Deborah L. Wolbrette, M.D.*

**Focus on fish.** Chicken or turkey was once thought of as the low-fat antidote to a diet of artery-clogging saturated fat. But if you have established heart disease, you need to take things one step further. Numerous studies now show that substituting fish for chicken and turkey at least two to three times a week greatly reduces heart disease, says Dr. Merz. Fish contains a heart-healthy type of fat—called omega-3 fatty acids—that makes your blood less sticky and acts directly on your heart muscle, helping it to beat normally.

**Delete trans fats.** Pay even closer attention to your intake of trans fatty acids, another unhealthy form of fat found primarily in fried and processed foods, such as doughnuts, crackers, and microwave popcorn. A study conducted in the Netherlands found diets that include trans fats lower the healthy

## VARICOSE VEINS: THREE OPTIONS FOR RELIEF

*You can probably blame your mother for those large, wormlike veins on your legs. Their primary cause is genetic, though standing all day can contribute to the problem.*

Veins contain valves that help prevent blood from flowing backward, especially as it travels against gravity from the legs back to the heart and lungs. A varicose vein forms when the valves weaken and aren't able to hold back the blood. Gravity pulls the blood down, causing it to flow backward, swelling the blood vessel and causing pain.

Varicose veins are not dangerous, but they can make your legs achy, tired, and even painful. Left untreated, they will continue to get worse.

Once you have varicose veins, no natural treatment will get rid of them. However, losing weight, wearing supportive stockings, avoiding standing for long periods of time, and exercising may slow their progression, prevent future varicose veins from forming, and keep existing veins from getting worse, says Lorrie J. Klein, M.D., a dermatologist in Laguna Niguel, California.

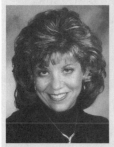

*Controlling your weight and exercising are two key tools to prevent and treat varicose veins, says Lorrie J. Klein, M.D.*

To get rid of a varicose vein, you need to do exactly that: Get rid of that section of vein with one of the common methods described here. Once the vein is removed, your blood finds an alternate route to travel, choosing nearby healthy veins to make its way back to your heart and lungs.

• **Sclerotherapy:** Despite the scary name, this procedure merely involves sticking a needle into your vein and injecting it with medication. The medication causes the vein to seal itself shut, like a straw after you've sucked out the air. This stops blood flow and shrinks the vein. Sometimes, instead of medication, a physician will use radio frequency energy delivered through a small tube to seal the vein shut. The procedure is quick and relatively painless but tends to work on only small varicose veins and spider veins.

• **Keyhole surgery:** In this minimally invasive surgery, a surgeon pulls the vein out through tiny incisions. This procedure is also called ambulatory phlebectomy. It's not as complicated or as scarring as other surgeries, but it does involve local anesthesia and some slicing.

• **Ligation:** Also called stripping, ligation is performed in an operating room under general or local anesthesia. This procedure involves tying the vein shut and then removing it from the leg. Ligation offers the highest success rate of all treatments but will leave a scar and may be painful. Reserve this option only for large veins that your doctor doesn't think will respond to other treatments.

• **Laser and light-source treatments:** This procedure requires a surgeon to use a light beam to seal off the vein. According to the American Venous Forum, light-based methods are most often used only for tiny facial spider veins and have limited value in treating varicose veins in the legs.

HDL cholesterol and harm blood vessels even more than diets that are high in saturated fats. Trans fats are also known to raise bad LDL cholesterol, a notorious artery-clogger. In the study, removing trans fats boosted healthy HDL cholesterol and made blood vessels more pliable, allowing blood to flow more easily.

Trans fats make up 4 to 7 percent of the dietary fat in most diets, and study author Nicole M. de Roos, M.Sc., Ph.D., a research fellow at Wageningen University in the Netherlands, recommends completely omitting them. To help eliminate trans fats, read labels. Foods that list hydrogenated or partially hydrogenated fats or vegetable oil on the ingredients list contain trans fats.

**Walk this way.** Exercise is healthy, but if you have heart disease or angina, you must listen closely to your body. When you exercise, your heart beats faster to supply your muscles with oxygen. If your arteries are narrow, this increased demand may mean that not enough oxygen gets back to your heart, triggering an angina attack.

But that's not an excuse to join the couch-potatoes club. Instead, choose your form of exercise wisely and monitor your symptoms carefully. "Walking is probably the safest thing," says Dr. Wolbrette. "Yoga is also fine. While exercising, if you start feeling angina symptoms, such as nausea or fatigue, stop." As soon as you quit exercising, the pain will subside as oxygen demand returns to normal and your heartbeat slows. You can take nitroglycerin if it has been prescribed by your doctor, but just ceasing the activity should make the pain subside.

## HIGH BLOOD PRESSURE: THE LOWDOWN ON BRINGING IT DOWN

Your blood pressure is highest when your heart beats and lowest when your heart relaxes between beats. That's why blood pressure numbers are expressed with both a high, or systolic, number (the pressure after the beat) and a low, or diastolic, number (the pressure when your heart is relaxed).

Your blood pressure during rest should be less than 140/90 mm Hg (millimeters of mercury). Anything above 140/90 increases your risk for heart disease, stroke, and other medical problems. In many cases, the following self-help tips will help you reach the target levels, but some women require prescription medication.

There are numerous pressure-lowering medications available, all of which act differently to achieve the same purpose. For example, a class of blood-pressure medications called beta blockers reduces heart rate. Angiotensin converting enzyme inhibitors, known as ACE inhibitors, and calcium channel-blockers help to relax artery walls, which, in turn, lowers blood pressure.

While these drugs have been proven to lower blood pressure, they unfortunately also come with a host of side effects, ranging from lethargy and leg cramps to insomnia and dizziness. You may react to various brands, types, and dosages differently. Be sure to talk with your doctor about how your medication makes you feel. Often, finding the right medication to lower your blood pressure—and help you feel better—is a matter of trying different drugs and dosages until you discover the one that works best for you.

*Eating fruits, vegetables, and low-fat dairy products lowers high blood pressure dramatically, reducing or eliminating the need for medication. Cut out salt for even better results.*
*—Liz Applegate, Ph.D.*

The following tips can help treat mild elevations in blood pressure without medication or reduce the amount of medication you need to take.

**Lay off the salt.** When researchers tested a diet rich in fruits, vegetables, and low-fat dairy products (known as DASH, which stands for Dietary Approaches to Stop Hypertension) on 459 people with hypertension, blood pressure dropped dramatically within two weeks. A subsequent study found pressure plummeted even more when the diet was coupled with salt restrictions. The main differences between the DASH diet and the one outlined earlier by the American Heart Association is the amount of fruits and vegetables. DASH recommends 8 to 10 servings, but Dr. Applegate suggests even more. "Eating 9 to 11 servings of fruits and vegetables really works as well as medication for some people," she says. Fruits and vegetables are rich in potassium, a mineral known to lower blood pressure, as well as plant-based chemicals that boost artery and heart health. Eating that many veggies also helps you naturally lower your sodium intake, says Dr. Applegate, because your appetite is satisfied—thus, you don't want to consume salty, processed foods. The DASH diet also recommends four to five servings of nuts, seeds, and beans a week, with only two to three daily servings of fats and oils.

**Meditate twice a day.** Several studies show that practicing transcendental meditation has the same pressure-lowering results as taking a single blood-pressure pill, such as a diuretic or beta blocker. "If they learned to meditate, women on two to three pills can go down to one, and women on one pill could probably get off the medication altogether," says Dr. Merz—as long as they have their doctor's approval. Learn more about transcendental meditation at www.tm.org.

**Cut back on alcohol.** Heavy drinking—four to five drinks a day—is linked to high blood pressure. Reduce your intake to one drink per day at most.

## MOTHER NATURE, M.D.: HEART DISEASE

*Many women with heart disease are already under the care of a cardiologist or family physician. Adding a naturopathic doctor to the health-care team can be a big plus.*

A naturopathic doctor can provide more specialized and specific advice, tailored to lifestyle, age, and personality, says *Sejal Parikh-Shah, N.D.,* assistant professor at the Canadian College of Naturopathic Medicine and a naturopathic physician in Toronto.

"You give me two patients with high blood-cholesterol levels, and I would treat them differently," she says. "In naturopathic medicine, we want to know the cause of the problem. In one patient, the cause might be diet; in the other, the cause might be stress. Age also comes into play. I would treat a postmenopausal woman differently than a woman in her 30s."

To determine the cause of a condition, Dr. Parikh-Shah conducts a series of both conventional and naturopathic tests. She also details an intense medical history. Then she spends numerous visits helping her patient learn to make strategic lifestyle changes to encourage the body's natural healing defenses to do their job, many of which are described throughout this chapter.

"When a woman comes to me with a complaint, she is my client for life," says Dr. Parikh-Shah. "Naturopathic medicine is a lifestyle change, especially when we're looking at heart disease. Once I get a client to a level where she is satisfied with her health, I usually continue to see her once or twice a year to make sure she's still progressing the way she wants to be."

Dr. Parikh-Shah makes the following suggestions for working with a naturopathic doctor to help heal heart-related problems:

**Don't look for a quick fix.** Many patients want one herb or supplement that will lower their cholesterol 20 points or drop their blood pressure to normal levels. Herbs and nutritional supplements—such as garlic, vitamin E, and B-complex vitamins—may help you along your way to wellness, but they are almost never the only answer. Managing heart disease involves larger lifestyle changes that include revamping your diet and reducing stress. "A pill is not going to treat lifestyle needs," says Dr. Parikh-Shah.

## SYNDROME X: TREATING A CLUSTER OF CONDITIONS

In some people, numerous risk factors cluster together—including obesity, low HDL, high triglycerides, and diabetes or its precursor, insulin resistance—forming a distinct condition known as syndrome X, also called metabolic syndrome.

Having syndrome X puts you at greater risk for heart disease than from any one of its risk factors alone. In fact, the latest cholesterol guidelines advise doctors to prescribe medication for people with syndrome X sooner than previously advised. You already know obesity, low HDL levels, and

**Write down what you eat.** Diet is often the first problem that people need to deal with. Yet, Dr. Parikh-Shah doesn't believe in one-size-fits-all diets. She tailors her advice to each person's lifestyle. Otherwise, a patient ends up with a plan on paper, but not in practice. To custom-tailor your heart-friendly diet, find out which foods you naturally grab—and when. Dr. Parikh-Shah recommends writing down everything you eat and drink for a week. Then examine your seven-day menu and look for healthful substitutions. For example, study your choices of fats. Could you have chosen olive oil instead of margarine? Do the same with carbohydrates. Could you substitute brown rice or quinoa for white rice and white bread? Only make substitutions you know you can stick with. Otherwise, your new diet will last as long as most people's New Year's resolutions.

**Pick the right exercise for you.** Conventional medicine recommends 30 minutes of cardiovascular exercise on most days of the week, but Dr. Parikh-Shah tailors that suggestion to patients, who usually fall into one of three categories:

- High stress, low fitness: For those who have never exercised before and lead pressure-filled lives, trying to fit in 30 minutes of cardiovascular exercise every day becomes one more stressful proposition. As an alternative, Dr. Parikh-Shah suggests a more meditative and calming type of exercise, such as tai chi, yoga, or deep breathing. Once a patient has stress under control, Dr. Parikh-Shah recommends a more cardiovascular exercise, such as power walking.
- Overweight, low fitness: Because obesity is a primary risk factor for heart disease, it's best to take on a form of exercise that will help drop weight. That's why Dr. Parikh-Shah suggests strength training and toning exercises along with cardiovascular exercise for overweight patients. Strength training not only builds muscle, which boosts metabolism and helps with weight loss, but also is easier on joints than many forms of cardiovascular exercise, making it a more comfortable choice for obese people.
- Normal weight, fairly fit: If a person has been exercising for a time, Dr. Parikh-Shah recommends pushing the pace to condition the heart even more. She suggests starting with walking and then advancing to jogging or another more vigorous exercise pursuit.

high triglycerides are bad for your heart. But diabetes and insulin resistance can be equally devastating. That's because the hormone insulin provides the key that allows blood sugar into your cells. People with diabetes or insulin resistance either don't make enough insulin or have cells that don't respond properly to insulin. In either case, sugar levels build up in your blood, damaging your heart, eyes, kidneys, and other organs.

If you have syndrome X, these are some precautions you should take.

**Make fat count.** You already know that replacing saturated and trans fats with carbohydrates reduces blood-cholesterol levels. But this is not true for people with syndrome X. "You put them on a high-carbohydrate, low-fat diet, and they respond with higher triglycerides," says Dr. Applegate. "They do much better on a 30- to 35-percent fat diet."

Before you race for the doughnuts, however, realize we're talking about healthy monounsaturated fats and essential fatty acids found in fish, flax seeds, and nuts. Any carbohydrates you eat must be the healthiest type: complex carbohydrates. Dr. Applegate says the best kinds, in order of preference for those with syndrome X, are vegetables, fruits, and whole grains. During every meal, strive to make healthier choices by picking fish instead of chicken, nuts instead of tortilla chips, quinoa instead of white rice, and flax- or soy-based cereals instead of refined sugar-based cereals.

**Scale back your servings.** If you've been diagnosed with syndrome X, you could probably stand to lose a few pounds, especially if you're carrying extra fat in your abdomen. Abdominal fat is another risk factor for heart disease. Stick to the lower number of servings in the DASH diet. (For more information, see page 193.)

**Put sugar in its place.** Easily digestible foods that hit the bloodstream quickly are most likely to raise blood-sugar levels, and refined sugar is the biggest booster of all. One of the easiest ways to cut back on sugar and other refined carbohydrates is to watch what you drink. Soda and flavored iced teas and fruit juices contain 15 to 20 teaspoons of sugar per 8-ounce serving—way over your daily allotment. Forget these beverages and brew your own iced tea instead. If you must sweeten it, use honey or molasses, both of which have heart-healthy antioxidants, says Dr. Applegate.

# 11 Immune System
## Beating What's Bugging You

*Imagine your immune system as a giant "Pac-Man" game: an army of voracious cells patrolling your body in search of unwanted invaders to consume.*

The immune system is an intricate network of organs and specialized tissue that protects you against infection. These sentinels work together to repel antigens, which include such foreign bodies as bacteria, viruses, pollen, and pet dander.

Your first lines of defense are on the surface: the oils of your skin, tears in your eyes, saliva in your mouth, and mucus in your nose and throat. Invading forces that sneak past your mouth are then attacked by stomach acid and intestinal bacteria. All other successful trespassers trigger your immune system's internal commandos, antigen-fighting cells called lymphocytes. The human body is home to close to a trillion lymphocytes, which either strike and obliterate antigens or mark them for destruction by other agents. More lymphocytes are produced as needed to resist infection.

These lymphocytes, a type of white blood cell, are found throughout the body, including in the lymph glands and blood. They are carried by lymph, a clear fluid that helps cleanse body tissues. The lymphocytes cycle from the lymph to the blood to the tissues and back to the lymph.

There are two main types of lymphocytes: B-lymphocytes, known as B cells, put the hit on invaders by producing antibodies, which are proteins that tailor themselves to destroy particular antigens. T cells are lymphocytes that help regulate the immune system and attack and destroy infected cells.

As any "Pac-Man" player can tell you, there comes a time in every game when the goblins get the better of the hero—and the human experience is no different. Bacteria, viruses, or other antigens sometimes outsmart the immune system's defenses. Statistics about two common infections—a cold and the flu—illustrate how vulnerable we are. Americans suffer through more than a billion colds a year. Approximately 35 to 50 million of us fall ill every flu season, resulting in some 100,000 hospitalizations and more than 20,000 deaths.

Infections aren't our only immune problem. Sometimes, the immune system misreads a threat and reacts violently to a commonplace irritant. Just ask any of the estimated 50 million Americans who suffer from allergies. Worse still, your immune system can turn on you, attacking your own tissue as if it were an antigen. An example of such an autoimmune disorder is lupus, a chronic, body-wide inflammatory condition that affects 1 out of every 185 people in the United States—the majority of whom are women.

Understanding the nature of *your* goblins can help tip the odds of the game in favor of your immune system.

## THE COMMON COLD: CONQUERING THE SYMPTOMS

It's a classic conundrum: If we can send a man to the moon, why can't we cure the common cold?

Part of the problem is that there is so little that's common about colds. There are about 200 viruses to blame, and these viruses mutate rapidly. Therefore, finding medication that works against one virus doesn't guarantee it will work against any of the others—or continue working for long, explains *Alice Chang, M.D.*, an instructor at Harvard Medical School.

*Women get colds three times as often as men, probably because they spend more time around children.*

According to the National Institute of Allergy and Infectious Diseases, women fall victim to colds three times more often than men. Why such a difference? Women, especially those between ages 20 and 30, are the primary providers of child care. And children—with their immature immune systems—are more likely to bring home a cold virus, which picks up strength from the small hosts before moving on to adult women.

## AVOIDING THE COLD BUG

Despite what your mother may have told you, the only connection between colds and cold weather is that chilly conditions tend to keep us indoors, where viruses and bacteria spread more easily, says *Catherine Shaner, M.D.* Dr. Shaner, a former pediatrician, is medical advisor for the American Safety and Health Institute, which trains worksite health-care professionals. Since colds are a major cause of lost work days, Dr. Shaner frequently deals with this illness.

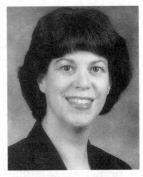

*Cold weather has nothing to do with making you sick, says Catherine Shaner, M.D. The only connection is in keeping you indoors where viruses lurk.*

Follow these tried-and-true tips for avoiding colds.

**Wash your hands.** Scrub up repeatedly throughout the day, even if you haven't had contact with someone who has a cold, advises *Birgit Winther, M.D.*, assistant professor of otolaryngology and pediatrics at the University of Virginia Medical School in Charlottesville. She suggests using regular hand soap instead of antibacterial cleaners, which actually don't kill cold viruses. Also, make a conscious effort not to touch dirty hands to your eyes, nose, or mouth.

> *Zap cold germs with plain old soap. Antibacterial cleaners don't kill cold viruses.—Birgit Winther, M.D.*

**Back it up.** If you must rub your face, use the back of your hand—or better yet, a clean tissue. Your palm and fingers are more likely to harbor cold viruses, says Dr. Winther.

**Keep your hands to yourself.** You might want to avoid shaking hands during winter months, when people often use their hands to shield coughs and sneezes.

**Stay hydrated.** When your skin is dry, it cracks, allowing viruses easy entry. Eight 8-ounce glasses of water every day will keep your skin supple and your mucous membranes moist and, thus, less susceptible to viral invaders, says Dr. Shaner.

**Clean surfaces.** Everything you touch, from tabletops to automatic teller machines, is teeming with viruses, says Dr. Shaner. The numerous germs responsible for colds can survive up to six hours on objects. Disinfect countertops and telephones at home and at your workplace with alcohol, a solution of ¼ cup ammonia to 1 gallon water, or a similar mixture made with bleach. Use a portable germicide on shopping cart handles, public toilets, and pay phones. Dr. Shaner recommends Virofree spray, which kills 120 assorted germs. Available at Linens 'n Things stores nationwide and online at www.virofree.com, this nonallergenic, odorless spray is safe for use in nurseries. And the small spray bottle is just the right size to carry in your purse.

## STRESS AND YOUR IMMUNE SYSTEM

*Can a bad day at work bring on a cold? Can marital strife make allergies worse? Bottom line: Does stress affect your immune system?*

Most definitely, says **Jesse Lynn Hanley, M.D.**, a California antiaging specialist, medical director of the Malibu Health and Rehabilitation Center, and author of *Tired of Being Tired*.

Research in psychoneuroimmunology—the fascinating connection between the mind and body—finds that positive and negative experiences directly affect the immune system, says Dr. Hanley. Stressful, sad, and scary experiences can suppress immune function for up to 24 hours after they occur, whereas lighthearted, happy, and entertaining experiences can boost the immune system's function for about three days.

So just a little bit of recreation every week can give you a consistently stronger immune system and improve your overall health.

Dr. Hanley isn't talking about dropping everything and going to the movies, nor does she encourage excess partying or obsessive exercising. "Fun activities are experiences that take you out of the trials and tribulations of daily life," she says. "Fun is whatever absorbs you so your mind is cleared of concerns and your body and mind are united and uplifted, even momentarily."

Finding a few minutes of amusement every day is essential, says Dr. Hanley. Otherwise, the stress of modern life puts many women in a state of adrenal overdrive. The two tiny adrenal glands, one above each kidney, secrete adrenaline and other stress hormones that influence nearly every bodily function. Time pressures, job demands, family responsibilities, and our own high expectations routinely trigger our bodies to release stress hormones. Our cave ancestors felt this rush perhaps once a week, but most of

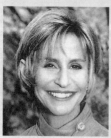

*Have a little fun every day to give your immune system a boost, says antiaging specialist Jesse Lynn Hanley, M.D.*

## COPING WITH A COLD

"A cold gets slowly better over a week, no matter what you do," says Dr. Winther. Over-the-counter medications may treat the symptoms to help you feel better, but they won't shorten a cold's duration. And, she notes, even non-prescription remedies may have side effects, such as dizziness or insomnia, and should, therefore, be taken with care. If you have hypertension, avoid decongestants, such as pseudoephedrine, which can increase your blood pressure.

If you must self-medicate, here's what our experts recommend.

**Stem that achy feeling.** Try acetaminophen or ibuprofen every four to six hours around the clock for the first two to three days. These nonsteroidal

us experience adrenaline surges several times a day, while stuck in traffic or rushing to meet a deadline at work.

And just as you can't rev your car's engine 24/7 without burning it out, your body can't withstand constant stimulation. You can't keep churning out stress hormones without giving your body a chance to recharge, says Dr. Hanley.

Wear and tear from stress may manifest itself as insomnia, weight gain, or fatigue. Unchecked stress is associated with recurrent infections, Type II diabetes, premature heart disease, and chronic depression. Adding to this adrenal overload are the cumulative effects of poor diet, environmental pollution, and the hurried pace of modern life. Learning to relax can reduce the burden on your body, giving it time to repair itself.

To help yourself wind down, try lifestyle changes, exercise, and relaxation techniques such as yoga or meditation:

**Breathe deeply.** When you're stressed out, your breathing is shallow. Stop for a moment. Draw air in through your nostrils until your lungs are full. Hold this breath for a count of five. Now exhale slowly through your mouth. Bringing oxygen into your lungs positively charges your biochemistry, literally feeding your cells with the breath of life, says Dr. Hanley. Just one conscious healing breath each day can make a difference to your health, although she recommends a series of three to five breaths, several times a day as needed.

**Avoid self-induced criticism.** All those should've, could've, and would've messages you beat yourself up with do nothing but erode your peace of mind, sending surges of stress hormones through your immune system and wearing you down. To break this cycle of self-flagellation, stop yourself midcrimination and substitute a positive message. Rather than, "I'm so disorganized, I always leave the office late," think to yourself, "Wasn't I clever to miss the crush of rush-hour traffic."

**Eliminate the expectations.** The biggest stressors are the high expectations you hold yourself to, says Dr. Hanley. You really don't have to have the perfect house, the perfect job, the perfect family. Realize that your life *is* perfect—for you.

anti-inflammatory drugs (NSAIDs) relieve the mild to moderate muscle pain associated with the early days of a cold.

*No matter what you've heard, there's no evidence that a large dose of vitamin C will do anything for your cold.*—Birgit Winther, M.D.

**Go easy on antihistamines.** Take an antihistamine at night to reduce nasal congestion. Antihistamines relieve inflammatory responses common to colds—such as a runny nose and watery eyes—but Dr. Winther does not recommend taking them during the day, since they are naturally sedating. If your nose is dripping like a faucet, you might try a nondrowsy formula for relief. Don't overdo it, though. You may hate blowing your nose all day, but that's nature's way of clearing the infection. Taking antihistamines too often thickens nasal secretions, setting you up for a bacterial sinus infection—and further misery.

## WASH YOUR HANDS THE RIGHT WAY

*You can't keep someone from sneezing on you, but you can rinse most potential viral illnesses down the drain.*

Doctors say that frequent hand washing is your best defense against infectious viruses. This advice may seem like a no-brainer, but most people don't wash their hands correctly, says **Catherine Shaner, M.D.,** medical advisor for the American Safety and Health Institute. They usually wash too fast. And that little squirt of soap, quick lather, and hasty rinse won't stop a cold, flu, or bronchitis virus.

Soap needs at least 30 seconds to suspend dirt, bacteria, and viruses, so you should lather up for at least that long. If you're not sure how long 30 seconds is without watching a clock, Dr. Shaner suggests singing the alphabet song or "Twinkle, Twinkle Little Star" in your head—or aloud, if you want some fun—while lathering. Then rinse your hands with warm water for at least 10 seconds. Whenever possible, dry your hands with a disposable towel, even at home. If someone has done a slapdash rinse and wipe of their hands before you, you don't want to rub their viruses off onto your clean hands. Wash your hands thoroughly several times a day, followed by an application of hand lotion. The skin is one of your immune system's first lines of defense, says Dr. Shaner. Keeping it supple reduces the cracks through which microorganisms can enter the body. (For more on skin care, see "Skin," page 434.)

**Be careful with vitamin C.** Many people are convinced that taking large doses of vitamin C will prevent colds or reduce their duration. To date, there has been no conclusive research that supports that megadoses of vitamin C do either. Dr. Winther cautions that taking too much vitamin C can cause severe diarrhea.

**Inhale steam.** Herbal steam can reduce congestion, and if the vapor temperature is 110 degrees or higher, it will kill cold germs on contact. Choose aromatic herbs with antiviral properties, such as eucalyptus or tea tree oil, to soothe your inflamed nasal passages. Place 20 drops of pure oil (available at health-food stores) in a bowl and pour in a quart of boiling water. Lean over the bowl and drape a towel over your head to create a steam tent. Breathe the vapors for 10 to 15 minutes. Repeat every four hours as necessary. Don't inhale steam if you have asthma, as it can cause lung irritation.

**Try an herbal remedy.** Taken at the first sign of symptoms, *echinacea purpurea* can reduce a cold's intensity and duration, says Dr. Shaner. Commonly known as purple coneflower, this Native American herb has been used to fight colds for centuries. It stimulates the immune system, enhancing your body's resistance to infection. Echinacea is most palatable in capsules, though it is traditionally taken in liquid form as a tincture. Both are available at health-food stores and most drugstores. Dr. Shaner suggests taking two 400-milligram capsules or 20 drops of tincture three times a day for the first three days of a cold—or until your symptoms subside.

*At the first sign of a sniffle, take two 400-milligram capsules of echinacea. It will reduce the intensity and duration of a cold.*—Catherine Shaner, M.D.

## THE FLU: FIGHTING BACK

You've probably heard people say, "I'm not sure if I have a cold or the flu. I just know I'm sick." Like a cold, influenza is a respiratory infection caused by a virus. In addition to nasal and chest congestion, flu symptoms include fever, headaches, and that feeling of being knocked off your feet.

The flu virus is propelled through the air by a cough or sneeze, and invades your body through your nose or mouth. The virus lingers on surfaces, such as a telephone or doorknob, where it can contaminate every passerby. Frequent hand washing is the strongest preventive measure you can take, along with disinfecting surfaces and avoiding people you know are sick, says **Catherine Shaner, M.D.**, medical advisor for the American Safety and Health Institute.

*A mild fever actually helps the body heal, so avoid taking aspirin when you have the flu. Instead, rest and get plenty of fluids.*—Catherine Shaner, M.D.

An annual flu shot is another powerful weapon against the flu. It is necessary to have a shot every year because strains of influenza continuously mutate, and new vaccines are created annually to combat variations of the virus. You may still get sick even after you get a shot, but you'll typically have a milder case. Always consult a doctor before getting a flu shot if you are allergic to eggs or have a history of Guillain-Barré syndrome.

## SHOULD I SEE A DOCTOR?

*A viral infection, such as a cold, the flu, or bronchitis, has a set life span. When it's over, you recover. Sometimes, however, these viruses set the stage for more serious problems.*

Lungs weakened by a cold or the flu are prime targets for a bacterial infection, which causes pneumonia, says *Birgit Winther, M.D.,* assistant professor of otolaryngology and pediatrics at the University of Virginia Medical School in Charlottesville. She recommends that you see a doctor if you experience any of the following:

• After a period of improvement from a cold or the flu, you suddenly get a high fever, shaking chills, chest pain with each breath, and a cough that produces thick yellow-green mucus.

• You vomit for more than a day or have severe abdominal pain. Prolonged vomiting can leave you dehydrated, and abdominal pain can be a sign of other problems, such as appendicitis.

• Your cough doesn't improve or worsens after one week. Sometimes, an X-ray is the only way to distinguish bronchitis from pneumonia in order to begin appropriate treatment.

• You are coughing up blood, are short of breath, have difficulty breathing, have a high fever (over 101 degrees), or have a fever that lasts more than three days.

• You're elderly and get a hacking cough or experience hoarseness or pains in the chest following a bout of bronchitis.

The vaccine is made from dead virus, so it cannot cause the flu. Within 6 to 12 hours of being inoculated, however, you may experience soreness at the vaccination site and a mild fever or aches that can last up to two days.

It takes about two weeks for the shot to start protecting you. To allow your immune system time to respond, those at high risk need to be inoculated six to eight weeks *before* flu season begins in November. According to the Centers for Disease Control and Prevention (CDC), you are at high risk if you or anyone in your household meet any of the following criteria.

- You are over 50 years old.
- You are living in a long-term care facility for the chronically ill, no matter what your age.
- You have a serious, chronic health problem, such as heart disease, lung disease (including asthma), metabolic diseases (such as diabetes), anemia or other blood disorders, or kidney diseases.
- You are less than 18 years old and are taking a long-term aspirin treatment that puts you at risk for Reye's syndrome if you get the flu.
- You are a doctor, nurse, visiting home nurse, volunteer worker, family member, or someone else who comes in contact with a person at risk of reacting seriously to the flu.
- You will be more than three months pregnant during the flu season, which runs from November to March.
- You have an immune system that is weakened because of HIV/AIDS or other autoimmune diseases, prolonged treatment with such drugs as steroids, cancer treatments that include X-rays or drugs, or bone marrow or organ transplants.

If you are not at high risk, wait until November to get your shot so those whose needs are more pressing can have priority. The CDC *encourages* flu shots for those who meet any of the following criteria.

- You provide essential community services (because you work for the police or fire department, for instance).
- You travel to the southern hemisphere between April and September or to the tropics at any time of year.
- You live in a dormitory or other crowded residence.
- You are in contact with children younger than age 2.
- You simply want to reduce your chance of getting the flu.

If you're in close contact with people who have the flu but you haven't been vaccinated, your doctor may prescribe one of three antiviral medicines:

amantadine, oseltamivir, or rimantadine. Any of these medications help prevent the flu if you take it for at least two weeks during an outbreak. If you come down with the flu, an antiviral drug can shorten the duration of the illness, but only if you take it within 48 hours of infection.

When the flu hits, symptoms come on quickly. You know the signs: dry cough, chills, body aches, stuffy nose, sore throat, headache, and a fever.

Dr. Shaner says these simple treatments are best to fight the flu.

**Use acetaminophen or ibuprofen for pain.** However, since either will also bring down your fever, it's better to do without. "Fever is our friend," says Dr. Shaner. "It fires up our immune system, allowing our body to fight off the infection naturally." Typically, a fever begins to decline on the second or third day. *Never* give aspirin to a child who has a fever, warns Dr. Shaner. It may cause a serious disease called Reye's syndrome.

**Soak in a lukewarm bath.** This is a natural remedy for easing body aches.

**Drink, drink, drink.** You need to stay hydrated when running a fever. Plus, fluids help thin nasal secretions. Fruit juices and water are your best choices.

**Avoid antihistamines.** You may want relief from nasal congestion, but these medications thicken secretions, leaving you vulnerable to a bacterial sinus infection. The flow of phlegm is nature's way of combating the infection.

**Take symptom-specific, over-the-counter medicines.** If you need something to suppress a cough, don't buy a multisymptom-formula medication. Look for a single active ingredient product for cough suppression, such as Delsym with 30 milligrams dextromethorphan.

**Stock up on antioxidants.** Chicken soup and green tea are super sources of antioxidants, the nutrients that bolster your immune system by zapping harmful compounds called free radicals. In addition, their warmth soothes your sore throat and clogged head.

**Go to bed.** Your body needs rest to fight off infection. If you try to be a brave solider, you'll just prolong the battle.

## SINUS PROBLEMS: UNSTUFFING YOURSELF

When a stuffy nose is accompanied with a terrible headache—or more accurately, a face-ache—you've developed a sinus infection, known as sinusitis. Sometimes, sinusitis follows on the heels of a cold or the flu and lasts about three weeks. But it can also continue intermittently for months or years, due to untreated or hard-to-control allergies. Chronic bronchitis is a long-term disorder that requires regular medical treatment.

Sinusitis is caused by nasal secretions that inflame the mucous membranes of the sinuses, those bony cavities in your skull surrounding your nose. The inflammation traps air and mucus, creating prime growing conditions for bacteria. Most healthy people harbor bacteria in their upper respiratory tracts without experiencing any problems—that is, until the body's defenses are weakened or sinus drainage is somehow blocked. Then bacteria that may have been living harmlessly in your nose or throat can multiply, causing sinus pressure, nasal congestion, weakness, coughing triggered by postnasal drip, and sometimes a fever.

A thick greenish gray nasal secretion is a sure sign of a bacterial infection. Doctors often prescribe an antibiotic to speed recovery. Decongestants, such as guaifenesin or pseudoephedrine, help reduce sinus pressure. Acetaminophen or ibuprofen can help relieve pain.

# *Clear your congestion with a neti pot, a gadget specially designed to flush the sinuses.*—Rebecca Wynsome, N.D.

To treat your sinusitus, try these self-care remedies recommended by *Rebecca Wynsome, N.D.*, a naturopathic doctor in Seattle.

**Steam it out.** Inhaling steam from a vaporizer or a cup of hot water can soothe inflamed sinus cavities. For best results, put a few drops of an antiviral oil, such as eucalyptus or tea tree oil, into a pan of boiling water and inhale the vapors for 10 to 15 minutes—but *only* if you don't have asthma.

**Press it out.** Soak a cloth in hot water, wring it out, then lay it across your face to help loosen sinus congestion.

**Flush it out.** Dislodge some of the gunk by using a neti pot to flush your sinuses with water. Available through www.gaiam.com and at most health-food stores, this specially designed pitcher lets you pour water into one nostril, where it then swirls through the sinuses and carries excess mucus out the other nostril. A neti pot comes with complete instructions, including tips on how to tilt your head to ensure a thorough cleaning. Its use is something of an acquired skill, so don't get discouraged if your first try isn't successful.

**Enjoy an enzyme.** Bromelain, a pineapple enzyme, can reduce the inflammation, nasal discharge, headache, and breathing difficulties associated with sinusitis. When naturopathic doctors recommend bromelain, they prescribe doses according to units of potency, either MCUs (milk-clotting units) or GDUs (gelatin-dissolving units). Most research that supports bromelain's effectiveness in treating sinusitis used doses of 500 MCUs taken four times a day. Some naturopaths recommend 3,000 MCUs taken three times per day for several days, followed by 2,000 MCUs per day.

**Harvest some horseradish.** This traditional mucus-dissolver has been used for centuries to reduce nasal stuffiness. One half to 1 teaspoon freshly grated root eaten three times a day will help clear things up.

## BRONCHITIS: LOOSENING THE CONGESTION

At some point in her life, nearly every woman will have a bout of bronchitis, an infection of the respiratory system's bronchial tubes. Acute cases are usually caused by a virus and clear up on their own within a week or two. In the meantime, you may have soreness or tightness in your chest, along with wheezing, chills, fatigue, or a slight fever. Sometimes, though, a bacterial infection is the culprit. While every bit as unpleasant as the viral variety, bacterial bronchitis clears up quickly once you take prescribed antibiotics. See a doctor if you are coughing up blood, are short of breath, have a high fever that lasts longer than three days, or have a cough that doesn't improve—or even worsens—after a week.

Acute bronchitis can produce thick yellow, white, or green phlegm. As the mucous membranes lining your air passages become irritated, your body makes secretions to coat the airways, causing that tight feeling in your chest. These secretions build up in your lungs and have to be expelled by coughing.

Dr. Wynsome recommends these steps to ease chest tightness and open up the tiny bronchi.

**Try an old-fashioned, castor-oil pack.** Soak a washcloth in castor oil so that it's saturated but not dripping. Position it on your bare chest, then cover it with plastic wrap. Place a heating pad on top of the plastic wrap. Set the pad to a comfortably warm temperature and leave it in place for 30 to 60 minutes.

**Drink up.** Take in plenty of fluids to make your mucus thinner and easier to cough up. Plug in a vaporizer so you're breathing moistened air, which helps loosen secretions.

**Go herbal.** Several herbs act as soothing expectorants. Coltsfoot may help loosen phlegm by relaxing bronchial tubes that are constricted or in spasm. Other expectorants appropriate for bronchitis include aniseed and garlic. "It's ideal to consult an herbalist or naturopath for proper doses," says Dr. Wynsome. "But if that's not possible, follow the dosage recommendations on the label, taking the herb until the bronchitis clears up." Take these herbal supplements in addition to any antibiotics your doctor prescribes, but *only* with your physician's knowledge and permission.

## ALLERGIES: TAMING OUT-OF-CONTROL REACTIONS

You're familiar with the stuffy nose, throbbing head, and itchy, watery red eyes that characterize most allergic reactions. But you may not realize that your immune system is as much to blame for your suffering as that dog dander or those dust mites.

In the case of allergies, antibodies intended for attacking viruses and bacteria react instead to such common irritants as pollen, animal dander, and dust. The immune combatants flood the affected area with histamines, those chemicals that encourage your tissues—most often in your nose and eyes—to fight back by becoming irritated and secreting fluids.

Researchers don't know why some people develop allergies, says *Arlene Schneider, M.D.*, chair of allergy and immunology at Long Island College Hospital in Brooklyn. Also a mystery is why certain children with allergies outgrow them—only to have them return in middle age.

In theory, avoiding allergy triggers seems like a good tactic. In reality, there's no way you can entirely avoid allergens because irritants are everywhere. You know you're outmatched when you realize that one ragweed plant can produce a billion grains of pollen every day.

*Air-conditioning is a blessing to allergy sufferers because it helps keep irritants out of your environment. Avoid activities that take you out-of-doors, advises Arlene Schneider, M.D.*

These are Dr. Schneider's suggestions for minimizing your allergen exposure.

**Get tested.** If you think you have allergies, get tested to find out exactly what your triggers are. There are two categories of allergy tests: those done on the body and those done in a lab. Skin tests, patch tests, and inhalation tests expose you to an allergen and gauge your body's reaction. Although state-of-the art for nearly a century, these tests are now being replaced by blood sampling profiles that measure the amount of histamine or allergen-specific antibodies in your blood.

**Demolish dust.** If dust mites are the bane of your existence, wash your bedding in hot water at least once a week to kill the microscopic critters. Use a damp cloth when cleaning so that you're actually picking up debris and not just shuffling it around.

**Check pollen.** Watch out for high-pollen days if you suffer from seasonal allergies. Avoid outings on sunny, windy days, when pollen counts are high.

**Filter air.** Fresh air brings myriad irritants with it. Use air-conditioning at home and in the car to cool, clean, and dry the air you breathe. Keep your windows closed, especially at night when symptoms are often worse.

*If allergies are a problem, keep your windows closed and stay indoors in the early morning when pollen levels are especially high.*

**Ditch early exercise.** An air-conditioned gym is the best place for allergy sufferers to work out. If you must exercise outdoors, don't do it between 5 and 10 a.m., when airborne pollen levels are at their highest.

**Give up gardening.** If you have seasonal allergies, yard work isn't for you. Mowing the lawn releases a cloud of grass pollen that takes at least 30 minutes to settle. Raking leaves stirs up irritating molds, as does digging in soil.

**Keep irritants out.** Don't bring pollen indoors. If you're outside for an hour or more during high-pollen season, wash your hands and change your clothes when you come inside. Rinse your eyes with cool tap water or artificial tears (available at drugstores) to remove irritants.

**Be sensible.** If you know you're allergic to cat dander, don't get a kitty. If wool makes you sneeze, learn to like cotton sweaters. Sometimes, women won't give up allergy-triggering things they love, thinking they can will their immune systems into submission. It's not going to happen.

# To ease congestion that's unmoved by antihistamines, your doctor may prescribe a decongestant or nasal spray.—*Arlene Schneider, M.D.*

**Choose the right medications.** If you have short-term seasonal allergies, over-the-counter antihistamines may be all you need for relief. Choose a non-drowsy formula so you're not trading the grogginess of allergy congestion for that of an antihistamine. For year-round allergies, most doctors prescribe such nonsedating antihistamines as Allegra (fexofenadine) or Claritin (loratadine), which provide 12- to 24-hour relief with few side effects.

Antihistamines do nothing to ease nasal congestion. That's why physicians frequently prescribe a companion decongestant, which reduces stuffiness by constricting the blood vessels in the nose. Since decongestants act throughout the body, not just in your nose, Dr. Schneider does not advise them for patients with heart disease, thyroid problems, or high blood pressure. If you suffer from any of these conditions, it is preferable to treat the congestion that accompanies allergies with a prescription corticosteroid nasal spray, like Flonase (fluticasone). Such a spray can reduce inflammation at the site, slowing the production of nasal secretions. It may be several days before you notice the spray's effects. Studies have found that corticosteroid nasal sprays are at least as effective as nonsedating antihistamines, so they are often recommended for people with allergic rhinitis, commonly known as hay fever. Don't refuse a prescription spray because you're afraid of steroids. Corticosteroids are not the same as athletic performance-enhancing anabolic steroids and have none of their dangerous side effects.

**Talk to your doctor about shots.** Depending on the complexity and severity of your allergies, your doctor may prescribe desensitization shots, which teach your body to change its response to specific allergens. Unfortunately, allergy shots are not a quick fix. Unlike vaccines, where one shot protects you, allergy injections take months—sometimes years—to be fully effective. Yet some people notice an improvement as early as two to four weeks after starting the shots. Until the shots kick in, though, you may need to take a daily antihistamine and decongestant to feel better, as well as use eyedrops or a nasal spray. For many people who struggle to control allergies or who experience significant side effects from medications, allergy shots can be extremely helpful and are worth the wait and trouble.

## HEPATITIS C: CONTROLLING THE HIDDEN SCOURGE

Is it possible to have a chronic, life-threatening illness and not know it? The answer is yes, especially if the disease in question is hepatitis C, says

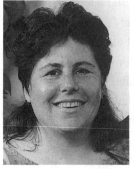

*Hepatitis C infects more than twice as many people as HIV, says Misha Ruth Cohen, O.M.D.*

*Misha Ruth Cohen, O.M.D.,* clinical director of Chicken Soup Chinese Medicine in San Francisco and author of *The Hepatitis C Help Book.*

*Hepatitis* is a generic term, referring to any liver inflammation. Most often caused by a viral infection, hepatitis can also result from certain medications or alcohol. Acute hepatitis A is spread through contaminated food and water. Hepatitis B and C are both caused by bloodborne viruses that can live in your body for years—even decades—without any outward symptoms. Vaccines are available for hepatitis A and B, but not for hepatitis C.

Dr. Cohen estimates that 4 million Americans have hepatitis C—and at least a third of them don't know it. Coupled with the absence of a vaccine, that makes hepatitis C "the pre-eminent public health threat of the early 21st century," says Dr. Cohen. Two to four times more people are infected with the hepatitis C virus than with HIV.

> *Over a million people don't know they are infected with hepatitis C. Because there is no vaccine, this potentially deadly virus could be the number-one health threat of our time.*
>
> —*Misha Ruth Cohen, O.M.D.*

Many people contracted hepatitis C through blood transfusions received before the discovery of this form of hepatitis in 1989. Hepatitis-C sufferers frequently have no symptoms, or their symptoms mimic other ailments, such as the flu or chronic fatigue syndrome. Therefore, the virus can persist unnoticed for years, causing irrevocable liver damage.

More than 70 percent of those infected with hepatitis C develop chronic liver disease, says Dr. Cohen. Approximately 15 percent develop cancer or cirrhosis (scarring of the liver that eventually erodes liver function) and eventually die from one of these diseases.

The good news is that today's sophisticated blood screens reduce the chance of contracting the virus through transfusion to about one in a million units of blood. New cases of infection come chiefly from blood-contaminated needles and sexual contact (the same is true of hepatitis B). Some people with hepatitis C can eliminate the virus without life-threatening consequences. Dr. Cohen has observed that women have a slightly better chance of ridding themselves of the virus, perhaps because they're more apt to seek treatment.

*Today's blood transfusions are safe, thanks to careful screening. Top causes of hepatitis infection are body piercing, tattooing, unprotected sex, and intravenous drug use.*

### PREVENTING EXPOSURE

Here's what you can do to reduce your risk of contracting hepatitis or to avoid passing the virus on to others.

**Shun intravenous drugs.** Don't share needles or other drug paraphernalia that may be contaminated with someone else's blood. It only takes one exposure to contract hepatitis B or C, says Dr. Cohen.

**Eschew the tattoo.** Both hepatitis B and C viruses can be passed along in the process of tattooing and body piercing, or by sharing a razor or toothbrush.

**Make sex safe.** Hepatitis B and C are transmitted by sexual contact, as well as by blood. *Never* have unprotected intercourse with an infected person or with anyone with whom you don't have a long history of honesty and trust.

## IF YOU'RE EXPOSED

Many people first discover they have hepatitis C after giving blood. All donated blood is screened, so the collecting agency will notify you if your blood tests positive for hepatitis.

If you suspect you have been exposed, get a blood test that checks for hepatitis antibodies. If the test comes back positive, Dr. Cohen recommends asking your doctor to do a liver biopsy to determine how much damage the virus has caused. No form of hepatitis is a universal death sentence, but you have to know *specifically* what the virus has done to your body in order to be treated effectively.

> *If you're diagnosed with hepatitis C, ask your doctor to do a liver biopsy to determine how much damage the virus has caused.*—Misha Ruth Cohen, M.D.

Therapy for chronic hepatitis is continuously evolving and may include interferon, a protein that keeps viruses from reproducing. You may also take antiviral and immune-strengthening medications. In later stages of the disease, a patient may need a liver transplant.

Dr. Cohen finds Western treatments for chronic hepatitis disappointing. The success rate among patients treated with interferon and antiviral drugs is only about 30 percent, she points out. In addition, many people experience devastating side effects that reduce their quality of life, damage other organs, or force them to discontinue therapy. Dr. Cohen advocates some of the principles of Chinese medicine, which views liver inflammation in terms of its symptoms and the corresponding impact on the whole body.

If you're infected with hepatitis C, Dr. Cohen recommends these self-care tips.

**Eat right.** Many hepatitis patients suffer from digestive disorders that can be eased by nutritional therapy. A low-fat, nutrient-rich diet that emphasizes vegetables and brown rice can strengthen the liver. Alcohol and recreational drugs accelerate liver damage and, therefore, must be avoided completely.

**Take selenium.** This mineral is essential for healthy immune function. Supplements have been shown to reduce the incidence of viral hepatitis in populations that are deficient in the mineral, presumably by stimulating the activity of white blood cells. Dr. Cohen recommends a daily supplement of 200 micrograms. Choose a supplement drawn from yeast, which the body absorbs better than selenite. Brazil nuts are a good source of selenium, as are yeast, whole grains, and seafood.

**Explore herbal remedies.** Dr. Cohen formulates treatments for hepatitis C using ginseng, ginkgo leaf, dandelion, salvia, and skullcap, among other natural ingredients. Only a qualified health practitioner should prescribe herbal remedies for this condition. "Taking recommendations from untrained personnel at health-food stores or from untrained practitioners is foolish at best and dangerous at worst," she warns.

## SHINGLES: CHICKENPOX REDUX

If you had chickenpox as a child, you'll remember the painful red rash, oozing blisters, and overwhelming urge to scratch. Well, with shingles, get ready for a nasty childhood flashback.

Herpes zoster, known as shingles, develops from the same virus that made you miserable with chickenpox. For years, the virus has been living quietly in the roots of nerves throughout your body. Stress, age, or some other ding to your immune system can bring it roaring back to life, shooting along the path of a nerve and causing excruciating pain.

An outbreak of shingles is signaled by pain, burning, tingling, or itching in one locale. These symptoms last one to three days and are followed by a red rash with blisters in the same area, enduring for two to three weeks before scabbing over. Generally, a blistering rash crops up on the affected side of your body, sometimes on your face or the back of your head.

At the first hint of shingles, see your doctor immediately for a diagnosis. Medications are effective only when started within 48 hours of the onset of symptoms. Your doctor may want to control the outbreak by prescribing an antiviral drug, such as acyclovir, famciclovir, or valacyclovir, which squelches the virus by halting replication of its DNA.

Shingles are contagious if someone who's never had chickenpox touches a weeping eruption, cautions *Catherine Shaner, M.D.*, medical advisor for the American Safety and Health Institute. Dr. Shaner suggests dressing any affected area with light gauze. Covering blisters also reduces chances of secondary infection, since any open sore invites bacteria.

*Shingles are caused by the same contagious virus that gave you chickenpox. Medication is effective only if you take it within 48 hours of the first symptoms.*—Catherine Shaner, M.D.

Once your doctor has diagnosed shingles, these treatments may ease the pain.

**Soothe with an antiviral ointment.** You can speed the healing of lesions by applying lemon balm or tea tree–oil ointments (available at health-food stores) or cold-sore ointment (found at drugstores), says Dr. Shaner. Check with your doctor before using any of these products. The U.S. Food and Drug Administration recently approved a topical antiviral gel, ViraDerm, for the treatment of herpes simplex viruses. It has been shown to kill the living virus, relieve pain, and reduce the time it takes an outbreak to heal. ViraDerm is available without a prescription at www.herpescured.com.

**Take ibuprofen.** This medication reduces inflammation and pain.

**Ice it.** A cloth-wrapped ice pack numbs the area and reduces itching. If pain from shingles continues even after blisters have healed, an ice pack can stun pain impulses.

Shingles may be less of a problem in years to come, says Dr. Shaner. With the advent of a chickenpox vaccine, there are fewer cases of the initiating virus, so it follows that there will be fewer cases of shingles. Unfortunately, this comes too late for most of us.

## LUPUS: LIVING WITH THE SYMPTOMS

Lupus is a chronic autoimmune disorder that affects about 1.5 million Americans, 90 percent of whom are females between ages 15 and 45. Lupus causes the body to attack its own tissues as if they were foreign substances, says *Catherine Shaner, M.D.,* medical advisor for the American Safety and Health Institute. Lupus can affect any organ or system in the body. Mild symptoms include achy muscles and joints, headache, and a characteristic butterfly rash on the face. Moderate symptoms include memory loss, hair loss, and photosensitivity. In the most serious cases, the effects of lupus can be devastating, causing anemia, triggering seizures, or impairing your heart, kidneys, and lungs. The disease is characterized by flare-ups interspersed with periods of improvement or remission.

No one knows the exact cause of lupus. Some researchers hypothesize that it is influenced by hormones because symptoms tend to be worse during pregnancy and menstrual cycles. Since lupus is a chronic disease with no known cure, those who have it need to learn what triggers attacks in order to best deal with them. "Wake up and listen to your body," says Dr. Shaner.

She has this advice for those living with lupus.

**Modify your lifestyle.** Preventive measures can reduce the risk of flare-ups. Accept your limitations. If you do something strenuous today, you won't be able to go grocery shopping tomorrow, so plan accordingly. If you are photosensitive, avoid sun exposure and always wear a sunscreen to prevent rashes.

**Tweak your thinking.** Physical and emotional stress often trigger outbreaks, so learn to let go of perfection. You don't have to be Superwoman. Let somebody else clean the toilet, bake the brownies for your child's class, or pick up the dry cleaning, if necessary.

**Take your medications.** Stick to the regimen prescribed by your doctor—even when you feel fine. While treatment is tailored to a person's specific needs and symptoms, commonly prescribed medications include nonsteroidal anti-inflammatory drugs (NSAIDs, like ibuprofen and naproxen), corticosteroids and other immune-suppressants (such as azathioprine, cyclophosphamide, and methotrexate), and medicines developed to treat malaria that also seem to reduce the skin and joint symptoms of lupus. To prevent specific complications associated with lupus, such as blood clotting too rapidly, some women need to take anticoagulants.

**Relish rest.** We are a culture of overscheduled overachievers. It's hard to admit we can't do everything and even harder to lie down when we need to. Ditch that outlook and learn to love quiet time and naps.

**Build stamina.** It's tough to get on a treadmill when you barely have the energy to get out of bed, but you need exercise to develop endurance. "You have to start slow and build up gradually," says Dr. Shaner. "Your body is worn out. You may only be able to exercise for a minute, but if you complete that minute, it will make your body stronger—and tomorrow you'll be able to do two minutes."

# 12 Life Crises

chapter

## Getting the Better of Turns for the Worse

*You will learn more from 10 days of agony than from 10 years of contentment. Pain can be your greatest teacher.*
—Debbie Ford, workshop leader, coach, and faculty member
The Chopra Center for Well Being; La Jolla, California

Deadlines. Divorce. Debt. Dependency. Domination.

The words themselves are fraught with distress. If you're suffering through any of these difficult situations, you're painfully familiar with the stress and grief that leave you feeling lost and unsure, with emotions spinning out of control. By turning to this chapter, you've taken that important first step by showing that you're willing to work to improve your life. You *want* help.

We tapped the keenest minds in the country for useful advice to prevent and deal with some of the most devastating crises a woman can face. Discover how to emerge from hardships stronger and wiser. Try to remember the observation of *Anne Wilson Schaef, Ph.D.,* author of *Meditations for Women Who Do Too Much:* "Obstacles are not personal attacks; they're muscle-builders."

## BURNOUT: BREAKING THE LIFE-DRAINING CYCLE

Many women work long and hard to get ahead, putting their careers before most everything else. They are driven, focused, competitive, tough. As feminist Gloria Steinem once said, "Some of us are becoming the men we wanted to marry." But professional success may come at too high a price if it robs a woman of peace of mind and a happy, centered life.

Even a workaholic can't be a nonstop producer. Often, it's a woman's unreasonable expectations of herself that bring her to the brink of collapse. *Anne Wilson Schaef, Ph.D.*, sees some patients who push themselves until they become so exhausted that they can't hold a pen or even get out of bed. The unwelcome result of such pressure? "A morass of procrastination," says Dr. Schaef. "The more they think about what needs to be done, the more leaden they feel." This lethargy can lead to black periods of self-recrimination and depression, she says. Other women respond to stress quite differently—though no more healthfully—by growing constantly edgy, irritated, and angry, or stifling their emotions to the point of becoming introverted and quiet. All these destructive reactions are signs of burnout.

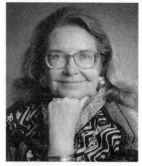

*Avoid burnout with this advice from Anne Wilson Schaef, Ph. D.: Take an occasional break from the daily grind. Give yourself a special treat—a shopping spree or massage, for example.*

In any form, pent-up pressure is toxic, overtaxing your heart and weakening your immune system. To make matters worse, many women turn to food, cigarettes, or alcohol in an effort to vent their frustrations or cope with perceived failures.

Knowing when you're on the verge of fizzling out is usually easy. Figuring out which stressors can be controlled or obliterated—and how to go about it—can be more difficult.

> *Trying to control everyone and everything in your life is futile and exhausting. Facing up to who and what you can't control is key to avoiding burnout.*—Anne Wilson Schaef, Ph.D.

If you are emotionally and physically spent, gain currency with these helpful tips from Dr. Schaef.

**Recognize the red flags.** Listen to your body because it will tell you when you need to take notice. For some women, the warning may be sobbing for no reason. For others, the wake-up call may be difficulty sleeping or waking. Heed nature's warnings and take action to eliminate the source of your stress.

**Focus on the inner you.** If all your waking hours are consumed with the welfare of others, it's likely you're unaware of your own needs. It's nearly impossible to pay proper attention to both at the same time. That's why it's so important to set aside at least a few minutes each day to center on yourself. Find a comfortable position, then breathe slowly and deeply. Turn your

## REDISCOVER THE HAPPIER YOU
*Even in the most troubled woman, there's a joyful person trying to get out.*

Under the burden of stress, you're actually a lighthearted person, says *Alexandra Stoddard,* author of *Choosing Happiness: Keys to a Joyful Life.* You just need to liberate your innocent, childlike self.

Here's what Stoddard recommends for developing a sunnier outlook:

**Describe yourself.** Choose about 10 words that sum up the real you. Some examples are *love, sunlight, food, home, gardens,* and *family.* Stoddard has given this exercise to countless people and, invariably, every word is positive.

**Become one with the words.** These words define what truly matters to you, who you want to be. Expand your list by elaborating on one or more of those words and then add 25 words to your inventory. Incorporate them all into an essay that celebrates what brings you cheer.

**Post it.** Put your word list in plain view—on the fridge, bathroom mirror, or dashboard—and check it every day. If you noted that you love to walk on the beach or hug your grandchildren, ask yourself, "When was the last time I did that?" Haven't gone to the museum in years, even though wandering its rooms is a favorite pastime? Well, maybe this is the perfect day to nurture your soul with art. "People worry about everything else but what makes them happy," says Stoddard. Make it a priority to live the life you desire.

**Be a slacker.** No one should be a total good-for-nothing, but you can strive to do less so that you can better enjoy each moment. "You create your own stress by trying to do too much in too little time," says Stoddard. So don't feel guilty about sleeping in on a Sunday morning or playing hooky one afternoon to go to the movies.

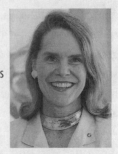

*Make a choice to live the life you desire, advises Alexandra Stoddard. Identify your passion and then pursue it.*

**Color your world.** Studies have found that hue affects mood. Red is invigorating, blue and green are calming, and cheerful yellow is great for mental clarity. A neutral, restrained decor could be contributing to your emotional rut. Put bright red towels in the bathroom, splash seafoam green on the walls of your kitchen, cover your bed with pretty sheets and a soft pink quilt. Trust your instincts as to which hues give you pleasure.

**Follow your fancy.** Write down three things you're in the mood for today and then have fun making your way through the list. Indulge your craving for deviled eggs or throw a tea party. Replace a quick shower with the treat of a bubble bath, complete with candles.

mind's eye and ear to your inner thoughts and feelings. Try to concentrate on the positive, banishing any negative thoughts that pop up. The more you practice this selective thought process, the easier it gets.

**Be good to yourself.** Applaud yourself for all that you've accomplished. Treat yourself now and then to a quiet stroll in the park, relaxing massage, colorful pedicure, or shopping spree. Whatever your chosen form of escape, give yourself an occasional time-out from the rat race. When you constantly worry about the next hurdle to leap, you lose perspective and gain stress.

**Walk away.** When you push to meet a deadline, sometimes you do a shoddy job because you're overwhelmed and distracted by the urgency of the task. Rather than charge through, the best thing you can do is to take a short break. The few minutes you spend away from the task will allow you to come back refreshed and more focused—and the work will show it.

**Learn to let go.** Trying to orchestrate the world around you is a major cause of burnout. "The illusion of control is exhausting," says Dr. Schaef. The only real change you can affect is with yourself. First, list the people and situations you don't have power over. Follow up with the reasons you can't change them. Ask yourself, "How would these people respond if I stopped trying to control them?" Then ask yourself, "How would that make me feel?" This exercise helps you recognize when your thoughts are irrational and see the benefits of letting go of control.

## DIVORCE: MAKING A NEW START

The dissolution of a marriage is almost always a devastating event. The guilt, uprooting, splitting of possessions, and loss of a partner can reduce even the most stoic woman to tears and self-doubt. Add to the mix the changing relationship with children and realignment of parental duties, and the toll is more significant still.

Even the most difficult breakup doesn't have to leave you emotionally scarred for life, assures *Lillian Glass, Ph.D.,* a psychologist and communications specialist with a bicoastal practice in Beverly Hills and New York City, and author of *Toxic People.* "In fact, some women see divorce as freedom," she

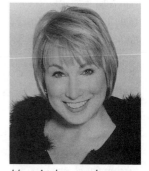

*It's a mistake to put down your spouse in front of the children, warns Lillian Glass, Ph. D. Make sure the kids know that both of their parents still love them.*

says. Divorce is never an easy path to tread, but it can be a stepping-stone to a stronger you.

Here's how you can turn a marital loss into a kind of personal victory.

**Expect mood swings.** Understand that you're not supposed to be okay at the outset. Allow yourself to mourn your divorce as you would a death, says Dr. Glass. Don't deny the agony. Instead, use this time to heal and fully release the sadness.

**Share the blame.** It usually takes two to dissolve a union. Recognize that perhaps you did things that contributed to the unraveling of your marriage. This realization will help you work through your anger at your former

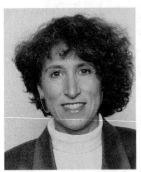

*Try not to react on the spot when your ex does something that makes your blood boil, advises Lois Gold, M.S.W. You don't really want to say or do anything that will heighten the hostilities unnecessarily.*

partner. But don't take *all* the responsibility, says **Lois Gold, M.S.W.,** marital therapist and author of *Between Love and Hate: A Guide to Civilized Divorce.* Assuming a burden of that magnitude can paralyze you with guilt. "Blame keeps us tied to the past," says Gold. "When we lessen blame toward others or ourselves, we can refocus our attention on how to improve situations—and life gets dramatically better." Start by noticing how you assign blame. Do you fault your children or ex for your anger? Do you point the finger at yourself for letting things get out of your control? Identify the beliefs that prevent happiness and teach yourself to change them. Then work to keep your new outlook on track.

**Get support.** Make friends with single or divorced women, suggests Dr. Glass. Join an organization that brings together divorced, separated, or widowed individuals. You might take a look at Beginning Experience (www.beginningexperience.org, 866-610-8877). Or go on a divorce retreat for women; check out Spa for the Soul at www.ariadnesthread.com. If you have children, network through the nonprofit support group Parents Without Partners (www.parentswithoutpartners.org) or take part in an online social club for divorced parents, such as www.soloparentsnetwork.com.

**Reassure your kids.** Don't bad-mouth your former spouse to your children, urges Dr. Glass. Talk openly and let them know that Mom and Dad have no wish to divorce *them.*

**Try something different.** A divorce can make you feel terrible about yourself, but only if you *allow* this to happen. You can either crawl in a deep hole or choose to reach new heights, to become an extraordinary person. Make a list of your daily routines and behaviors. Then jot down ideas of what would bring interest and fulfillment to your life: challenges, risks, possibilities. Make a point to try at least two of these broadening opportunities every week for the next month. You might do yoga for the first time, get a makeover, or splurge on a new wardrobe. Take an acting or photography class, purely for the fun of it. Just think of all the people you'll meet. More importantly, you'll keep busy and start breaking out of your shell.

*Whether it's directed at your ex or yourself, blame keeps you focused on the past. When you let go of recriminations, you can move on.*

*—Lois Gold, M.S.W.*

**Take another vow.** Solemnly promise yourself that your actions will be consistent with the kind of person you desire to be. For example, if you want to become a better parent, pledge to spend at least an hour a day of quality time with your kids. Plan a monthly excursion to somewhere special, like a planetarium or national park. Share your resolution with two people you're sure will help you stay true to your vision.

**Keep a cool head.** Don't make important decisions when you're angry, hurt, or reacting to something your ex has done or said. If he is late dropping off the kids after their weekend visit or announces that he's moving in with his new girlfriend, give yourself some time and distance before reacting or responding. Snap judgments may only escalate any existing hostilities, says Gold.

**Remain a parenting team.** A 2002 study showed that children of parents who have arranged to share custody experienced less anxiety and depression, as well as fewer behavioral problems, than those who live with one parent and have little or no contact with the other. Researchers found that joint-custody kids are almost as well-adjusted as children from two-parent homes. Of course, there are exceptions: Spouses who are abusive or mentally ill are obviously not good influences.

# FINANCIAL GRIEF: CRAWLING OUT OF DEBT

"First, we form habits; then they form us. Conquer your bad habits or they'll eventually conquer you," says sports psychologist Rob Gilbert, Ph.D.

This axiom certainly holds true when it comes to spending. Being loose with your money may end up defining—and ruining—your life. Eventually, credit-card bills get so high you're barely able to pay the interest. Bill collectors

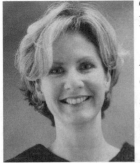

call daily. Guilt consumes you every time you shop. Fights with your partner break out over every penny.

"Money is the leading cause of divorce," says *Karen Casanova,* author of *Letting Go of Debt.* Her own marriage fell apart after her husband racked up almost $200,000 in gambling debt. Casanova eventually worked her way back to financial stability, becoming an expert on digging out from under.

*Cut up your credit cards, advises Karen Casanova. She learned the hard way that paying those interest charges will only put you deeper in debt.*

Here's what she did—and advises you to do, too.

**Own up to it.** You can't solve a fiscal problem until you acknowledge that it exists and then accept the responsibility for it. Don't fault others or credit-card companies. "Blaming others is a waste of energy," says Casanova. "Instead, seek serenity and positive, workable solutions."

**Ask for guidance.** Find someone—a friend, family member, therapist, or financial planner—to help you devise a spending plan. If you're truly in desperate financial straits, steer toward a nonprofit debt-management agency, such as www.metrodebtconsolidation.com, www.myvesta.org, or A Family Budget Counseling (800-887-3328). These services provide free one-on-one consultations. They're able to negotiate lower rates on high-interest credit cards and determine an affordable amount to pay each month to cover all your creditors. In many instances, such an arrangement can go a long way toward improving your credit rating. To get help from a nonprofit group, you will have to fill out an application to prove that you are a hardship case. Be wary of any debt-manager that requires a big enrollment fee up front; they are probably *not* a not-for-profit company.

**Write bigger checks.** If you owe $2,500 on a credit card that charges 20-percent interest and you only pay $25 each month, it will take you more than 25 years to pay off the balance. Blame it on the interest charges you'll accumulate each month. Always try to pay as much as you possibly can each month to pare the debt down, recommends *Christina Koenig*, president of A Family Budget Counseling in Bellrose, New York. You may have to forgo nonessential purchases as a result, but it's the wisest course.

**Transfer your balance.** Most of us receive offers in the mail for credit cards all the time. Don't be so quick to throw the next one away. If you find a card that offers 0- to 3-percent interest for nine months, jump at the chance to shift your total balance from a card with a higher finance rate, advises Koenig. Then divide your balance by nine to find the amount you need to pay each month in order to be out of debt by the time the introductory offer expires. Once that deal is dead and gone, the formerly attractive low rate can jump to as high as 22 percent. So if you're not paid up, look for another low-interest card.

**Think green.** Stop racking up more debt and cue in to using cash. If you can't pay in full for a purchase, then perhaps you shouldn't buy it. Even if this approach requires you to draw from your savings, you'll still come out ahead because most savings accounts earn less than 3-percent interest anyway. Koenig points out that if your creditors charge an interest rate higher than that, you're losing money by keeping yours in the bank.

> *Cut up your credit cards and do everything you can to pay off your balance. Buy only what you can purchase with cash.*—Christina Koenig

**Curb spending.** Do you really need to stop for gourmet coffee every morning? Look for ways to subtract expenses that can really add up: Bring your lunch to work. Buy generic products. Discontinue premium cable channels. Use vinegar instead of expensive cleaning solutions.

**Cut up credit cards.** Leave one piece of plastic for major purchases and emergencies. Go a step further and put that card in a cup of water, then freeze it. If the urge to splurge hits, the thawing time will give you a chance to think twice.

**Be a skeptic.** Ignore those scams that offer to erase any negative—yet accurate—credit history from your record. The Federal Trade Commission says that there's no legal way this can be done. Also be wary of advance-fee loans that promise to provide money for free, regardless of your past credit history. These proposals are probably not legitimate or charge such high interest rates that they're not worth the bother.

## AGING PARENTS: THE BURDEN OF CAREGIVING

About 22 million American households care for an elderly relative. Add in the demands of caring for dependent children, a marriage, and career, and thus is born what experts refer to as the Sandwich Generation, made up of those caught in the middle of competing responsibilities.

The stark reality is that life spans have lengthened considerably. By 2030, nearly 70 million people in the United States will be over age 65—that's double the statistics for 1995. Today, one in four families has a member who tends an elderly or chronically ill parent. Not surprisingly, almost 75 percent of these caregivers are female. If you're a baby boomer (born between 1946 and 1965), you may spend more years ministering to your parents than you did rearing your children.

Such a commitment takes its toll. When caring for a relative becomes a top priority, then stress, anger, and resentment can result. You may feel guilty, suffer physical reactions, or find your lifestyle becoming restrictive. Nip such unproductive tendencies in the bud. Pay attention to yourself, or you won't be much good to anyone else.

Consider this advice for making elder care easier on everyone, as well as more effective for the one in need.

**Reach out.** You can get free information, referrals, and support from such nonprofit groups that specialize in elder-care issues as the following.

- Area Agency on Aging: Visit www.n4a.org or check the phone book for the number of your local agency.
- Children of Aging Parents: www.caps4caregivers.org, 800-227-7294
- National Family Caregivers Association: www.nfcacares.org, 800-896-3650
- Aging Parents and Adult Children Together, a branch of the Federal Trade Commission: www.ftc.gov/bcp/conline/pubs/services/apact/, 877-382-4357
- Caregivers-usa.org offers a nationwide database of services, from financial aid to transportation and disability services.

**Initiate talks.** If your parents are still of sound mind, there's no time like the present to openly discuss how to prepare for any possible decline, says *Alexandra Kennedy, M.A.*, a psychotherapist in Santa Cruz, California, and author of *The Infinite Thread: Healing Relationships Beyond Loss.* This provides an opportunity for family members to air fears and preferences. Involve your siblings, even the long-distance ones. Decide ahead of time who will be the principal caregiver and which responsibilities others will have.

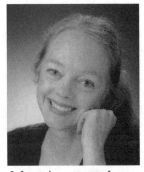

*Safeguard your parents from falls and broken hips. Rid their home of potential tripping hazards, such as dangling cords, and fix loose handrails, suggests Alexandra Kennedy, M.A.*

**Get the picture.** Know the facts about your parents' income: Is there a private pension? How much Social Security do they receive? Do they have direct deposit? Have they arranged for survivor's benefits?

## ONE WOMAN'S STORY: ELDER CARE

*Alexandra Kennedy found a way to provide good care for her parents—without neglecting herself.*

Psychotherapist Alexandra Kennedy's 89-year-old stepfather became seriously ill in January 2002 and required surgery. He was suddenly no longer able to look after himself or Kennedy's mother, also age 89, who had begun to show signs of Alzheimer's disease.

Even though Kennedy lived two hours away, she had to step in when her parents' bills began to pile up and other household needs were neglected. "It didn't take long for the round-trip emergency journeys to become exhausting," she recalls. With her mother fighting to remain at home and not move into a nursing facility, finding a solution that everyone could live with wasn't easy.

In time, Kennedy was able to convince her mother to try a local caregiving agency, which offered 24-hour assistance with cleaning, cooking,

and driving. Resistant at first to any loss of privacy, her mother didn't click with the first few aides, who were all female. Kennedy kept trying to achieve a successful fit. She soon figured out that her mother's personality was best suited to male attendants who challenged her and worked crossword puzzles with her.

With a caring person in her mother's house around the clock, Kennedy no longer has to take on so much or worry constantly. Instead, she puts her energies into simply relishing her mother's company. "I'm trying to put a positive spin on her health situation," says Kennedy. "With my mother no longer remembering things from days—or even minutes—ago, we can just be in the moment together. There's no focus on regrets or a spat we had hours ago. We simply enjoy the time and love each other."

Make a list of their assets, including their locations and value. Grasp the full extent of your parents' debts, itemizing such expenses as mortgage and car payments. Consider hiring a daily money-management service to help with writing checks, balancing accounts, and establishing a budget, as well as organizing and keeping financial records. Costs vary, but $25 to $100 a month buys not only their expertise, but also your peace of mind, especially if your parents have numerous credit cards, lose track of income or checkbooks, or make unusually large charitable donations. Contact the American Association of Daily Money Managers (www.aadmm.com, 301-593-5462) for more information.

*Talk with your parents and make a plan for their long-term care* before *it becomes a necessity. Be familiar with their finances and the resources in your area.*—Alexandra Kennedy, M.A.

**Help prevent accidents.** To avoid falls, make sure your parents' home is easy to maneuver, thus protecting them and giving you one less thing to worry about. Put kitchen items where they can be reached without having to stand on a chair or stool. Remove such tripping hazards as dangling cords and throw rugs. See that handrails are securely fastened on both sides of stairways. Place a fire extinguisher near the stove. You can request a safety checklist from Aging Parents and Adult Children Together at 877-382-4357.

**Explore housing options.** There are numerous alternative-living arrangements from which to choose. Some offer recreational and social programs but may not provide services that will become necessary if a parent's health declines. Many provide transportation to stores and medical appointments. Think about your parents' requirements now, as well as potential future needs. Before deciding on a location, visit the premises and talk to the staff, residents, and residents' family members, recommends Kennedy. Consider having a lawyer review any contracts before you sign. For more information on housing choices, contact the American Association of Homes and Services for the Aging (www.aahsa.org, 800-675-9253).

**Lay the past to rest.** Discuss any unresolved issues with a parent before it's too late. If a subject is potentially emotionally charged, diffuse the situation by first consulting a therapist or writing out your thoughts, says Kennedy. Then decide what you really want to convey, making sure the points serve the best interests of your relationship.

## ABUSE: GETTING OUT BEFORE IT'S TOO LATE

Mistreatment by a supposed loved one is an overwhelmingly female problem—90 to 95 percent of victims are women. Count it out: Every nine seconds, a woman is beaten in the United States. Every year, about 4 million women are physically abused by their partners, including those involved in lesbian relationships.

It may not be easy to know if you're in an abusive relationship. "It's not always as black-and-white as a black eye," says *Elaine Weiss, Ed.D.*, clinical professor in the department of family and preventive medicine at the University of Utah School of Medicine. Abuse can be psychological, as well as physical. "Abuse is not about anger; it's about power and control," says Dr. Weiss, who chronicled her own experiences in her book, *Surviving Domestic Violence: Voices of Women Who Broke Free.*

*Abuse doesn't always involve physical violence. You should take a close look at the health of your relationship if your partner is very controlling or is constantly criticizing you, advises Elaine Weiss, Ed.D.*

Too often, women convince themselves that their partners will mellow in time. That's just not going to happen, warns Dr. Weiss. In fact, such situations tend to escalate in severity. "To change, abusers have to take responsibility. But they don't—they blame their partners," says Dr. Weiss. " 'She spent too much money.' Or 'she wouldn't have sex with me.' They'll say anything they can use."

Dr. Weiss offers this counsel on how you can recognize an abusive relationship—and get out.

**See the signs.** A free-and-equal partnership defines a healthy relationship. If your significant other completely dominates you, then he has achieved total control. Be on guard if you find yourself being isolated from family and friends, kept in the dark about household finances, left out of all decisions, forced to dress a certain way or have sex when you don't want to, or constantly criticized.

**Dispel myths.** Abuse is not about a disagreement getting out of control, but rather a constant state of warfare. Remember that *anyone* can end up in a violent relationship. Having a good education, impressive income, or solid upbringing doesn't grant you immunity. The only thing female victims of abuse have in common is the standard two X chromosomes, says *Alexandra Kennedy, M.A.,* a psychotherapist in Santa Cruz, California, and author of *The Infinite Thread: Healing Relationships Beyond Loss.*

**Know when to escape.** Abused women think about walking out every day, but many obstacles keep them from actually going through with it: money, housing, and fear for their kids, to name a few. A woman doesn't leave an abusive relationship but escapes it. Most women can't make that break for freedom until they finally accept that their partners will never change.

*The first step to ending an abusive relationship is accepting that it will never get better. Get help and make a plan for you and your children to get away.*—Elaine Weiss, Ed.D.

**Do it for your kids.** Witnessing or experiencing violence can permanently alter a child's brain chemistry. Studies show that girls are especially vulnerable to the effects of abuse. The ramifications are long-lasting: These children often grow up to experience depression or anxiety disorders. And since violence begets violence, such kids are more aggressive while they're young and continue to be so when they're older.

**Get help.** If you decide to get out of an abusive situation, plan carefully and seek the assistance of a trained professional. Remember that a woman is in more danger during the six months *after* she leaves than at any time during the relationship. Her departure tells her abuser, "You no longer control me"—and that message can provoke a desperate response. Call your local shelter for abused women. You don't have to stay there to take advantage of their support. Or contact the National Domestic Violence Hotline (www.ndvh.org, 800-799-7233).

# 13 Menopause
## The Power of
## Personal Change

*Let's set the record straight: Menopause is* not *a disease, it does* not *make you crazy, it does* not *end your sexuality, and it's* not *the first step toward decrepitude. However, it* is *non-negotiable.*

Is there a woman's health event more shrouded in myth and misapprehension than menopause? Probably not, even though it's a natural passage for every woman. Most menopausal women don't consider themselves lucky, but they might if they realized that as recently as a century ago, few women lived long enough to even experience menopause. Today, women can expect to live three to four decades beyond their childbearing years. And they will live well, thanks to the many options available for easing women through "The Change."

Conventionally considered a tumultuous journey lasting many years, menopause is really just a single day—the day that marks 12 months without menstruation. It can come as early as age 35 or as late as 55, but the average age of menopause is—and has been for all of recorded history—age 51.

What you may think of as menopause is actually the years that doctors call perimenopause. That's the time when you have more frequent menstrual cycles without ovulation, and you start to experience symptoms typically associated with menopause, such as hot flashes and mood swings. This transition period can begin 10 to 12 years before menopause, with erratic and dramatic shifts in hormone levels coming four to five years before menstruation stops, says **Larrian Gillespie, M.D.,** a urogynecologist in Beverly Hills.

Every woman's perimenopausal journey is different. Some pass through with minimal discomfort. Others experience life-disrupting symptoms: hot flashes, night sweats, anxiety, depression, irritability, insomnia, headaches, palpitations, and irregular or very heavy periods.

Perimenopause begins when your menstrual cycle's delicate hormonal ballet slows and eventually stops as your ovaries run out of eggs, usually around age 50. A woman is born with millions of eggs. But they immediately begin disintegrating, leaving about 300,000 available for fertilization by the time she reaches puberty—less by the time she's ready to try conceiving. As aging ovaries start to produce less estrogen, your pituitary gland releases more and more follicle-stimulating hormone (FSH) to encourage greater estrogen production. That's why high levels of FSH are the best indicator of whether you're actually perimenopausal. Eventually, both estrogen and progesterone levels decrease dramatically, periods cease, and menopause occurs.

For some women, menopause simply means the end of menstrual periods. But for others, it's an unwelcome reminder that they're aging. In our youth-centered society, this realization can trigger anxiety about the future and a sinking feeling that the best years are behind them. That's nonsense, says *Elizabeth Lee Vliet, M.D.*, a women's health specialist in Dallas and Tucson. "Menopause, like puberty, is a natural benchmark, a new beginning. As with any new phase of life, you have to understand your options to maximize your experience."

*Women who embrace the changes of midlife, rather than dread them, find menopause to be an empowering event.—Elizabeth Lee Vliet, M.D.*

In her book, *Screaming to Be Heard: Hormone Connections Women Suspect ... and Doctors Still Ignore,* Dr. Vliet says that the years following menopause can be fulfilling if women make informed choices about what's right for them. Midlife is a good time to pause and take stock of your life journey. Women who embrace these changes, rather than dread them, find menopause to be an empowering event. Even unpleasant perimenopausal symptoms, such as hot flashes, can trigger many women to improve their health, perhaps for the first time in their lives. This pro-active self-care can lead to all kinds of positive results. "Menopause is a time when many women realize the personal power they possess," says Dr. Vliet.

# HOT FLASHES AND NIGHT SWEATS: HANDLING THE HEAT

More than 70 percent of perimenopausal women in the United States experience hot flashes—that internal heat wave that turns the face, neck, and arms red. These surges last anywhere from three to six minutes and can happen several times a day. Hot flashes that occur while you're sleeping and are accompanied by drenching perspiration are called night sweats. Night sweats can have other medical causes—such as cancer, acquired immune deficiency syndrome (AIDS), or a side effect from a medication—so it's important to tell your doctor if they frequently disturb your sleep.

Hot flashes are caused by fast declines of estrogen that interfere with the body's natural thermostat, located in the hypothalamus of the brain. Blood vessels dilate to help cool the body. The increased blood flow to your skin makes you feel hot and become red or flushed. In other words, as your core body temperature decreases, your skin temperature increases. Hot flashes usually have a consistent pattern, though each woman's pattern is different. Some hot flashes are easily tolerated, others are annoying, and a few are downright debilitating. Once they start, hot flashes can erupt for as long as three to five years before tapering off—and there's no way to know when they'll stop. Add to that the fact that hot flashes and night sweats can disrupt your sleep, even if they're not strong enough to actually wake you.

Some women put a positive spin on hot flashes by calling them personal power surges, but they're still tough to live with. Fortunately, you can take these steps to control the heat waves.

**Explore estrogen.** The standard medical treatment for hot flashes—and the only one approved by the U.S. Food and Drug Administration (FDA)—is hormone replacement therapy (HRT). (You should note that in October 2002 the National Institutes of Health announced a name change, since HRT implies a full restoration of hormones, which does not occur. The new name is menopausal hormone therapy, which you are likely to start seeing referred to as HT.) A considerable body of research has established the effectiveness of HRT in combating hot flashes, says *Elizabeth Lee Vliet, M.D.,* author of *Screaming to Be Heard: Hormone Connections Women Suspect ... and Doctors Still Ignore.* Of course, there are pros and cons to HRT. (For more information, see our special section on HRT, page 251.) If your FSH test is not high enough to indicate that you're in menopause, you may consider taking birth control pills to help control perimenopausal symptoms.

"If you use a low-dose oral contraceptive in the premenopausal years, you typically do not experience the hot flashes and other symptoms that mark the endocrine transition to actual menopause," says Dr. Vliet. "That's why I often say the pills help you 'sail over the turbulent waters' of perimenopause."

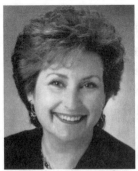

*Reduce the frequency of your hot flashes with regular exercise, suggests Larrian Gillespie, M.D. A brisk walk on most days helps regulate your body temperature.*

**Avoid triggers.** Identify the factors that bring on hot flashes. These can include overly warm rooms, strong emotions, hot drinks, spicy foods, sugar, alcohol, and caffeine. Then try to avoid those triggers whenever possible, says *Larrian Gillespie, M.D.,* a urogynecologist in Beverly Hills.

**Check your medication.** Some drug therapies, such as Evista (raloxifene) for osteoporosis and Nolvadex (tamoxifen) for cancer, can also cause hot flashes, says Dr. Vliet. If you think one of these triggers your hot flashes, check with your health-care provider about switching to an alternative medication.

**Breathe deeply.** When a hot flash starts, take slow and deep abdominal breaths to keep it from reaching full-blown proportions, says Dr. Gillespie. Deep breathing may also decrease the frequency of hot flashes, as well as shorten the duration of the flush. Practice taking slow, deep breaths—deep enough to make your stomach rise—whenever possible. (For more information on deep-breathing techniques, see page 283.)

> *When a hot flash starts, take slow and deep abdominal breaths to shorten the duration of the flush.*
> *—Larrian Gillespie, M.D.*

**Exercise regularly.** Routine physical exercise can significantly lower the number of hot flashes you experience, says Dr. Gillespie. This is possibly due to the effects exercise has on the brain chemicals that regulate body temperature. She suggests at least 30 minutes of moderately challenging exercise, such as a brisk walk, five days a week.

## ONE WOMAN'S STORY: MENOPAUSE

*At age 51, Olga Haley, of Beaverton, Oregon, found herself heading into "the gray cloud of menopause."*

Olga Haley began noticing perimenopausal symptoms at age 46. By the time she turned 51, she was feeling many of the distressing effects associated with this natural, but sometimes thorny, passage.

For Haley, insomnia was the worst symptom. Lying awake about three hours every night contributed to other maladies, including headaches, exhaustion, and lethargy bordering on depression. "Finally, I went to see my gynecologist, who prescribed hormone replacement therapy (HRT), telling me that the safeguards it provided for my heart outweighed the dangers of breast cancer." Haley admits, "I was dubious, but I took the prescription and got it filled anyway."

She also decided to resign from her position as a vice president at a public relations firm and begin working from home so that she could manage her life and menopause better. Although her workload was still fairly heavy, at least she could schedule rest breaks once or twice a day to make up for the insomnia.

About four years later, Haley felt a stinging in her left breast. She went for a mammogram, white with fear that she had breast cancer. Fortunately, the problem turned out to be cysts. Soon after, she heard a report that estrogen given as part of HRT was linked to a 40-percent increase in breast cancer. "I was so frightened that I literally threw my prescription away and quit cold turkey," says Haley.

Abruptly stopping HRT caused massive headaches for a few days, but they eventually subsided. Haley decided to quit seeing her male doctor and found a female gynecologist who encouraged the use of alternative treatments. Rather than advocating the one-size-fits-all approach that her other doctor took, Haley's new physician worked with her to design a program geared to her unique needs.

Haley began using herbal products, such as Pro-Gest, a natural progesterone, and valerian root, to help her sleep. She also took vitamin E, an antioxidant thought to have heart protective benefits, as well as vitamin D and calcium to stave off osteoporosis.

Vigorous exercise is now part of Haley's health regimen. She had been taking walks for years, but then she committed to a more regular routine and now pushes for longer distances. She started with small weights, doing 20 repetitions of six exercises every day, then added sit-ups. And unless it's a Friday- or Saturday-night splurge—when she doesn't care if she's a little sleepless—Haley avoids alcohol and caffeine late in the day.

Listening to her body and charting her own course of wellness enabled Haley to return to work downtown. Today, at age 57, she owns a successful public relations firm and is as active as she ever was. Yet she doesn't regret stepping out of the mainstream and taking time to evaluate her life.

"Menopause brought with it a real sense of loss," says Haley. "I would feel down in the dumps, even though I had everything I ever wanted: a great husband, wonderful home, good job. Then I realized that my life was far from over, despite all the foolishness women are fed by our society. I have a good third of my life ahead of me, so I started thinking about all that I could still contribute."

**Reduce stress.** Daily exercise also reduces stress, a known trigger for hot flashes, says Dr. Gillespie. You might also find relief from meditation, yoga, visualization, or biofeedback. Splurge on a massage or take a leisurely bath.

**Keep your cool.** Dress in layers so that you can easily remove clothing to bring down heat. Keep your room cool at night. Carry a spray bottle of cold water and mist yourself whenever a flash starts. Keep a minifan on your desk turned on high and directed toward your face, says Dr. Gillespie.

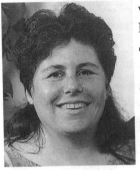

Consider this fragrant tip from Chinese medicine practitioner Misha Ruth Cohen, O.M.D.: Put out the fire of a hot flash with a soothing soak in a cool bath enhanced with peppermint tea.

**Soak in mint.** A cooling peppermint soak can help quell hot flashes, says *Misha Ruth Cohen, O.M.D.,* who practices Chinese medicine in San Francisco. Make ½ gallon peppermint tea by boiling ½ cup fresh peppermint leaves in 1 gallon water for 10 minutes. Strain the tea. Draw a cool bath and add the tea. Slip in and soak until you begin to feel cool. If fresh peppermint isn't available, you can substitute any kind of fresh mint, which is generally available at grocery stores.

**Try some herbs.** Traditional herbal medicines offer a variety of treatments to ease hot flashes, says *Rebecca Wynsome, N.D,* a naturopathic physician practicing in Seattle. (Always check with your health-care provider before taking any herbal supplements, as they may have side effects or interact with other medications. Because some of these herbs have estrogen-like effects, they can potentially increase the risk of certain reproductive cancers.) Dr. Wynsome recommends the following natural remedies.

- Black cohosh: Used by Native Americans to treat gynecological problems, this herb has estrogen-like compounds that cool the heat. It's available in a tablet or tincture (liquid) at health-food stores. Follow dosage directions on the bottle. Don't take black cohosh if you have heart disease because it can decrease your heart rate. And since there's no scientific data on the safety of long-term use, don't take it for longer than six months, advises *Alicia M. Weissman, M.D.,* assistant professor in the Department of Family Medicine at the University of Iowa College of Medicine and Hospitals and Clinics in Iowa City.

- *Vitex agnus-castus* or chasteberry: This plant also contains estrogen-like compounds. Recommended by Hippocrates in the fourth century B.C.

for "feminine discomforts," chasteberry is believed to act on the hypothalamus, the part of the brain where the body's natural thermostat is located. It also acts on the pituitary gland, regulating progesterone levels. Available at health-food stores as a tincture, the recommended daily dose is 40 drops in a glass of water, depending on the strength of the tincture. Check the bottle for details.

- Dong quai: This Chinese herb is commonly used to treat menopausal symptoms and has pain-relieving, antispasmodic, and anti-inflammatory qualities, according to clinical studies conducted in China. Herbalists believe dong quai revitalizes the female body by correcting hormonal imbalances, says Dr. Cohen. And when hormone levels are in balance, you don't experience hot flashes. Dong quai is available as a tincture, extract, pill, or powder; choose the form that appeals to you. Follow the dosage recommendations on the package.

    Although often recommended for hot flashes, taking dong quai is not without risks, warns Dr. Weissman. Don't use it if you take Coumadin (warfarin), since it can increase the effect of this blood thinner. The herb contains psoralens, cancer-causing chemicals that can also make you extra-sensitive to sunlight, causing a rash. And if a brand contains bovine tissue, it could pose a risk for variant Creutzfeldt-Jakob disease, the human form of mad cow disease. (Although a supplement's label may state that its cow extracts come from countries certified to be disease-free, keep in mind that the FDA does not monitor supplement content.) Talk with your doctor about the possible benefits and risks of using this herb.

## INSOMNIA: FINDING SWEET SLEEP

Menopause-related insomnia has two hormonal causes: The drop in estrogen can disrupt patterns of healthy, deep sleep. As you age, your body also produces less melatonin, a hormone from the pineal gland that regulates the sleep-wake cycle. This reduction of estrogen *and* melatonin keeps many women from reaching and maintaining the deepest levels of sleep, says *Larrian Gillespie, M.D.,* a urogynecologist in Beverly Hills. Hot flashes can make this fitful slumber even worse. So while it's a myth that menopause itself makes a woman irritable, there's no doubt that weeks of sleep deprivation and the resulting fatigue can shorten anyone's fuse.

# Don't eat or work out within three hours of bedtime, since doing either can keep you awake.—*Larrian Gillespie, M.D.*

Fortunately, simple lifestyle changes can alleviate most menopause-related sleep disturbances, assures Dr. Gillespie. However, if the following tips don't help, see your doctor to rule out other medical conditions—such as thyroid abnormalities, allergies, sleep apnea (breathing problems), and anemia—that can cause sleep problems and fatigue.

**Settle down.** Treatment of insomnia should first focus on improving your sleep routine, says Dr. Gillespie. Give yourself enough time to wind down before you get in bed. Once there, do relaxing things, such as read; don't balance your checkbook or bring work to bed. Developing a routine that emphasizes quiet, relaxing activities an hour before turning in can make a big difference in your ability to get a sound sleep.

**Eat early.** Avoid heavy meals in the evening. And whatever you eat, don't have it within three hours of bedtime. Too much gastrointestinal activity can keep you awake, says Dr. Gillespie.

**Set the scene.** Noise, temperature, and light can interfere with sleep, so be sure all are adjusted to your liking. If disturbing outside noises are creeping in, apply seals to windows and doors, or hang sound-muffling drapes. Or mask noises with a sound machine that simulates ocean waves or a peaceful forest.

**Avoid stimulants.** Stay away from alcohol, caffeine, and nicotine—not just in the evening, but all day, advises Dr. Gillespie. These substances stimulate the central nervous system. Keeping them out of your body increases sleep efficiency and total sleep time. Watch out for less obvious sources of caffeine, such as chocolate, soft drinks, and green tea.

**Exercise daily.** Working out reduces stress and promotes better, more restorative sleep, says Dr. Gillespie. Plus, it simply tires you out. Most perimenopausal women who partake in some form of regular, rigorous exercise report less sleep disturbances. Just be sure not to work out within two to three hours of bedtime, since it may stimulate you.

**Try estrogen.** The U.S. Food and Drug Administration has not approved hormone replacement therapy for insomnia, but the therapy has been shown to improve sleep for some menopausal women. With supplemental estrogen, hot flashes and night sweats decrease or disappear.

If you choose to pursue alternative methods, consider the following.

**Mellow with melatonin.** Women experiencing menopause-related insomnia should try a melatonin supplement, says *Adelaide Nardone, M.D.*, a gynecologist from Providence, Rhode Island, and medical consultant to the Vagisil Women's Health Center. She recommends taking 1 to 3 milligrams two to three hours before bedtime. Start with 1 milligram per night and see how you do for a month. Then, if necessary, step up to a higher amount—say, 2 milligrams—for a month. Taking too much melatonin can make you feel groggy the next day, so it's best to take the smallest effective dose. Melatonin tablets, in varying strengths, are available at drugstores without a prescription.

**Go herbal.** Half an hour before bedtime, drink calming chamomile tea, suggests *Rebecca Wynsome, N.D*, a naturopathic physician practicing in Seattle. You can buy prepared tea bags or make your own brew by steeping 2 teaspoons chamomile flowers in 8 ounces piping hot water for 10 minutes.

Valerian is another herb that can help you fall asleep and stay asleep, says Dr. Wynsome. Try taking about 20 drops valerian tincture in water at bedtime. You may need more or fewer drops; experiment to find the dosage that suits you best. Do not take valerian with conventional tranquilizers or sedatives because it can amplify their effects, cautions Dr. Wynsome.

## FATIGUE: REGAINING ENERGY

If you're not sleeping well, naturally you're going to be tired. But other issues related to menopause might be making you feel like you need a nap by lunchtime. You might want to talk with your doctor about getting tested for hypothyroidism and having your adrenal glands checked.

**HYPOTHYROIDISM** Thyroid hormone is a must for physical and mental energy. An underactive thyroid gland produces too little of this key hormone and can lead to a condition called subclinical hypothyroidism, a common problem in perimenopausal women and even more common in postmenopausal women. Dr. Gillespie says that by age 70 nearly 70 percent of women have this condition. Typical medical tests don't detect subclinical hypothyroidism, which can sabotage energy levels. If you're sleeping well but are still tired, ask your doctor to test you for levels of thyroid stimulating hormone. Levels above 5.0 microIU/mL may mean your body is trying to correct for hypothyroidism, and you may need synthetic thyroid hormones.

Here are some self-help strategies to supplement thyroid medication.

**Avoid salt with iodine.** Iodine can further suppress thyroid function in someone with subclinical hypothyroidism, says Dr. Gillespie.

**Go easy on the soy.** "Too much soy can turn off your thyroid," she says. Limit yourself to one portion a day, about 1.5 ounces tofu, 3 tablespoons soy powder, 4 ounces soy ice cream, or 8 ounces soy milk.

**ADRENAL EXHAUSTION** Your adrenals are two pinto bean–sized glands that sit atop your kidneys and produce hormones that help you cope with the stresses of daily life. Stress can wear you down as your body releases

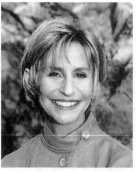

increasing amounts of two stress hormones: cortisol and dehydroepiandrosterone (DHEA). This leaves you fatigued and susceptible to a variety of illnesses, says *Jesse Lynn Hanley, M.D.,* an antiaging specialist in Malibu, California, and author of *Tired of Being Tired.*

While adrenal exhaustion can happen to anyone—not just perimenopausal or postmenopausal women—stress can make some change-of-life discomforts more acute. Too much cortisol, for example, suppresses female hormones, which could trigger more frequent hot flashes. Or the release of adrenal hormones, such as adrenaline, at night can trigger night sweats.

*Stress leads to fatigue. Energize your body by taking vitamins and eating a diet high in whole fruits and vegetables, advises Jesse Lynn Hanley, M.D.*

If you've been battling a barrage of life stresses and find you are frequently fatigued, Dr. Hanley recommends these steps to help your glands recover.

**Eliminate unnecessary obligations.** Don't do anything that's going to leave you feeling depleted. Listen to your mind and body, and respect their needs—especially about when enough is enough.

**Eat healthfully.** Consume more fruits and vegetables, preferably those grown organically. Pesticides and herbicides are pollutants that your body has to work overtime to eliminate, thus draining your energy and vitality. If organic produce is not available, wash fruits and vegetables well to remove pesticides and other toxins. Eat whole, not processed, foods as often as possible. Reduce the amount of refined sugar in your diet and avoid caffeine, which may give you quick energy but will leave you more fatigued than before.

*Your body has to work overtime to eliminate pesticides, draining your energy and vitality. Avoid them by choosing organic produce.*

—*Jesse Lynn Hanley, M.D.*

**Take vitamins and minerals.** Vitamins and minerals are the catalysts of cellular function. Without an adequate supply of these elements, your vitality fades. Rather than taking one megadose tablet every day, she recommends small doses of multiple vitamins and mineral supplements from forms that can be taken two to six times a day with food. Taking these supplements throughout the day gives your body a better chance of absorbing what it needs. Dr. Hanley recommends products made by Ethical Nutrients, New Chapter, Rainbow Light, and Solray, all of which are available at health-food stores.

## DEPRESSION: BATTLING THE BLUES

Among the many myths associated with menopause is the idea that mental problems, such as depression, are inevitable as hormone production decreases. New scientific studies show that declining estradiol (the main type of estrogen produced by the ovaries) may contribute to milder forms of depression and anxiety symptoms. However, lower hormone levels don't necessarily cause the more severe forms of major depression, says *Elizabeth Lee Vliet, M.D.*, of Dallas and Tucson, who specializes in menopause.

Yet many women during midlife do suffer from feeling blue or discouraged. Some begin questioning past life decisions or grapple with unfinished emotional business. Others suffer from sleep deprivation and overwork, leading to fatigue and irritability—conditions that may be mistaken for depression. And hormonal fluctuations, though normal, can contribute to mood swings. When hormone-related changes coincide with other life stresses, many women feel overwhelmed, angry, or out of control.

How do you know if what you are experiencing are common blues or clinical depression? The duration of symptoms is one important key, says Dr. Vliet. If you remain down, discouraged, or hopeless for more than two weeks—despite pleasant events in your life—you probably have clinical depression. Thoughts of death or suicide are extremely serious symptoms and should never be ignored, particularly if you think about specific ways of taking your life. Seek qualified professional help immediately.

Even if your blues are transitory, they can interfere with your life. Again, action is key to keeping funky feelings at bay.

**Try therapy.** If your doctor recommends counseling or psychotherapy to help you cope more effectively with life stresses, don't let self-consciousness hold you back, says Dr. Vliet. Family or factors other than menopause cause most stress for women during midlife. Talking to an objective third party can help bring your concerns into manageable focus.

**Improve your habits.** Eating healthfully, exercising regularly, and practicing relaxation techniques can help alleviate depression, says Dr. Vliet. Conversely, drinking alcohol, smoking, and taking recreational drugs all make depression worse.

*Do you have more than the blues? If you feel discouraged or hopeless for more than two weeks—despite some pleasant events—you probably have clinical depression.*

*—Elizabeth Lee Vliet, M.D.*

**Investigate estrogen, reconsider progesterone.** As part of a comprehensive treatment plan, hormone therapy helps some depressed women. In contrast, progestin, a synthetic progestogen, can worsen funky feelings, particularly in women who experienced negative mood changes prior to each menstrual period in previous years. The same result can come from using wild yam progesterone creams, says Dr. Vliet. That's because too much progesterone can cause an imbalance of brain chemicals that triggers depression. If you have this reaction, talk to your doctor about changing your medication.

**Look to herbs.** If you have mild to moderate depression and don't want to go the prescription antidepressant route, you may find relief by taking Saint-John's-wort. Herbalists have used this herb for centuries to help ease depression. *Rebecca Wynsome, N.D,* a naturopathic physician practicing in

Seattle, suggests taking 300 milligrams three times a day with meals. Look for a standardized 0.3-percent formulation.

*Unless you want a late-in-life baby, St. John's-wort may give you more stress then it relieves—it can halve the Pill's effectiveness.*—Elizabeth Lee Vliet, M.D.

Be careful if you're taking birth control pills, warns Dr. Vliet. Research from the National Institutes of Health found that Saint-John's-wort can decrease the Pill's effectiveness by as much as 50 percent. "Unless you want a late-in-life baby, this herb may give you more stress than it relieves," she says.

**Nurture yourself.** Maintaining emotional health during perimenopause requires a balance between your obligations to others and your self-nurturing needs. While many women can identify their sources of stress, they often find it difficult to take care of themselves. As primary caregivers to families, women often put their own needs last, says *Adelaide Nardone, M.D.,* a gynecologist from Providence, Rhode Island, and medical consultant to the Vagisil Women's Health Center. Learn to put yourself first—at least some of the time.

## MEMORY PROBLEMS: SURVIVING THOSE MENTAL LAPSES

You go upstairs to get something ... but what? Oh, where did you put those bills? And now that you think about it, what's happened to your memory?

Most women in midlife have moments—known as meno-fog—when even the simplest details elude them. Many perimenopausal women complain of mental fuzziness, especially when it comes to recalling something that happened recently. But is there really a menopause connection?

Absolutely, says *Elizabeth Lee Vliet, M.D.,* of Dallas and Tucson, who specializes in menopause. Several recent studies indicate the direct effect of estrogen on memory, specifically on verbal memory. The brain is an important target organ for estrogen, and as estrogen levels decline, brain function is bound to be affected.

Research into the effects of estrogen on brain tissue shows that different forms of the hormone regulate either the development or functioning of various nerve cells in the brain, says Dr. Vliet. For example, estradiol, the main type of estrogen produced by the ovaries, promotes growth of new dendrites, the branchlike extensions of cells that shorten the space between cells. New growth enhances communication between cells.

Estrogen can also benefit the brain's long-term health by improving blood flow and oxygen delivery, as well as protecting nerve cells from damage. Studies of women taking estrogen replacement therapy (ERT) have found improved verbal memory and performance on cognitive tests. But ERT certainly isn't the only route available to improve your memory and clarity of thought.

**Use it.** The old adage, use it or lose it, definitely applies to brain function, says *Arianna Staruch, N.D.,* a naturopath in Portland, Oregon. Mental challenges, such as learning to play a musical instrument or working crossword puzzles, act like weight training for the brain. There are even specific exercises, called neurobics, developed by Lawrence C. Katz, Ph.D., and Manning Rubin, that can help stimulate your brain and keep it active. These include such tricks as brushing your teeth with the hand you don't normally use or driving a different route to work.

*Practicing such little tricks as brushing your teeth with the hand you don't normally use can stimulate your brain and keep it active.*—Arianna Staruch, N.D.

**Destress.** Women often think they're suffering from age-related cognitive decline, when they're actually just stressed out, says *Larrian Gillespie, M.D.,* a urogynecologist in Beverly Hills. Women in midlife are often responsible for both children and aging parents. They're doing their utmost to excel at work as well as at home, and so they run from dawn to dusk—with nary a pause. "No wonder you're stressed out!" she says. Juggling so many demands results in brief mental blips that often make women think they are beginning to slide toward Alzheimer's disease or senile dementia. Take a deep breath and realize that stress-induced memory lapses can be controlled *if* you reduce the stress.

**Get moving.** Physical fitness helps with memory, since exercise increases the amount of oxygen and nutrients going to the brain, says Dr. Vliet. She recommends a simple aerobic workout, such as walking for 30 minutes a day, several times a week.

**Eat well.** A diet high in antioxidant-rich fruits and vegetables may be helpful in reversing nerve-cell aging in the brain, says Dr. Staruch. Focus on such colorful foods as leafy greens, red peppers, strawberries, blueberries, and grapes. Also reduce the fat in your diet, recommends Dr. Vliet. Dietary fat contributes to plaque deposits in the arteries, which block blood flow to the brain.

**Socialize.** Humans are social beings, and social interactions stimulate the brain, says Dr. Staruch. Taking steps to avoid isolation, especially later in life, may improve not only your quality of life, but also your mental functioning.

**Consider supplements or herbs.** Talk with your doctor about taking one of these herbal remedies. Remember that even so-called natural treatments require medical supervision, because they can interact with other medications or treatments.

- Acetyl-L-carnitine: This amino-acid derivative has shown promise for improving memory by protecting nerve cells, says Dr. Staruch. A typical dosage is 250 milligrams a day. Check with your health-care provider to be sure that's appropriate for you.

- Antioxidants: These include vitamins C and E, which provide protection from nerve-cell damage. Dr. Staruch suggests 500 milligrams vitamin C and 400 International Units vitamin E every day.

- Ginkgo: Research conducted in Europe over the past three decades indicates that leaves from ginkgo biloba, the world's oldest living species of tree, can improve short-term memory and concentration, says Dr. Vliet. That's particularly true among people with age-related impairment. Most clinical trials have used between 120 to 240 milligrams ginkgo biloba extract per day, generally divided into two to three portions. Ginkgo biloba extract acts as a vasodilator, meaning it improves blood flow in the brain. However, ginkgo may interact with certain medications, especially blood thinners.

- Huperzine: Derived from a Chinese moss, *Huperzia serrata* prevents the breakdown of acetylcholine, a substance that the nervous system needs to transmit information from cell to cell. Studies conducted in the United States and China found that huperzine enhanced memory in adolescents, as well as older patients with memory impairment, says Dr. Staruch. Researchers generally had participants take 100 to 200 micrograms huperzine two to three times a day. Check with your primary physician before trying this herb to be sure that it won't interact with any prescription medication you're taking.

# SEXUAL DYSFUNCTION: RETHINKING YOUR SEX LIFE

Comedian Bill Maher once defined menopause as "men on pause—it's when women just aren't interested in sex anymore." Although good for a laugh, this is certainly not true, says *Adelaide Nardone, M.D.*, a gynecologist from Providence, Rhode Island, and medical consultant to the Vagisil Women's Health Center. Some of the changes women go through at midlife *do* leave them feeling less than sensual, though, and many women experience some form of sexual dysfunction during this phase of life.

Decreasing hormone levels can affect your interest in sex. So can changes in your vagina, including dryness (also related to declining hormone levels), which can make intercourse painful, says Dr. Nardone. Add to this mix a passel of life stresses, concern over body image, and sleep deprivation from hot flashes, and it's not surprising that many perimenopausal women are simply not in the mood.

Sexual problems in perimenopause seem to be linked to whether women have the threshold level of estradiol, the main type of estrogen produced by the ovaries, says *Elizabeth Lee Vliet, M.D.*, a women's health specialist in Dallas and Tucson. Studies conducted at the Yale University Menopause Center found that women with estradiol levels greater than 50 pg/mL reported minimal adverse changes in their sexual function. Women whose estradiol levels were below 50 pg/mL, however, had a dramatic increase in sexual problems of all types, including decreased lubrication, burning and pain during intercourse, difficulty having an orgasm, and diminished quality of orgasm. While there isn't an established norm for estradiol levels as you move through menopause, Dr. Vliet says a desirable target range for women during this time is 90 to 100 pg/mL. (As a comparison, an estradiol level of 200 pg/mL is normal in the first half of a menstrual period before a woman reaches menopause.)

Since testosterone governs arousal in men *and* women, a woman's sex drive is affected as aging ovaries produce less of this so-called male hormone. Progesterone, which is often part of a hormone replacement regimen, interferes with your body's ability to use what little testosterone is available, says Dr. Vliet. However you look at it, the less testosterone the lower your sex drive.

These are Dr. Nardone's suggestions for keeping your sex life vital.

**Don't ignore vaginal changes.** In perimenopause and the years following menopause, many vaginal changes occur due to decreasing estrogen levels. If the tissues of the vulva and vaginal lining become thin, dry, and less elastic, the result is a condition known as vaginal atrophy. Over time, as vaginal walls become thinner, the tissues may become easily inflamed or abraded, then may bleed. At some point in their lives, at least one-third of women will experience vulvovaginal problems, and vaginal atrophy will affect almost all postmenopausal women.

Waning estrogen levels and vaginal dryness may hinder your ability to become aroused, making intercourse uncomfortable and even painful, says Dr. Nardone. If this occurs often, you may begin to associate pain with sex, which is a real turnoff. Discuss your situation with a gynecologist and consider using an over-the-counter, water soluble, hormone-free vaginal lubricant.

**Explore ERT.** If vaginal atrophy is still interfering with your sex life, then the best treatment is supplemental estrogen, says Dr. Nardone. Estrogen replacement therapy (ERT) restores the thickness and elasticity of vaginal tissues and also relieves dryness. All ERT forms approved by the U.S. Food and Drug Administration are effective for this use, but symptoms respond more quickly to the vaginal forms of estrogen, such as creams, suppositories, or rings. If you have a severe case, you may need several weeks of treatment to restore the vagina to a healthy condition.

Apart from sexual problems, women with vaginal atrophy may experience episodes of bacterial vaginitis and urinary tract infections. Thinning vaginal tissue and an increase of vaginal alkalinity can trigger these conditions. Fortunately, ERT helps, as it thickens and restores elasticity to vaginal tissue.

**Accept yourself.** Your perception of your body is an important component of your sexual health. The physical changes that menopause brings, such as a thicker waist and sagging breasts, may alter your self-image. It's important to break out of our culture's Barbie-doll concept of beauty and accept that desirability comes in many shapes and sizes. If you maintain a positive outlook about your body and are comfortable with yourself, you'll probably experience greater sexual enjoyment. Practice the same attitude when it comes to your partner's appearance, which is also typically changing, suggests Dr. Nardone. Keep in mind that regular exercise will help you and your partner remain more energetic and youthful. In fact, most partners that work out report having more satisfying sexual relations.

**Stay healthy mentally.** Depression, stress, and anxiety may affect a woman's primary erogenous zone—her mind—which can undermine sexual desire. Talk to your doctor or therapist if mental burdens impede your sex life.

**Make time.** Late meetings, soccer games, and chores can interfere with emotional and physical intimacy, since couples often take their sex lives for granted. Good communication is key to uncovering the roots of sexual changes. Physical changes at midlife may mean that it takes longer for one partner—or both—to become fully aroused. Don't rush the process; make time for quality sexual encounters, advises Dr. Nardone.

> *Need another reason to exercise? It can improve your sex life. Most partners that work out report having more satisfying sexual relations.*
> *—Adelaide Nardone, M.D.*

**Start Kegels.** Kegel exercises, the repeated contraction and relaxation of the genital-pelvic muscles, improve sexual function. They also have the added benefit of toning the muscles that control urine flow, preventing leaks. Urinary incontinence can be caused by weakened pelvic muscles, resulting from childbirth, aging, or declining estrogen levels. When done correctly, Kegels are highly effective in strengthening the paravaginal tissues and may even improve sexual relations, but you must continue these exercises indefinitely.

So get started today: While urinating, contract your vaginal muscles to stop the flow. Hold this contraction for a slow count of 5, then release. Once you're familiar with it, you can do this exercise anytime, anywhere: waiting at a stoplight, talking on the phone, folding clothes. Dr. Nardone suggests starting with 10 a day and building up to 50.

**Check your meds.** Many medications, such as those for high blood pressure and depression, can create problems with sexual desire and orgasmic capacity. If you think a medication may be affecting your sex drive, talk with your doctor about an alternative drug.

**Try something different.** Intercourse does not have to be the primary sexual activity you enjoy, says Dr. Nardone. Devote more attention to other sexually satisfying behaviors: oral sex, massage, sensual baths, manual stimulation, and caressing. Women without partners can explore masturbation, a normal and healthy expression of sexual interest, she suggests.

## MENORRHAGIA, OR HEAVY BLEEDING: STANCHING THE FLOW

During a normal menstrual cycle, estrogen increases, causing a buildup of the uterine lining. Ovulation occurs halfway through the cycle; that cues your body to produce progesterone, which in turn makes estrogen production decline. If there is no ovulation, as is often the case in perimenopausal women, then estrogen doesn't decrease and the lining of the uterus keeps building. So when the lining eventually sheds, you have very heavy bleeding during your period, a condition known as menorrhagia. Aside from the menstrual discomfort, menorrhagia may lead to anemia (too few red blood cells) unless you get enough iron in your diet to offset the blood loss. If your monthly flow increases in your perimenopausal years and you start feeling rundown, get checked by your doctor.

Sometimes, excessive menstrual flow is caused by fibroids, which are noncancerous growths in or around the uterus, says *Adelaide Nardone, M.D.,* a gynecologist from Providence, Rhode Island, and medical consultant to the Vagisil Women's Health Center. While fibroid tumors often have no symptoms, they can produce dramatic menstrual changes, such as prolonged and heavy bleeding, intense cramps, and back pain. The cause of fibroids is unknown, but their growth can be stimulated by perimenopausal estrogen surges. Once you enter menopause, your fibroids should shrink and the symptoms should abate. In some cases, estrogen replacement therapy can also stimulate their growth, so consider this fact when deciding on therapy, says Dr. Nardone.

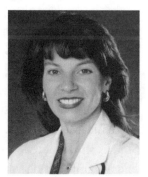

*Consider hormone therapy and supplements to stem the tide of heavy menstrual bleeding, suggests Adelaide Nardone, M.D.*

Other causes of heavy flow are such noncancerous growths as polyps in the uterine lining, called the endometrium. Problems with blood clotting can also be the culprit. In a minute percentage of cases, some types of cancer in the uterus, vagina, or cervix can cause abnormal bleeding from the uterus or vagina, says Dr. Nardone. Regular pelvic exams and Pap smears are particularly helpful in diagnosing these serious diseases at an early stage, when treatment is most effective. If you're using more than four overnight pads a day for more than two days or saturating more than two maxipads an hour, call your doctor for an evaluation, says Dr. Nardone. If you start feeling less energetic after two or three extremely heavy periods, have your physician check you for anemia. Menorrhagia can be exhausting and embarrassing, as any perimenopausal woman who's overflowed two tampons and an overnight pad within an hour of arriving at work can attest.

*If you're using more than four overnight pads a day for more than two days or saturating more than two maxipads an hour, call your doctor for an evaluation.*

*—Adelaide Nardone, M.D.*

Fortunately, there are choices you and your doctor can make to stem the tide.

**Consider hormones.** When heavy bleeding is caused by changes in estrogen and progesterone levels, it can often be regulated with prescription hormones, such as low-dose contraceptives. Other prescription hormonal drugs, such progestogens, are also sometimes used for short-term treatment.

**Consider supplements.** To treat heavy menstrual periods, try vitamin A. Studies show that women who took vitamin A for at least three months had a significant decrease in the amount of blood flow or length of the period, or both. In her book *Women's Encyclopedia of Natural Medicine,* Tori Hudson, M.D., recommends that you take 60,000 International Units (IUs) per day for one to three months, if your doctor approves. If ongoing treatment is necessary, drop to between 10,000 to 25,000 IUs after three months because higher amounts or extended use can lead to vitamin-A toxicity in some people. Research also suggests that 2,000 to 4,000 milligrams vitamin C per day and bioflavonoids from such foods as grapes, cherries, blackberries, blueberries, and citrus fruits can reduce menstrual blood loss by strengthening capillaries. Use nutritional supplements only with the approval and supervision of your doctor.

**Consider surgery.** Several surgical procedures can eliminate menorrhagia. Ask your doctor for more information.

# A Totally Up-to-the-Minute Guide to Hormone Replacement Therapy

Results from the Women's Health Initiative (WHI)—the largest research study ever conducted on the effects of hormone replacement therapy (HRT)—burst upon the world in July 2002 ... and blew up decades of standard medical practice.

The randomized, controlled clinical-trial portion of WHI—underway since 1993 and sponsored by the National Institutes of Health's National Heart, Lung, and Blood Institute—follows more than 68,000 women, between ages 50 and 79, for 8 to 12 years. These women have chosen to enroll in one, two, or all three of the following components: Calcium/Vitamin D, Dietary Modification, or HRT. The women in the HRT component are being examined for the effects of HRT on endometrial and breast cancers, heart disease, and osteoporosis.

## THE WHI RESULTS, SIMPLIFIED

Part of the Women's Health Initiative (WHI) study was halted early when it became clear that women taking Prempro, a form of hormone replacement therapy (HRT), faced an increased risk for breast cancer that surpassed the potential benefits of the treatment. Contrary to beliefs held for more than three decades, the study also found that HRT does *not* prevent heart disease—in fact, it may slightly increase the risk for heart attacks and stroke.

Overall, the study discovered that HRT *increased* the risk for invasive breast cancer by 26 percent, coronary heart disease by 29 percent, and stroke by 41 percent; it also doubled the rate of pulmonary embolisms (blood clots in the lungs). Consider this WHI comparison of two groups of 10,000 women: The first group is women who are not taking hormones. The second group is postmenopausal women who still have their uteruses and take estrogen plus progestin. In one year, of the women taking hormones, 8 more will have invasive breast cancer, 7 more will have heart attacks, 8 more will have strokes, and 18 more will have blood clots, compared to the first group.

Some positives emerged from the study, including the discovery of a 34-percent reduction in hip fractures and a 37-percent drop in colorectal cancers. Still, because the risks were greater than the benefits for women taking Prempro, the trial ended after only five years.

The risks were not increased for women who had had a hysterectomy and were taking estrogen alone, so that part of the WHI study continued. The results also do not necessarily apply to lower doses of Prempro or to other delivery methods of HRT—such as the patch or vaginal cream. These types of HRT need to be studied separately.

## HOW TO RESPOND TO THE NEWS

The study led to an outpouring of conflicting advice and frightening headlines, which—not surprisingly—prompted many women to throw up their hands in bewilderment and resign themselves to menopausal experiences like those of their great-grandmothers.

But as with most news reports about hormone replacement therapy (HRT) over the years, those from the Women's Health Initiative (WHI) were incomplete and often incorrect, says hormone specialist *Elizabeth Lee Vliet, M.D.* For a woman to stop taking HRT on the basis of any single study—or worse, any single news story—is tantamount to throwing the baby out with the bathwater. It just doesn't make sense, says Dr. Vliet.

*For a woman to stop taking HRT on the basis of a single study—or worse, a single news story—is tantamount to throwing the baby out with the bathwater. It doesn't make sense.*

*—Elizabeth Lee Vliet, M.D.*

The WHI study presented women with a different set of criteria with which to weigh the risks and benefits of HRT. It also gave women and their physicians a strong reason to revisit the reasons HRT is prescribed. It will still be recommended to treat symptoms of menopause, such as hot flashes, but doctors will no longer prescribe HRT to prevent or treat heart disease.

Still, some women may wish to continue HRT longer to reap other potential benefits, such as preventing and/or treating osteoporosis or because they believe it keeps them feeling and looking younger. In most cases, however, a physician will try to keep a woman on the lowest possible dose of estrogen and progestin.

Another variable in the HRT discussion is the type and form you take. The WHI study found adverse outcomes with only one type of HRT: Prempro, a combination of mixed estrogens harvested from horse urine and a potent, synthetic progestin. This combination is not natural to the human female body, although there are many types like this on the market that are approved by the Food and Drug Administration (FDA). "Different estrogens can be as different as night and day," says Dr. Vliet. "The 1920 Model T and the 2003 Thunderbird are both Fords, but they're hardly the same car."

Putting this recent flap into perspective, Dr. Vliet points to public reaction a few years ago when the common antihistamines Hismanal (astemizole) and Seldane (terfenadine) were taken off the market because of adverse effects. "The FDA did not recall all antihistamines," she notes, "nor did the media claim risky effects from every other antihistamine." Similarly, despite the frightening headlines about Prempro and other horse-derived therapies, other HRT choices (such as estradiol) are still considered safe.

## DECIDING IF HRT IS RIGHT FOR YOU

Along with safety concerns, the question of hormone replacement therapy (HRT) brings up other issues: If I want to take hormones, what hormones should I take? In what amounts?

Unfortunately, many women are confused or uninformed about their HRT choices. (It's likely that you will start seeing HRT referred to as HT, short for menopausal hormone therapy. In October 2002, the National Institutes of Health announced the name change because HRT implies a full restoration of hormones, which does not occur.) They don't know what to ask their doctor to determine which hormonal regimens—if any—would best suit them, says *Larrian Gillespie, M.D.*, of Beverly Hills, a menopause specialist who posts a free Internet newsletter on hormone therapy. (Visit www.menopausediet.com and click on "Newsletter.") As a result, these women suffer needlessly. So before you make any HRT decision, empower yourself with knowledge. "For too long, women have taken the word of their doctors—who are usually men—when it comes to HRT," says Dr. Gillespie. Instead, she advises you to take an active role in the decision, working with your health-care provider to fine-tune an individual approach that works for you.

*The Women's Health Initiative study found adverse outcomes with only one type of HRT: Prempro, a combination of mixed estrogens and a synthetic progestin. There are many other hormones available.*

## ONE SIZE DOES NOT FIT ALL

Tailoring hormone replacement therapy (HRT) to the individual woman is vital to minimize side effects and control symptoms, says **Elizabeth Lee Vliet, M.D.**, author of *Screaming to Be Heard: Hormone Connections Women Suspect ... and Doctors Still Ignore.* About 40 percent of American women between ages 50 and 74 try HRT to alleviate menopausal discomforts. Yet roughly 25 percent quit taking HRT within a month; up to 80 percent quit within two years because the symptoms they experience—such as migraines, nausea, and breast tenderness—seem worse than the menopausal problems they were trying to solve.

These problems stem from a one-size-fits-all approach to HRT, says Dr. Vliet. For decades, estrogen derived from pregnant mares' urine (Premarin and Prempro) accounted for more than 85 percent of HRT prescriptions. This is mainly due to the fact that most doctors get their primary menopause information from pharmaceutical companies looking to protect their share of the $2 billion-a-year HRT market.

No doctor would give every patient with an infection the same antibiotic. Yet in the world of medicine, there's been one basic recipe for menopausal complaints, says Dr. Vliet. She says that what each woman needs is *individualized* hormone therapy, using hormones identical to what her body makes *before* menopause—a concept that makes intuitive sense to women. "Hormone therapy is like a hat: Not all types suit every woman," says **Larrian Gillespie, M.D.**, a urogynecologist in Beverly Hills.

*(special section)*

# Each woman needs individualized hormone therapy, using hormones identical to what her body makes before menopause.—Elizabeth Lee Vliet, M.D.

Fortunately, today, there are menopause specialists trained in the nuances of individualized hormone therapy, says Dr. Vliet. The daily discomforts associated with HRT can be avoided if your doctor closely follows your personal fluctuations in estrogen and progesterone, the two key female hormones.

Dr. Vliet recommends that every perimenopausal woman consult a menopause specialist, rather than a general practitioner or gynecologist. A menopause specialist will take the time to listen to your specific symptoms, take blood tests to obtain information on a variety of health measures, test your serum hormone levels, and then tailor treatment to your individual needs. Finding this type of doctor may take some work. Dr. Vliet suggests asking women you know for personal recommendations or looking for a likely candidate at the Web site of the North American Menopause Society. (Visit www.menopause.org and click on "Consumers," then "Referral Lists.")

## UNDERSTANDING ESTROGEN

Estrogen isn't a single hormone; it's actually a group of hormones. Your body produces three principle forms: estradiol, estrone, and estriol. Prior to menopause, estradiol is the main type of estrogen manufactured by the ovaries. After menopause, your body primarily produces estrone. Estriol, present in our bodies all the time and produced by the placenta during pregnancy, is the weakest and most cancer-protective form of estrogen, says *Rebecca Wynsome, N.D,* a naturopathic doctor in Seattle who specializes in menopausal health.

Each type of estrogen can be administered differently: tablets, gels, patches, and creams. Tablets—the most popular form used in the United States—are made of estradiol and estrone, with doses ranging from 0.3 to 1.25 milligrams. To minimize side effects, your best bet is to start with the lowest dose and increase it gradually until you get relief from your menopause symptoms. Some women find that the smallest dose of 0.3 milligrams works for them.

A potential drawback to supplemental estrogen in tablet form is that the hormone's potency lessens as it moves through the digestive system, says *Elizabeth Lee Vliet, M.D.*, author of *Screaming to Be Heard: Hormone Connections Women Suspect ... and Doctors Still Ignore*. To avoid this,

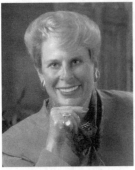

researchers created transdermal estradiol. Patches are the primary form of transdermal delivery in the United States, but gels or creams are also prescribed. These allow estrogen to be absorbed through the skin directly into the bloodstream, as it would be if the ovaries were producing it naturally.

Another benefit of the patch is that it dispenses estrogen continually, rather than in one large burst. This more closely resembles your body's own estrogen production, says Dr. Vliet.

One advantage of the estrogen patch is that it resembles your body's own natural estrogen production by dispensing the hormone continuously, says Elizabeth Lee Vliet, M.D.

The patch resembles a small, rounded bandage. You place the patch on the skin of your abdomen, buttocks, torso, or hips (never on your arms or legs) and change it according to your individualized dosing schedule. You can keep it on while you shower, bathe, or swim. Unlike the estrogen pill, there is not as much flexibility of dosage. The patch is available in four basic doses, ranging from 0.0025 to 0.1 milligrams.

Estrogen cream is primarily applied to the vagina to prevent atrophy and the breakdown of tissue caused by a lack of natural estrogen. Though estrogen is absorbed from the vaginal mucosa into the bloodstream, only a very small amount circulates in the body. Therefore, the effects tend to be undependable for any menopause symptom other than vaginal dryness.

## PICKING THE RIGHT ESTROGEN

Knowing your specific need for additional estrogen is important, says Dr. Wynsome. This is because, even after menopause, your body continues to make some estrogen through the adrenal glands and fat cells. Dr. Vliet recommends using estradiol to replace the estrogen that's lost at menopause, rather than adding estrone, which your body continues to produce. Estrone has more potential adverse side effects, she says.

How much supplemental estrogen you need depends on how much your body is already making, and the only way to know that is by undergoing an annual saliva or blood test. Dr. Wynsome suggests tracking estrogen levels with at-home saliva tests that check the ovarian output over a month's time. Ask your health-care provider for the test. You spit into a different test tube every third day for 30 days and send each to the lab for testing. Women who have not menstruated for five years can use a one-day saliva test. Dr. Vliet recommends having a blood test when you start hormone replacement therapy, followed by a test every three months to keep track of your hormonal needs.

*The only way to know how much supplemental estrogen you need is to know how much your body is already making. And the only way to know that is to take an annual saliva or blood test.*—Rebecca Wynsome, N.D.

After evaluating a woman's unique hormone profile, Dr. Vliet prescribes a plant-based estrogen. Estrace, for example, is a native form of the primary human estrogen, 17-beta estradiol, which is derived from soybeans.

Don't confuse "bioidentical" with "natural" hormones, cautions Dr. Vliet. Any product that comes from a biological source is natural, including estrogen from a pregnant mare's urine (like that old standby Premarin), but that doesn't mean it has the same molecular makeup as estrogen made by the human body.

Many natural plant estrogens are available at your local drugstore, but some plant-based products are bioidentical and others are not. In some cases, Dr. Vliet says she may ask a compounding pharmacy—which mixes doses on a patient-by-patient basis—to blend a customized bioidentical formula that meets a woman's specific needs. Compounding pharmacies are becoming the pharmacies of choice for many menopause specialists, says Dr. Vliet. Check your local Yellow Pages for pharmacies that offer compounding services.

Dr. Wynsome uses a compounding pharmacy when she prescribes an alternative formulation to synthetic hormone replacement therapy called Bi-est, which is 80-percent estriol and 20-percent estradiol. Or depending upon the customization a woman needs, she may prescribe Tri-est, which is 80-percent estriol, 10-percent estradiol, and 10-percent estrone.

*Many menopause specialists prefer using compounding pharmacies that mix customized estrogen doses for each prescription.*—Elizabeth Lee Vliet, M.D.

## PROGESTERONE: THE OTHER HORMONE

Progesterone is the other hormone your ovaries make. It prompts your body to shed its uterine lining and, thus, have a menstrual period. If your uterus is intact, your doctor will probably prescribe hormone replacement therapy (HRT) combining estrogen and progesterone. Why? Because the cue to shed your uterine lining reduces the increased risk of endometrial cancer that occurs with estrogen replacement therapy alone. If you get only estrogen, your uterine tissue continues building up and receives no hormonal cue to stop. If you've had a hysterectomy, you can take estrogen alone because you run no risk of getting uterine cancer.

"A woman who has not had her uterus removed should always follow *natural* hormone replacement therapy (nHRT) that includes bioidentical progesterone, at least 10 to 13 days each month," says *Rebecca Wynsome, N.D.*, a naturopathic physician practicing in Seattle. (Progestins are the synthetic forms of progesterone that have been indicted in numerous studies as increasing risks of breast cancer and heart disease.) For example, you can take one estrogen and one oral micronized progesterone pill every day as part of a 30-day cycle; or you can take estrogen for the first 25 days and add one progesterone tablet from Day 14 to 25. You don't use nHRT during the final five days of the 30-day cycle, when the uterus sheds its lining through what appears to be a menstrual period. (Of course, it's not a *true* menstrual period because ovulation has not occurred. But if you take nHRT, you may have a regular monthly period, depending on the dose prescribed.) Oral micronized bioidentical progesterone is preferred because it doesn't produce the side effects that synthetic progestins often do. Initial testing and monitoring assist the physician to prescribe the type, strength, and nHRT ratios that are right for each woman.

You can also get natural progesterone replacement in the form of a cream, which is absorbed into the bloodstream through the skin. Unlike synthetic progestins, there are few reported side effects. To get maximum absorption with the fewest side effects, natural progesterone should be used vaginally, recommends **Larrian Gillespie, M.D.,** a urogynecologist in Beverly Hills.

Many over-the-counter wild yam creams claim to provide the same benefits as prescriptive progesterone cream, says Dr. Wynsome—but they don't. Wild yam doesn't contain actual progesterone, and your body cannot convert wild yam extract into progesterone. If any of these creams do have progesterone, it's because their manufacturers add the hormone. Even if you follow label directions, you may get too much progesterone because hormones applied to the skin are absorbed erratically, causing you to perhaps get too much at once. "So I'm not in favor of the creams. Testing shows creams overdose patients even if the label specifies the amount and application method," says Dr. Wynsome.

*Don't be fooled by the claims of wild yam creams. Wild yam doesn't contain real progesterone, and your body can't convert wild yam extract into progesterone.—Rebecca Wynsome, N.D.*

## HOW MUCH HRT DO YOU NEED?

When it comes to hormone replacement therapy (HRT), it appears less is more, says **Margery Gass, M.D.,** director of the Menopause and Osteoporosis Center at University Hospital in Cincinnati. Commenting on the Women's Health, Osteoporosis, Progestin, Estrogen (HOPE) trial, which examined HRT in more than 2,600 postmenopausal women over a two-year period, Dr. Gass says that low doses of estrogen and progestin seem to work as well as higher doses in many circumstances with the added benefit of fewer side effects, such as breast tenderness, bloating, and bleeding.

The study, which released its findings in 2001, gave one group of women the most common daily dose of horse-derived estrogen—0.625 milligrams conjugated equine estrogens—either alone (in the form of Premarin) or in combination with 2.5 milligrams progestin (in the form of Prempro). Other study participants were given 1.5 milligrams progestin with either 0.3 or 0.45 milligrams conjugated equine estrogens daily.

The lower dose treatments were just as effective in reducing such menopausal symptoms as hot flashes and thinning of the vaginal lining. "We finally have good evidence that lower doses can be satisfactory," says Dr. Gass. This is an important advance for women who are considering HRT but are uneasy about possible adverse impacts, most of which have been reported at higher doses. "It is always good to review the current list of risks and benefits of HRT with a knowledgeable clinician," says Dr. Gass.

*Studies show that lower dose HRT treatments reduce menopausal symptoms effectively.*—Margery Gass, M.D.

## ENDOMETRIAL AND BREAST CANCERS: ARE YOU AT RISK?

In August 2003, the headlines screamed: HRT Tied to Breast-Cancer Deaths! News reports on the findings of the Million Women Study in Great Britain seemed to imply that all forms of hormone replacement therapy (HRT) are a sure prescription for breast cancer. But those reports painted a needlessly harsh and incomplete picture that frightened women already wary of HRT's link to breast and endometrial cancers, says *Elizabeth Lee Vliet, M.D.,* author of *It's My Ovaries, Stupid!* Unfortunately, many women base their decision on such alarming news reports or an out-of-context statistic, instead of evaluating their personal risk factors with their health-care providers.

What did the media leave out about the Million Women Study?

- It wasn't a controlled clinical trial. Rather, it was a health questionnaire survey about hormone use and other health issues.
- Detailed conclusions focused on only two types of estrogen, one of which is far more potent than estrogens generally prescribed in the United States, says Dr. Vliet. No data was given for the bioidentical (human) form of estradiol.
- British health-care standards may have contributed to the rate of breast-cancer deaths. The British National Health Service provides mammograms for women over 50 only once every three years (rather than

annually as in the United States) and not at all for women younger than 50. "In the Million Women Study, average time between diagnosis and death was only 1.7 years," says Dr. Vliet. "It's just unheard of here for death to occur so quickly. Many of those women must not have been diagnosed until they had late-stage cancer. This makes me question the validity of any conclusions about hormones based on this questionnaire."

On average, American women have a 3.3-percent cumulative lifetime risk of developing breast cancer, says *Larrian Gillespie, M.D.,* a urogynecologist in Beverly Hills. This calculation is based on a lifespan of 95 years, with the risk of developing breast cancer increasing from 1 in 52 at age 50, to 1 in 9 at age 85. So if you read a study that says HRT increases risk of breast cancer by 8 percent, understand that the risk may be more or less for you, based on your age and such factors as a family history of the disease, she advises.

You also need to consider how long you plan to be on HRT and at what dose, says Dr. Gillespie. The risk appears to increase the longer you're on it and the higher the dose. The Women's Health Initiative study found that breast cancer risk increased with additional years of combined estrogen-progestin use and only became truly significant after five years of use.

*Average lifetime risk for breast cancer is 3.3 percent, but your individual risk may be more or less.*—Larrian Gillespie, M.D.

Before you make a decision about HRT, Dr. Vliet recommends taking a computerized risk assessment test—called the Gail Model Risk Index—that calculates your personal risk of developing breast cancer, based on five known predictors. A risk index higher than 1.67 percent means you are at high risk and should talk with your physician about ways to reduce your risk. You can take the test online at http://calc.med.edu (search for "breast cancer").

Additionally, many women don't realize that the type of estrogen they take may make a difference in these cancer risks, says Dr. Gillespie. Premarin, the most commonly prescribed estrogen tablet, has been available since 1941 and has been the focus of virtually all research linking HRT to breast cancer. But the estrogen in Premarin and Prempro—conjugated esterified estrogens—contain about 17 compounds that are foreign to the human body. These foreign elements increase the body's inflammatory response, increasing your risk for cancer and heart disease. Also, these stock formulations provide "way more estrogen than needed," says Dr. Gillespie, and this overload may also increase cancer risk. In studies using physiological amounts (the amounts you'd normally have in your body) of bioidentical estradiol with natural progesterone, in dosages tailored to individual women, researchers have not found a striking increase in breast-cancer risk with HRT, says Dr. Vliet.

*Individualized dosages of bioidentical estradiol with natural progesterone do not appear to significantly increase breast-cancer risks.*—Elizabeth Lee Vliet, M.D.

In 1975, research linked sustained high levels of estrogen to endometrial cancer. That's why doctors now prescribe estrogen with progesterone: It stops the endometrium (the lining of the uterus) from overgrowing into a cancer-prone state. Risk of endometrial cancer from HRT is reduced to less than 1 percent by the added progesterone or progestin. Dr. Vliet notes that obesity after menopause is a greater risk factor than HRT because high sustained levels of estrone in body fat are then unopposed by progesterone from the ovaries.

## THE BENEFITS OF HRT

Now that research shows long-term use of hormone replacement therapy (HRT) may increase the risk of breast cancer and cardiovascular disease, talk to your doctor about whether you should take it.

It's good to remember that the risk of osteoporosis is also reduced by estrogen replacement. In the Women's Health Initiative (WHI) study, both Prempro and estrogen alone reduced the risk of hip fractures, which is common in women who have osteoporosis. Osteoporosis is the leading cause of pain in later life, with complications causing about 52,000 deaths every year. However, doctors can treat it with nonhormonal drugs—such as Actonel (risedronate), Evista (raloxifene), and Fosamax (alendronate)—that retard bone loss, without increasing the risk of developing breast cancer. So while HRT remains a useful weapon to prevent and treat osteoporosis, doctors may no longer recommend it as their first choice.

Some studies suggest postmenopausal estrogen replacement may protect women against such age-related eye ailments as macular degeneration, as well as colon cancer, cognitive function, wrinkles, and tooth loss. Significant reduction in colon cancer risk has been confirmed in the WHI study results so far.

## WHAT'S THE ANSWER?

Scientists may have some definitive answers to the complicated risks and benefits of hormone replacement therapy (HRT) between 2006 and 2010, when all the findings from the Women's Health Initiative study are released. Additional studies are needed to examine other forms and doses of HRT.

Not only are types of HRT under scrutiny, but also method of delivery seems to make a difference. Whereas studies show the risks of synthetic hormones in tablets, other research suggests that transdermal (patch or gel) delivery of 17-beta estradiol (bioidentical to the human body's dominant estrogen) does not significantly increase risk of cancer, heart disease, or blood clots, says *Larrian Gillespie, M.D.,* a urogynecologist in Beverly Hills. In fact, estradiol may help to prevent these conditions, she says. The key is to talk with your doctor about the best HRT form, dosage, and delivery method for *you.*

Some women feel that the benefits they gain from HRT are too good to give up, so they continue taking it with no stop date in mind. Again, this is a personal decision, based on your specific health risks and how you feel. "I can't say what anyone else should do, but speaking for myself, I want to think well and feel well, so I'm probably going to take it the rest of my life," says *Elizabeth Lee Vliet, M.D.,* a women's health specialist in Dallas and Tucson.

*Any medical treatment has some particle of risk. But don't let fear keep you from feeling the best you can.*—Larrian Gillespie, M.D.

"Make an informed choice. Don't let blind fear keep you from feeling the best you can," says Dr. Gillespie. "There's no medical treatment that doesn't have some particle of risk. But women are intelligent. They can sift through alarmist headlines, fear-mongering drug advertisements, and the reams of research out there to make a decision that's best for them."

# 14 Menstruation
## Is Your Period a Question Mark?

*Chapter*

*Many women have more trouble finding a good gynecologist than Stanley had tracking down Livingstone.*
—Niels Lauersen, M.D., and Steven Whitney
*It's Your Body: A Woman's Guide to Gynecology*

My little visitor. Aunt Flo. Red menace. The curse. Riding the cotton bicycle. Hundreds of euphemisms exist for a woman's menstrual period and, over the centuries, more than a few wacky notions have thrived. For instance, not so many decades ago, shampooing was taboo for menstruating females. Swimming was out, bed rest was in. Exercise was okay, as long as you didn't overdo it. And bathing? Forget about it: As recently as the 1950s, some doctors advised a menstruating woman to stay out of the tub.

Lucky for us, the medical community in the new millennium has a more rational and scientific view of menstruation, as well as better methods of helping women cope when problems do occur with that time of the month.

## PREMENSTRUAL SYNDROME: THE JEKYLL-AND-HYDE PHENOMENON

The symptoms that are collectively known as premenstrual syndrome (PMS) were first described in 1931. More than 70 years later, we still don't know what causes the bloating, irritability, and assorted aches and pains that come on just before menstruation and fade once a woman's period actually begins.

The most widely accepted medical theory of the cause of PMS: an ongoing imbalance in the levels of serotonin, a brain chemical that affects mood, sleep and other critical functions of mind and body, says **Adelaide Nardone, M.D.,** an obstetrician and gynecologist in Providence, Rhode Island, and a medical advisor to the Vagisil Women's Health Center. Imbalances in the levels of serotonin in turn cause imbalances in estrogen, progesterone, and testosterone, the sex hormones that control the menstrual cycle. "Women—indeed, all people—need to view PMS and related menstrual concerns as imbalances, not diseases," says **Bonnie Mackey, M.S.N.**, a holistic nurse practitioner and president of Mackey Health Institute, a complementary health-care practice and training center in West Palm Beach, Florida. And those imbalances can produce an array of physical and emotional symptoms.

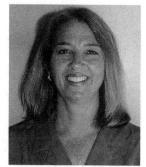

*PMS may make you feel lousy, but it is shouldn't be treated like a disease, says nurse practitioner Bonnie Mackey.*

Common physical symptoms include:
- Appetite changes, food cravings
- Breast tenderness
- Headache, muscle or joint aches
- Nausea, gastrointestinal upset
- Clumsiness
- Hot flashes, dizziness
- Fatigue, low energy
- Fluid retention, bloating

Emotional symptoms include:
- Irritability, anxiety
- Depression, crying spells
- Mood swings
- Sleep disturbances
- Forgetfulness, difficulty concentrating
- Social withdrawal
- Decreased libido

Few women escape PMS. The American College of Obstetricians and Gynecologists estimates that as many as 85 percent of menstruating women struggle with one or more symptoms of PMS each month. About one-sixth of those women are affected seriously enough to seek help, making PMS the most common premenopausal disorder for which women see a doctor, says **Susan Thys-Jacobs, M.D.**, an endocrinologist at St. Luke's-Roosevelt Hospital Center in New York City.

That leaves a whopping five-sixths who don't get medical help for PMS. "Many women become so used to their symptoms that they don't seek help or even talk about them," says Dr. Thys-Jacobs. "They simply endure the discomfort until days pass and they return to normalcy." A woman may even be ashamed of her symptoms. But the problem doesn't lie with a woman's personality or lack of willpower, rather within her body—beyond her control, she says. Women need to realize that treatments for PMS can cancel a woman's monthly trip to hormone hell.

# Is it PMS or something else? Get tested to rule out thyroid problems, anxiety, and depression, which have symptoms similar to PMS.—Marla Ahlgrimm, R.Ph.

First, a woman should make sure that what she's experiencing is actually PMS and not another condition. Some underlying health problems can masquerade as PMS—or make it worse, notes pharmacist **Marla Ahlgrimm, R.Ph.**, founder and chairman of Women's Health America and co-author of *Self-Help for Premenstrual Syndrome*. Most women with PMS claim that once their periods start they feel as if a cloud has lifted. However, women who suffer instead from depression, obsessive-compulsive disorders, anxiety, and even thyroid problems might maintain that they feel a little better but ... "That 'but' indicates a need to dig deeper to identify and treat the underlying problem," says Ahlgrimm. If there's a "but" in your story, talk to your doctor about testing and treatment for other conditions.

Some women experience the more serious form of PMS, known as premenstrual dysphoric disorder, or PMDD, which requires treatment by a health-care provider. (For more information, see page 272.) Others can ease PMS symptoms on their own with a variety of supplements and lifestyle adjustments.

These expert tips can help you avoid many of the pitfalls of PMS.

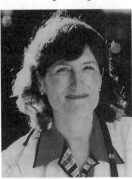

Salt and caffeine can aggravate PMS symptoms. Avoid foods with these the week before your period, recommends Mary Jane Minkin, M.D.

**Keep track.** No definitive medical tests exist to diagnose PMS, so how do you determine if you really have it? The best method is to chart your symptoms, says *Mary Jane Minkin, M.D.,* clinical professor of obstetrics and gynecology at Yale University. Your doctor can give you a chart to complete. Or you can find samples online at www.estroven.com/PMS/images/tracker.pdf or www.pampermesoftly.com/tracking/symptom-tracking.htm. To create your own chart, write the days of the month across the top of a piece of paper, then list your symptoms down the side of the page. Indicate the days on which each symptom occurs and rank its severity on a scale from 1 to 5, with 5 being the most intense. Fill out charts for at least three months to see if a pattern emerges and any remedies you tried have worked. Ahlgrimm advises you to be patient: It takes three to four months for nutritional and lifestyle changes to yield benefits.

## SHOULD I SEE A DOCTOR?

*Practically every woman suffers some discomfort during menstruation. You need to determine if your symptoms are tolerable or if they are severe enough to require medical help.*

See your physician if you experience any of these menstrual difficulties:

**PMS interferes with your life.** You should seek help if you're so depressed, anxious, edgy, irritable, tearful, or otherwise overwhelmed by symptoms of PMS that you're avoiding situations and people you used to enjoy or your job performance is affected. Consult with an endocrinologist, a doctor who specializes in hormones. The solution to your problem might be as easy as correcting a thyroid imbalance or calcium deficiency, or getting a prescription for an appropriate medication.

**You have abnormal bleeding.** See your doctor immediately if you have any of these red-flag symptoms, advises **Mary Ciotti, M.D,** an associate professor in the department of obstetrics and gynecology at the University of California at Davis:

- Spotting between periods
- Increasingly irregular periods
- Bleeding so heavy you're going through more than one pad or tampon every two hours or if a maxipad plus a tampon isn't enough to get you through the night

**You're constantly depressed.** It may be tempting to blame all depression on PMS, but that condition's symptoms ebb and flow with your menstrual cycle. If you find you're depressed

all the time—not just premenstrually—then you should seek medical help.

**You have increasing pain.** Ask your doctor about endometriosis, a condition in which tissue of the uterine lining grows outside your uterus, advises *Nanette Santoro, M.D.,* professor of obstetrics and gynecology at the Albert Einstein College of Medicine and director of the division of reproductive endocrinology and fertility at Montefiore Medical Center in New York City. This condition could be

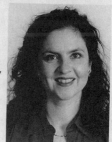

*If you have constant pelvic or lower back pain that can't be explained, ask your doctor to check you for endometriosis, says Nanette Santoro, M.D.*

a possibility if you have any of the following symptoms:

- Cramps that begin more than a few days before your menstrual cycle, last well into the cycle, and even persist after its completion
- Pain during intercourse
- Pelvic or low-back pain that's been getting worse for the last couple of years
- Infertility

For more on endometriosis, see page 384.

Charting takes the unpredictability out of PMS and provides a sense of control, says Dr. Minkin. Some women whose symptom charts show that they have only one or two difficult days each month decide not to treat their PMS medically but just rearrange their schedules. If you decide to seek help, your charts will help your doctor determine the best treatment for your individual symptoms.

*Track your PMS symptoms for several months. The charts will help you decide whether to seek medical care.*
—*Mary Jane Minkin, M.D.*

**Stabilize blood sugar.** Anxiety, mood swings, fatigue, and depression can all be triggered by changes in blood sugar, says Ahlgrimm. To keep your blood sugar on an even keel, eat such complex carbohydrates as vegetables, whole-grain breads and pastas, and brown rice. Steer clear of sugars and refined carbohydrates, including white bread, pastries and candy. Even fruits can pose a problem because the body absorbs their sugars so rapidly. "If eaten alone, fruits can act like candy," warns Ahlgrimm. Solution: Have a slow-burning whole wheat cracker or peanut butter with that fast-burning fruit to keep your blood sugar stable. You might want to divide your daily calories into six small meals a day and snack on fruits, veggies, nuts, and yogurt. But don't buy low-fat yogurt without checking the label for sugar content, Ahlgrimm warns. Too many low-fat yogurts are loaded with sugars to improve taste.

**Exercise away PMS.** "Of all the PMS remedies that a woman can try, vigorous aerobic exercise is the simplest, cheapest, and most available," says Dr. Nardone. Activity that makes you perspire relieves bloating, water retention, and related weight gain. It boosts your metabolic rate, thus fighting PMS lethargy and helping prevent weight gain. Exercise also combats premenstrual depression by triggering endorphins, the opiate-like brain chemicals that produce a natural high. Outdoor exercise has the added benefit of exposing you to sunlight, a proven treatment for seasonal affective disorder, which may worsen PMS symptoms. A brisk 20- to 30-minute walk, two to three times a week, helps reduce anxiety and fluid retention as well, says Ahlgrimm. Even if you don't exercise at any other time, try to get about a half hour of vigorous activity on each of those days of the month when your PMS symptoms flare up.

Working out with a partner or in a group provides even greater protection from PMS symptoms, since it promotes companionship, communication, and sharing. "This practice is certainly a good antidote to the feelings of loneliness and despondency that women experience with PMS," says Dr. Nardone.

**Beef up your Bs.** B-complex vitamins can help reduce the symptoms of PMS, says Ahlgrimm. Choose a B-complex supplement that balances all the major B vitamins proportionately, including thiamin, riboflavin, niacin, folate, $B_6$, and $B_{12}$. Dr. Minkin advises that $B_6$ is particularly good for relieving water retention, but cautions you not to exceed 100 milligrams a day. Taking more can put you at risk for nerve damage.

**Mine the benefits of magnesium.** This mineral helps your body utilize B vitamins and also relaxes muscles. Ahlgrimm recommends 350 to 500 milligrams magnesium daily. "Start with a low dose—100 or 200 milligrams a day—and gradually increase to 500 milligrams," she says. (The safe upper limit is 600 milligrams, says Dr. Nardone.) If you develop diarrhea, you're getting more magnesium than your body can absorb. Cut back to a dose that doesn't trigger this side effect.

**Oil up.** Gamma-linolenic acid (GLA) is an essential fatty acid (a component of fat) found in evening-primrose, borage, and black currant oils. The two days before your period begins, take 500 to 1,000 milligrams each day. This may help relieve cramps, breast pain, fluid retention, depression, and some other PMS symptoms, says *Lucinda Messer, N.D.,* a naturopathic physician in Kirkland, Washington, who specializes in women's health. You should not take GLA if you have epilepsy or take antipsychotic medication or anticoagulants, says Dr. Nardone.

**Cut back on salt.** When you eat salt, your body retains water. Since water retention is a part of so many PMS problems, Dr. Minkin recommends lowering your intake considerably. You don't have to eliminate every speck from your diet, but you should avoid salty foods in the week before your period. Be particularly wary of processed foods, which are high in sodium.

**Curb caffeine.** If anxiety and irritability plague you the week before your period, Dr. Minkin suggests limiting your caffeine intake, since it is a stimulant and can exacerbate these symptoms. Make your morning coffee decaf and go easy on the chocolate.

**Combine chocolate with cheese.** Chocolate, candy, and other confections aggravate symptoms of PMS by causing a spike in blood sugar, which is quickly followed by an energy crash. If you can't live without candy—and

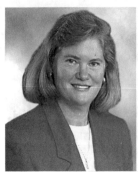

*Eating chocolate may aggravate your PMS symptoms, but you can offset its effects if you follow it up with a few bites of cheese, says Marla Ahlgrimm, R.Ph.*

who among us is immune to the temptation of chocolate?—eat cheese at the same time, suggests Ahlgrimm. She explains that the protein and fat in cheese (or other high-protein foods) can counteract the candy's effects to prevent the spike in blood-sugar levels that chocolate otherwise causes. "It's better not to eat chocolate," says Ahlgrimm, "but if you must, choose better quality chocolate products. They're better for your blood sugar and overall health than cheapo choco-fixes because they're higher in fat," she says. The higher fat content means you can satisfy your cravings with less candy, which will limit the amount of sugar released into your bloodstream.

**Avoid tenderness.** Studies show that women who take 400 International Units vitamin E daily may experience less breast soreness, says Dr. Minkin.

**For swelling and bloating, consider a diuretic.** A diuretic is a medication that removes water from the body by increasing urine flow, explains Dr. Nardone. Discuss with your doctor if it's the right medication for you. And if you decide to take it, ask your doctor to start you on the lowest dose possible, since diuretics can deplete the body of potassium, an essential mineral.

**Keep a journal.** Instead of dismissing PMS as something negative you need to get over, look at its positive side, urges *Jesse Lynn Hanley, M.D.,* a women's wellness specialist and author of *What Your Doctor May Not Tell You About Premenopause.* She points out that this is a time of month when women are often their most sensitive and creative. Use that sensitivity to listen to your inner voice by keeping a journal. If you don't feel like jotting down thoughts every day, aim for when your symptoms are at their worst. "Never stop writing at the first page," adds Dr. Hanley, "because women usually start out with things that aren't really important." If you keep writing, you get past those superficial complaints to reveal underlying problems. So when you're feeling better, you'll have a clearer picture of how you can fix those problems. For example, if, during a surge of PMS-related anger, you shout to your family, "I'm sick of cooking dinner for you every night!" Talking out this situation with yourself in your journal may reveal the real issue to be that you feel you're doing the majority of the housework. And once you know what actually triggered the outburst, you can do something about the problem.

**Rub on progesterone.** Dr. Hanley recommends the calming, hormone-balancing effect of plant-based progesterone cream to help ease PMS symptoms. Use a dose of ⅛ to ¼ teaspoon of cream. Measure carefully because this is powerful stuff. Start using the cream on Day 14 of your cycle (Day 1 is the day you begin menstruating). You can rub it anywhere on your skin, but your body will absorb the hormone faster if you apply it to an area with relatively little fat, such as your face or neck. If you have cramps, zero in on that painful area. Some women apply the cream at bedtime (it lasts 12 to 24 hours); others split the dose and apply it two or three times during the day. Continue using the cream until your period starts. On rare occasions, breast tenderness or spotting may occur when using the cream, but these side effects typically disappear in subsequent cycles.

## PMS: IS IT A CALCIUM DEFICIENCY?

*Researchers are exploring the intriguing possibility that PMS is linked to an imbalance or deficiency of calcium in the body. If they're right, an effective treatment could be just over the horizon.*

For 16 years, *Susan Thys-Jacobs, M.D.,* has been studying the connection between calcium and PMS. An endocrinologist affiliated with Columbia University and St. Luke's-Roosevelt Hospital Center in New York City, Dr. Thys-Jacobs is convinced that balancing a woman's calcium levels may be a simple and effective approach to treating the disorder.

Dr. Thys-Jacobs and researchers at 12 U.S. medical centers conducted one of the largest studies on calcium and its effects on PMS. Half of the participants took 600 milligrams supplemental calcium twice a day. The remaining test subjects took a placebo. Within two to three months, the women who took the calcium experienced a 48-percent reduction in the severity of their symptoms, with 15 out of 17 typical PMS symptoms relieved.

Calcium plays a key role in regulating many of the body's processes. Dr. Thys-Jacobs theorizes it may reduce PMS symptoms by interacting with and helping to balance hormones. Most women don't get enough calcium from their diets because they cut calories or fat, avoid dairy, or don't like calcium-rich foods. That's why Dr. Thys-Jacobs recommends calcium supplements. You can take Tums, calcium citrate, OsCal with vitamin D, or Caltrate + D (all available at most grocery stores, drugstores, and health-food stores). Take 600 milligrams in the morning along with 100 to 200 International Units vitamin D, which is essential for the absorption of calcium. Take the same dose before going to bed.

Don't expect an immediate change when taking such supplements, since they work gradually. "You will start seeing an effect within one to two months," says Dr. Thys-Jacobs. If you don't, she recommends you get a complete evaluation by your doctor. Certain medical conditions may prevent your body from using calcium properly.

**Get to know Yasmin.** If natural, over-the-counter remedies provide no relief, you may want to consider prescription medications. Dr. Minkin says one of the most promising choices is Yasmin (drospirenone/ethinyl estradiol), a birth control pill approved by the U.S. Food and Drug Administration in 2001. Yasmin blocks the hormones that cause the bloating and mood swings associated with PMS. It also acts as a diuretic, further decreasing bloating and tenderness. It can cause side effects and interact with other medications, so make sure you inform your physician immediately if any new symptoms appear after starting the medication.

## PMDD: WHEN THE MONSTER GETS OUT OF CONTROL

Are your PMS symptoms really severe? You're not only tearful, blue, achy, and bloated, but also you fly into rages, plummet into the pit of depression, trash relationships, kick the dog, and are unable to function normally even with the help of some or all of the PMS remedies we've talked about? If so, you may be one of the 3 to 5 percent of women who have premenstrual dysphoric disorder (PMDD). Think of it as PMS on steroids.

Researchers don't know what causes PMDD but suspect it's linked to low levels of serotonin, the brain chemical that plays a key role in mood, appetite, and sleep. They've found that PMDD occurs most often in women who have a history of mood disorders, such as clinical depression, postpartum depression, obsessive-compulsive disorder, or anxiety. Treatments for PMDD's physical symptoms are similar to those for PMS. The same can't be said for PMDD's emotional symptoms—the usual remedies just aren't effective for the intense symptoms of this disorder.

An important breakthrough in treating PMDD came in the 1990s when it was identified as a separate condition from PMS, explains *Mary Jane Minkin, M.D.*, clinical professor of obstetrics and gynecology at Yale University. The breakthrough in treatment came with the introduction of selective serotonin reuptake inhibitors (SSRIs), a class of medications used to treat depression. Even though women with depression may take several weeks to respond to an SSRI, women with PMDD often feel better within a day of taking one, says Dr. Minkin. This is a clear indication that serotonin is somehow involved in the disorder.

Prozac (fluoxetine) and Zoloft (sertraline) are the two SSRIs that the U.S. Food and Drug Administration has approved for PMDD. If neither of these is effective for you or they produce side effects, ask your doctor about other SSRIs, such as Celexa (citalopram) or Paxil (paroxetine), says *Adelaide Nardone, M.D.,* an obstetrician and gynecologist in Providence, Rhode Island, and a medical advisor to the Vagisil Women's Health Center.

When marketed for PMDD, Prozac goes by the brand name Sarafem. You can take it daily or just when your symptoms are a problem, such as the seven days before your period, says Dr. Nardone. With any SSRI, you and your doctor should work out a dosage that controls symptoms while also preventing or minimizing side effects.

## CRAMPS: ALLEVIATE THE ACHE

Got cramps? Join the crowd. More than half of all menstruating women suffer from them at least one to two days during their periods.

The medical term for menstrual cramps is primary dysmenorrhea, but whatever you call them, cramps can make you miserable. They're caused by contractions of the uterus that are triggered by hormones called prostaglandins. The result is that all-too-familiar aching fullness or heaviness of an impending or beginning period. They're also the bad guys that induce intestinal cramps and bring on diarrhea. Feel lightheaded? It's probably those prostaglandins again, kicking a few points off your blood pressure and making you dizzy. The cramps of secondary dysmenorrhea—an uncommon condition—are caused by reproductive problems, such as fibroids or endometriosis, says *Mary Jane Minkin, M.D.,* clinical professor of obstetrics and gynecology at Yale University in New Haven, Connecticut.

Most women experience their worst menstrual cramps during their teens. The pain tends to diminish after childbirth (perhaps because the cervix expands) or as women get older, when blood is able to pass more easily during menstruation, says Dr. Minkin.

Don't try to tough it out. It's easier to prevent pain altogether than to reduce it. Here's what you can do to prevent cramps.

**Block prostaglandins.** You can disrupt the process by which prostaglandins cause cramps with over-the-counter (OTC) nonsteroidal anti-inflammatory drugs (NSAIDs), says Dr. Minkin. The key is to stop prostaglandin action early, *before* you hurt. So take aspirin, ibuprofen, or naproxen at the first twinge. If these OTC drugs don't work, talk to your doctor about more powerful

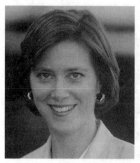

Nancy Lonsdorf, M.D., suggests you soothe menstrual cramps with a hot water bottle on your abdomen or lower back.

medicines, suggests **Mary Ciotti, M.D.**, associate professor in the department of obstetrics and gynecology at the University of California at Davis.

**Try vitamin E.** Research shows that vitamin E may inhibit the formation of prostaglandins. A study found that menstrual pain was reduced in women who took 100 International Units vitamin E five times a day for five days, beginning two days before menstruation.

**Apply heat.** Gently massage your abdomen, then cover it with a hot water bottle to relieve discomfort, advises **Nancy Lonsdorf, M.D.**, medical director for the Raj Ayur-Veda Health Center in Fairfield, Iowa, and author of *A Woman's Best Medicine for Menopause.* Or put the soothing heat on your lower back.

**Mellow out with magnesium.** This mineral is nature's muscle relaxant, says woman's wellness specialist *Jesse Lynn Hanley, M.D.* Soak it up by adding old-fashioned Epsom salts to a soothing bath or take magnesium supplements to ease muscle cramps. Dr. Hanley recommends taking 400 milligrams magnesium oxide a day, beginning the week before your period, until your period starts. The main side effect of overdosing is diarrhea, so you'll know if you need to cut back.

**Be good to yourself.** Make time to rest when your flow is heavy, usually on Days 2 and 3 of your period. You don't have to take to your bed, but you should slow down. "This is a time to be kind to your body," says Dr. Lonsdorf. Plan your schedule to include only light work or chores on these days. Turn in for the night at a decent hour.

**Talk to your doctor about the Pill.** Many gynecologists are recommending women take birth control pills continuously, eliminating the "dummy pills" in the last week of the pill pack. "This type of regimen eliminates the monthly bleeding that occurs during that week—and many of the annoying symptoms of menstruation," says **Adelaide Nardone, M.D.**, an obstetrician and gynecologist in Providence, Rhode Island, and a medical advisor to the Vagisil Women's Health Center. However, there can be irregular bleeding with this regimen, so discuss its pros and cons with your doctor, she says.

Another potential option—in clinical trials at the time of this book's publication—is Seasonale, a new type of low-dose birth control pill that blocks menstruation for three months.

# AMENORRHEA: THE CASE OF THE MISSING PERIOD

*After all the hassle of having periods, shouldn't we be relieved when they just go away? Not necessarily.*

There are times when having no period is normal: before you even start menstruating, during pregnancy, and after menopause. In addition, breast feeding can put your period on pause, and accelerating perimenopause may result in fewer periods. But when you've been menstruating regularly and then suddenly stop, it could be a warning sign. Here are some conditions that can cause your period to cease:

- Stress
- Medicines and birth control pills
- Polycystic ovarian diseases
- Pituitary or thyroid problems
- Excessive weight loss or weight gain
- Chronic illness

Consult your doctor if you've gone two to three months without menstruating, recommends *Nanette Santoro, M.D.,* professor of obstetrics and gynecology at the Albert Einstein College of Medicine and director of division of reproductive endocrinology and fertility at Montefiore Medical Center in New York City. "For a woman in her 40s or 50s, ascribing the absence of her period to menopause can be a mistake," she cautions. So see your doctor if you've stopped having periods but don't have any menopausal symptoms, such as hot flashes, vaginal dryness, sweats, or sleep disturbances.

Strenuous exercise can cause athletes to not have periods. Working out to the point of amenorrhea is most common with women in their 20s and 30s. But it can happen to a woman at any age if she burns off more calories than she consumes, even if she doesn't appear to lose weight, says *Nancy I. Williams, Ph.D.,* assistant professor of Kinesiology and Physiology at Pennsylvania State University at Philadelphia. Her studies suggest that the body adapts to taking in fewer calories and using more, a typical scenario for a woman who diets and exercises. This can cause the body to produce lower-than-usual levels of thyroid hormone, which in turn affects estrogen levels, thus disrupting ovulation and menstruation.

Dr. Williams hopes to determine the exact calorie intake that can prevent exercise-induced amenorrhea and maintain healthy estrogen levels. "Estrogen is a key hormone in the body for many physiological systems, influencing bone strength and cardiovascular health, not just reproduction," she says. For now, Dr. Williams recommends adding about 300 calories of healthful foods to your daily diet to reverse exercise-induced amenorrhea.

And for women in their teens, it's important to do reverse exercise-induced amennorhea *as soon as possible,* says *Adelaide Nardone, M.D.,* an obstetrician and gynecologist in private practice in Providence, Rhode Island. "They need estrogen for normal reproductive development and normal growth," she points out. "If you have a daughter with this problem and it persists for two to three months, see a gynecologist and discuss whether or not she should take birth control pills or hormone replacement therapy."

# 15 Mind and Emotions
## Smart and Sensitive
## Advice for the Inner You

*Reality is the leading cause of stress
among those in touch with it.*
—Lily Tomlin, actress and comedienne

Remember this television advertisement? A phone rings, kids scream, a dog barks, and a pot boils over on the stove—and in the midst of all the chaos, a frazzled woman moans, "It's another Excedrin headache." That commercial aired years ago, and the marketing pros behind it knew then what most of us know today: The bustle of daily life can have a significant bearing on our health, both emotionally and physically.

The relationship between mind and body is powerful and complex,

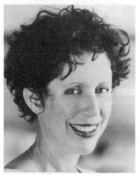

says *Jessie Gruman, Ph.D.,* executive director of the Center for the Advancement of Health in Washington, D.C. Stress, anger, and anxiety cause the release of stress hormones and raise blood pressure and heart rate. Although those changes aren't harmful in the short run, over time unrelieved stress can lead to a variety of physical ailments, including adult-onset diabetes, impaired memory, slower healing of wounds, and heart disease.

*Stress and negative emotions can push women into such destructive activities as smoking, overeating, drug use, and excessive drinking, says Jessie Gruman, Ph.D.*

Beyond the direct links between stress and health, however, are indirect effects. To cope with troubling feelings, some women turn to such unhealthy behaviors as smoking, overeating, using recreational drugs, or abusing alcohol—all of which can harm a woman's health and life, says Dr. Gruman.

There are several ways to better manage stress and emotions so that you can live a healthier life, says **Helen Grusd, Ph.D.**, past president of the Los Angeles County Psychological Association. They include changing your attitudes, improving your diet, and increasing your workouts.

Dr. Grusd should know: She holds a clinical faculty appointment at University of California at Los Angeles Medical School, where she teaches biopsychosocial medicine. In simple language, that means treatment of body, mind, and relationships. And, she says, the best way to ensure the wellness of your biopsychosocial being is to be in touch with yourself. Too many women only realize something is wrong when they've reached 10 on the severity-of-symptoms scale. "Don't wait until you get to that point," she counsels. "Catch yourself when you're still a 4."

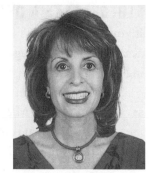

Healthy lifestyle choices, such as a balanced diet and regular exercise, help manage stress and negative emotions, says Helen Grusd, Ph.D.

*Many women don't realize the severity of their problems until they're ready to boil over. Don't wait until you reach that point—be in touch with yourself and recognize the warning signs.*

*—Helen Grusd, Ph.D.*

So just as you monitor the oil and gas levels in your car, you need to keep a check on your feelings, says Dr. Grusd. Ask yourself the following questions: How high is my anxiety level? Am I running low on patience? Is my anger in danger of boiling over? How do these emotions compare to how I felt yesterday ... last week?

The first step toward this kind of awareness is deepening your understanding of stress and emotional problems. The second step is managing these difficulties with self-treatment, professional help, or a combination of the two. Which means your immediate next step is this: Keep reading!

## STRESS: TAKE A DEEP BREATH

If you're like most women, your life sometimes feels like a frantic juggling act. The faster you juggle, the more balls get added to the mix. You're dealing with the modern problem of chronic stress.

Stress can bring on a host of physical diseases and behavioral symptoms, says *Nassim Assefi, M.D.,* women's health attending physician in the departments of medicine and obstetrics and gynecology at the University of Washington School of Medicine in Seattle. By-products of stress include:

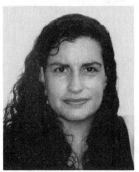

*Today's woman deals with more pressures than her sisters of previous generations, says Nassim Assefi, M.D. Chronic stress can be the cause of debilitating health problems, including ulcers, back pain, eating disorders, and insomnia.*

- Physical problems: irritable bowel syndrome, nausea, abdominal pain, heartburn, ulcer, loss of appetite, heart palpitations, headache, back pain, high blood pressure, frequent illnesses
- Eating disorders: binge eating, anorexia, or bulimia
- Lifestyle difficulties: substance abuse, frequent minor accidents, difficulty functioning at school or on the job, family conflicts, relationship problems, social withdrawal
- Emotional troubles: anxiety, irritability, anger, depression, insomnia, difficulty concentrating, fatigue, negative thinking

If you experience any of these concerns, see your doctor to rule out a physical cause, says Dr. Assefi. If stress is the reason for the problem or is responsible for worsening symptoms of an ongoing condition, your doctor may refer you to a qualified mental-health professional.

Even if you decide to seek professional help, there are numerous steps you can take on your own. There are no hard-and-fast rules for coping with stress. It's simply a matter of finding what works for you. Your best friend may find her morning jog a necessary pressure-buster, while you feel that getting up an hour earlier to exercise only adds to your stress.

Experiment to find the best combination of stress-relievers for you. Here are some useful recommendations.

**Find a friend.** Women seem to naturally seek out pals as a response to stress, says *Shelley E. Taylor, Ph.D.,* a psychology professor at the University of California at Los Angeles. Dr. Taylor refers to this as the tend-and-befriend pattern. She says that females of many species—including humans—respond to stressful conditions by protecting and nurturing their young (the tend response) and by seeking social contact and support from others, especially other females (the befriend response). Think about the last time you had a fight with your husband or teenager. Did you stew about it alone? Or did you reach for the phone to call your best friend? Even asking for directions when you get lost (a typically female response) is an effort to reach out and touch someone socially, says Dr. Taylor.

She and her fellow researchers believe this tend-and-befriend pattern may have a biological basis, due in part to women's high levels of the hormone oxytocin. Oxytocin has been studied largely for its role in childbirth, but both men and women secrete it in response to stress. Animals and people with high levels of oxytocin are calmer, as well as more relaxed and social.

## Don't let everyday annoyances add to your stress. Learn to tolerate things you can't change.—Annette Annechild, Ph.D.

**Join a support group.** As Dr. Taylor's theory shows, it's important for women to talk to one another. "We need to connect with people who can relate to our experiences and reinforce how valuable and worthwhile our contributions are," says *Joan Broderick, Ph.D.*, assistant clinical professor of psychiatry in the Applied Behavioral Medicine Research Institute at the State University of New York at Stony Brook. A group provides support, whether formally (through a mental-health organization or hospital) or informally (like a monthly book group or stock club).

**Accept what you can't change.** This applies not only to serious situations, but also to minor annoyances that aggravate you every day, says *Annette Annechild, Ph.D.*, director of Healing Arts Center of Georgetown in Washington, D.C. For instance, there's little you can do about a traffic jam. Instead of drumming your fingers on the steering wheel and sending your blood pressure soaring, you might listen to a favorite CD, read a book you keep in the car for

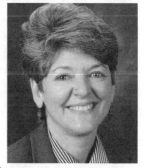

*Women need to lean on each other in times of trouble, says Joan Broderick, Ph.D. Finding a support group will link you with people who can relate to your experiences.*

such times, fantasize about your next vacation, or simply take a few deep breaths. (For more on deep breathing, see "Stress-Busters," page 283.)

**Know when to change.** On the other hand, there are times you need to make alterations in your life, says Dr. Annechild. If you're overcommitted and can't handle one more responsibility, just say so. Politely decline when you're nominated to serve on a committee. See if you can arrange a flextime schedule at work. Get your family to give you more help around the house. Unless you ask for—and make—changes, you can't expect to see results.

> *You're in charge of making changes in your life, so learn how to say no to impossible demands.—Annette Annechild, Ph.D.*

**Step it up.** Take an aerobics class, jog, walk, skip rope—just get moving, says Dr. Annechild. Aerobic exercise increases the heart rate and releases feel-good hormones, called endorphins, that help you manage stress. At the University of Illinois at Urbana-Champaign, researchers recently found that regular exercise—as little as 30 minutes a day, three times a week—is not only good for your body, but also good for your mind.

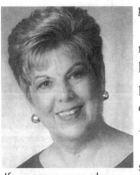

If your nerves are on edge, rethink your choice of beverage. Lay off the caffeinated coffee, tea, or soft drinks, advises Shoshana Zimmerman, N.D. Try herbal tea instead.

**Skip Starbucks.** Caffeine only adds to your jangled nerves by acting as a central nervous–system stimulant, says *Shoshana Zimmerman, N.D.*, a naturopathic physician in Palo Alto, California, and co-author of *My Doctor Says I'm Fine … So Why Do I Feel So Bad?* Opt for herbal tea.

**Keep laughing.** Humor helps keep things in perspective and defuses stressful situations, advises Christiane Northrup, M.D., author of *The Wisdom of Menopause*. To regain a sense of well-being, watch *I Love Lucy* or some other comedy you enjoy. Go see a funny movie. Check out humorous books, magazines, or videos. Dr. Northrup recommends humorist and stress expert Loretta LaRoche. Watch LaRoche's video *How Serious Is This?* or read her book *Relax—You May Only Have a Few Minutes Left.*

## SHOULD I SEE A DOCTOR?

*Everyone experiences some depression and anxiety in life. But when "sometimes" becomes "all the time," go to the doctor.*

**Hinda Dubin, M.D.,** clinical assistant professor of psychiatry at the University of Maryland School of Medicine in Baltimore, recommends seeing your physician immediately if you experience any of the following symptoms for more than two weeks:

- Sadness or anxiety
- Lack of interest in activities you formerly found pleasurable
- Feelings of hopelessness or pessimism
- Sleep disturbances
- Changes in appetite; weight loss or gain
- Decreased energy or fatigue
- Difficulty concentrating
- Physical symptoms, such as digestive upsets that don't respond to treatment

Your doctor may refer you to a qualified mental-health professional. Before your first appointment with a therapist, write down your feelings and how you've been managing those feelings. Keep track for a week and see if you notice any change, recommends **Jessie Gruman, Ph.D.,** executive director of the Center for the Advancement of Health in Washington, D.C.

An emotional time line of your life may also help you and your therapist identify patterns: When did you get married? When did you start drinking? When did you first feel depressed? "Therapy is much like 'X marks the spot,'" says **Annette Annechild, Ph.D.,** director of the Healing Arts Center of Georgetown. "How did we get here? And where are we going?"

If you choose to see a mental-health professional, it's important to find someone you trust, whether that's a psychiatrist, psychologist, social worker, or pastoral counselor. A psychiatrist is a medical doctor and can prescribe medications, such as antidepressants. The others can't write prescriptions, although they frequently work in conjunction with psychiatrists.

Interview at least two or three therapists before settling on a choice, suggests Dr. Gruman. Before you choose one, she recommends asking yourself these crucial questions: Does this person seem to understand me? Am I—or could I become—comfortable in his or her presence? Could I develop confidence in this person's ability to help me? Is this person judging me or cutting me off before really hearing my story? Does this person use language and have ideas that make sense to me?

Remember that you don't have to be in therapy for the rest of your life. Short-term care focused on problem solving is often quite effective. Most women do fine seeing a therapist for 6 to 10 sessions, then checking back in periodically, says Dr. Gruman.

If you find that the therapy isn't working or that the therapist isn't sympathetic or experienced with your particular problems, try someone else. "Be a savvy consumer," says Dr. Gruman. "Just because someone studied psychology in school doesn't mean she has all the answers or is the right therapist for you."

*If you don't know how to have fun,
then you're probably not fun to be
with. Find something that gives you
pleasure—a hobby or sport, perhaps.*
—*Annette Annechild, Ph.D.*

**Find your bliss.** "Women so rarely know what their pleasure is," says Dr. Annechild. And when we don't have enough merriment in our lives, we can become martyrs and nags—which is no fun for us or anyone else. Don't remember what amusement is? Think back to your childhood. Did you enjoy ice skating … finger painting … jigsaw puzzles? Pick a favorite activity and try it again. Or check out adult-education classes at a local community college. Choose something you've never done before, like painting or quilting or auto mechanics. You may discover a completely new side of yourself.

**Check in each hour.** Get a watch with an alarm and set it to go off every hour, says Dr. Annechild. Each time it beeps, ask yourself, "What's the best thing I can do for myself right now?" The answer could be as basic as taking the time to go to the bathroom, getting a drink of water, or walking around the block. Even giving yourself a spritz of perfume can do wonders for your mind-set and feelings about yourself.

**Get your finances in order.** Fiscal worries are a common cause of stress, says **Virginia B. Morris, Ph.D.**, author of *A Woman's Guide to Personal Finance*. If you're drowning in debt, curb your spending, seek help from a financial planner, or call a credit counselor who will work with you and your creditors to come up with a plan to help you dig out from under. To find a counselor in your area, contact the National Foundation for Credit Counseling at 800-388-2227 or online at www.nfcc.org.

**Revisit your priorities.** Are you working overtime to buy a bigger house, a better car, a more stylish wardrobe? Think about what's really important to you, advises Dr. Annechild. Write down the priorities in your life and set goals to achieve them. Then whenever something stressful intrudes, ask yourself where it fits in on that list. If it doesn't, find a way to eliminate it.

**Ask for help.** You don't have to go it alone, says Dr. Annechild. When life gets a bit much to handle, ask family and friends to pitch in. Their input could be as simple as picking up the kids from school or taking the dog to the vet, or as complex as taking over your life for a couple days while you check into a hotel for a much-needed getaway. Promise your rescuers you'll do the same for them when they feel stressed to the max.

**Learn stress-relieving techniques.** These skills include visualization, deep breathing, progressive muscle relaxation, and meditation, says Dr. Annechild. (To learn more, see "Stress-Busters" below.)

## STRESS-BUSTERS

*Annette Annechild, Ph.D.,* director of the Healing Arts Center of Georgetown, teaches stress-reduction techniques to the harried—and often high-powered—clients she sees in her Washington, D.C., practice. These are some of the pressure-relievers she recommends.

**Visualization:** Also called guided imagery, you practice this technique by making mental pictures of relaxing situations. Accompanied by deep breathing, visualization can lower heart rate and blood pressure. To get started, sit down and get comfortable. Take several slow, deep breaths. Close your eyes and imagine yourself in a tranquil setting, perhaps at your favorite beach. Picture the scene with all your senses: Feel the warm sand between your toes; smell the salt air; hear the waves crashing on the shore; sip a cool fruit drink, watch seagulls coast on the breeze. The more you put yourself into the scene, the more your body can convince itself that it's actually there. When you're ready to return to the present, stretch your fingers and toes, then your entire body, and slowly open your eyes.

**Deep abdominal breathing:** Controlled breathing can reduce the release of stress hormones in your body and slow your heart rate. The increased oxygen that is brought in by deep abdominal breathing also causes your body to release endorphins, which are natural mood-enhancing hormones. To practice such deep breathing, lie on your back in a quiet room free from distractions. Place your hands on your abdomen. Take a slow, deep breath through your nostrils. If you're breathing correctly, your hands will rise as your abdomen expands. Then exhale. Now inhale again and count to five. Pause for three seconds, then exhale to a count of five. Do this exercise 10 times the first time you try it. Gradually increase to 25 repetitions, twice a day.

**Meditation:** A 1992 study published in the *Journal of Transpersonal Psychology* found that people who meditated on a regular basis were more relaxed, better able to control negative thoughts, and calmer in stressful situations. The meditation that Dr. Annechild recommends can quiet your body and mind. She suggests meditating for about 20 minutes, twice daily—but even five minutes a day will work wonders.

**A pleasing word or sound, sometimes referred to as a mantra:** Repeat it over and over. Focus on the word or sound itself. Don't become distracted, frustrated, or upset if other thoughts intrude. Acknowledge them and refocus on your chosen mantra. The traditional Sanskrit word used in meditation is *om,* but you can select a word or sound—or even a phrase—such as *peace* or *love,* anything, in fact, that makes you feel comfortable and relaxed.

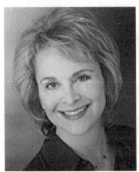

**Think herbal.** Plant remedies, such as kava and valerian, may ease symptoms of anxiety, says *Hyla Cass, M.D.*, assistant clinical professor of psychiatry at the University of California at Los Angeles School of Medicine and author of several books on herbal remedies, including *Kava: Nature's Answer to Stress, Anxiety, and Insomnia.*

Kava is often used as a sleep aid and muscle relaxant. In recent scientific research, it has been shown to be as effective as some prescription antianxiety medications, without the side effects of lethargy and fuzzy thinking. However, in both Europe and the United States, there are warnings about the potential for liver toxicity (such as liver failure) caused by the use of kava. The U.S. Food and Drug Administration's current recommendation is that anyone who has known liver problems or who takes drugs that affect the liver should not use kava.

*If you don't want to take a prescription anxiety medication, ask your doctor about natural remedies like kava and valerian, suggests Hyla Cass, M.D.*

Sold over the counter in most health-food stores and drugstores, kava is available in tablets, capsules, tincture, and even sprays. The taste of kava is quite strong, so most people prefer tablets or capsules, says Dr. Cass. She recommends taking a dose that contains 60 to 75 milligrams kavalactones (the active ingredient), two to three times daily. Also effective for anxiety, says Dr. Cass, is the herb valerian, which acts as a mild tranquilizer. The capsule form of valerian is your best bet, since the herb has an unpleasant taste and odor. Dr. Cass suggests using a standardized extract (0.8-percent valeric acid) and taking 50 to 100 milligrams, two to three times daily, for relaxation. This word of caution from Dr. Cass: Valerian can interact with alcohol and certain antihistamines, muscle relaxants, psychotropic drugs, and narcotics. If you're on any of these medications, you should take valerian only under the supervision of a health-care practitioner.

*Kava is as effective as some antianxiety drugs but doesn't make you feel tired or loopy. It's not for you, though, if you have liver problems.*

## DEPRESSION: BEYOND THE BLUES

As Susanna, a 60-year-old public-relations executive in Baltimore, describes it, her lifelong bouts with clinical depression leave her feeling like she's "swimming through mud." But clinical depression is more than a simple case of blahs. It's a serious illness that affects twice as many women as men, usually striking between the ages of 18 and 44. The first step toward recovery from depression is admitting that you have it. That's often difficult for today's always-in-control woman to do, says *Helen Grusd, Ph.D.,* past president of the Los Angeles County Psychological Association.

*Depression affects twice as many women as men, and younger women more than seniors. Hormones and genetics are key factors.—Helen Grusd, Ph.D.*

Depression hits for many reasons, says *Hinda Dubin, M.D.,* clinical assistant professor of psychiatry at the University of Maryland School of Medicine in Baltimore. It may be caused by an imbalance in the brain chemicals, known as neurotransmitters, that send messages between brain cells and affect behavior, emotions, and thought. It could be triggered by stress, grief, or other difficult situations. In women, depression may also result from hormonal changes that go along with birth control pills, premenstrual syndrome (PMS), and postpartum depression, says Dr. Dubin.

Family history also comes into play. If you have a parent, sibling, or other close relative who has suffered from depression, you're likely to experience it yourself. Your psychological makeup also determines your propensity for the condition. Women with low self-esteem who are pessimistic and easily overwhelmed by stress are more prone to depression than optimistic women with high self-esteem who are upbeat and handle stress well, says Dr. Grusd.

Depression can also be a by-product of serious illness, such as stroke, diabetes, or cancer, as well as of certain medications, such as those prescribed for high blood pressure, arthritis, and acne, says Dr. Dubin. In some cases, the pain and frustration of an illness causes depression; in others, the condition—or the medication used to treat it—causes changes in the body's chemistry, resulting in depression.

## ONE WOMAN'S STORY: DEPRESSION

*Leslie Preston, age 54, is a single woman living near Washington, D.C. She works in the real-estate field. Preston experienced her first case of serious depression 16 years ago, after ending a serious relationship.*

It came on slowly, over a period of four to six months. Unlike many women who suffer from depression, Leslie Preston (not her real name) slept fine and continued functioning well at her job. But she lost a lot of weight and felt increasingly blue. The thought crossed her mind that she was becoming depressed, but since she'd never been so down before, she figured maybe she just had a lingering case of the flu.

Finally, though, there was no escaping how low she felt. "I knew something was wrong, and I wanted to take care of it," says Preston. She made an appointment with a therapist.

Preston saw the therapist once a week for several months but didn't notice any improvement. In fact, she felt worse. The therapist said that if Preston didn't feel better soon, she would recommend Preston see a psychiatrist, who would be able to prescribe antidepressants.

That January, Preston hit her lowest point. "I felt alone and desperate," she recalls. "It felt like I was at the bottom of a black hole and couldn't find my way out. I saw only blackness. There was no light, no hope." To make matters worse, all of Preston's friends and relatives were out of town at the time. When Preston reached her parents, they heard how desperate she sounded and flew home immediately. They took her to see a psychiatrist who, unbeknownst to Preston, had previously treated family members. It turned out that depression runs on both sides of her family. With that biological fix in, the psychiatrist told her "there was little chance I could have escaped."

After evaluating Preston's condition, the psychiatrist decided that he wouldn't admit her to a hospital since she wasn't suicidal. "I never wanted to kill myself," Preston says. "All I wanted was to feel better."

To diagnose depression, says Dr. Dubin, your doctor will look for four to five of the following symptoms.

- Sleep disturbances: You may wake early in the morning and be unable to get back to sleep, or sleep too much or too little.
- Lack of interest: People suffering from depression often lose interest in activities that they previously enjoyed.
- Feelings of guilt: We all heap blame on ourselves from time to time. But if you're experiencing such guilt most of the time, that may signal depression.
- Low energy: Lack of vitality is frequently a symptom of depression.
- Lack of concentration: When you're depressed, you may have difficulty focusing your mind.
- Appetite disturbances: Lack of appetite is a common symptom of depression, but increased appetite can also be an atypical sign.

Preston saw the psychiatrist six days a week for several years and began taking an antidepressant. For the first month, she counted relief in seconds. "One day, there were 20 seconds when I didn't feel like there was no hope," she says. "Then there was a minute, then a minute and a half. "It was six months before Preston began feeling that she was no longer in the dark, a year before she felt normal. But normal isn't quite the right word.

"I never did get back to feeling the way I had before," she says. "This was starting all over. It was the worst thing that had ever happened to me, but in equal measures also the best."

Looking back, Preston thinks the depression was her body's way of telling her to focus on her life. "I'd never been an introspective person, and I had never really examined my life," she says. "I wasn't listening to what was going on in my life and relationships. So my body said it was time to shut down and start paying attention."

For years, Preston was terrified that the depression would return. But that fear has faded. Still, she doesn't take any chances. While she no longer takes antidepressants, she continues to see a therapist once every six weeks "to touch base and make sure I'm on the right track. "She has also learned to recognize some of her triggers for depression—one taboo is spending too much time alone. "Going for long periods without seeing someone is very bad for me," Preston says. "I make sure I'm as busy as possible."

Today, she keeps a list of people she can contact if she's having a bad day. "I've learned that just because one person isn't available when I call doesn't mean that I'm alone in the world," she says. "It just means that not everyone can be there for you at the same time, in the same way, so I just go down the list until someone's around."

Preston's personal guideline? If she's feeling seriously out of sorts for more than 48 hours, it's time to do something about it. That usually means calling a friend. "But I wouldn't hesitate to start seeing the therapist more often or taking antidepressants again," Preston emphasizes. "It's hard to reach out when you're feeling so bad, but it's the most important thing you can do."

- Psychomotor changes: Being unable to motivate yourself to move or, alternately, being restless, fidgety, and unable to sit still can be symptoms of depression.
- Thoughts of suicide: Thinking of killing yourself—or a preoccupation with death, in general—is a strong indication of depression. (If you're feeling suicidal, call 911 immediately.)

If you think you may be suffering from serious depression, call your physician, says Dr. Dubin. She will evaluate you for physical conditions that can cause similar symptoms. If you are diagnosed with depression, you can start therapy with your primary-care doctor. Or you may be referred to a mental-health professional who can offer a variety of treatments, from cognitive behavioral therapy (which helps you reframe how you think about yourself and your life) to lifestyle changes, hypnosis, or antidepressant medications.

Of course, not all cases of depression require medical help. Sometimes, you're just suffering from the blues—you know, those days when life really isn't a bowl of cherries. Whether it's caused by a looming deadline at work, a fight with your husband, or cabin fever from being stuck in the house with sick kids, you're in a funk. It's not a fun way to feel, but it's fleeting—simply a part of the rhythm of life that we all go through.

## BOUNCING BACK FROM THE BLUES

You've probably developed your own ways of coping with mild depression, from watching a weepy movie to spooning through a pint of Rocky Road. Here are a few more coping mechanisms you might try on a down day.

**Accept the fact that you're depressed.** If you don't feel comfortable talking about your depression to family or friends, Dr. Grusd suggests that you join a support group. Call a local hospital or state agency to find an organization in your area. Meeting people who are going through the same thing will help you realize that you're not alone and that depression is nothing to be ashamed of. Whether your condition is caused by a chemical imbalance or life-changing event, don't bottle up your feelings. Most therapists agree that acceptance is necessary before healing can take place.

## ANTIDEPRESSANTS: WHEN DRUGS MAY BE PART OF THE SOLUTION

*For serious depression, drugs are often recommended as an adjunct to psychotherapy.*

To ease mild to moderate depression, talk therapy and self-help techniques may be all that's needed, says **Hinda Dubin, M.D.**, clinical assistant professor of psychiatry at the University of Maryland School of Medicine in Baltimore. But more serious cases may require the assistance of medication.

Two symptoms of clinical depression, explains Dr. Dubin, are lack of energy and impaired concentration, which can keep you from making the most of therapy. The right antidepressant may improve vitality and focus so that you can center on your treatment. It can also help to boost your appetite, ease sleep problems, and correct the chemical imbalances in the brain that can cause depression.

Dr. Dubin says three categories of antidepressants are most commonly prescribed for depression:

- Tricyclic antidepressants, which include such drugs as Elavil (amitriptyline) and Tofranil (imipramine)
- Monoamine oxidase inhibitors (MAOIs), which include Nardil (phenelzine) and Parnate (tranylcypromine)
- Selective serotonin reuptake inhibitors (SSRIs), which include such drugs as Celexa (citalopram), Luvox (fluvoxamine maleate), Paxil (paroxetine), and Prozac (fluoxetine), as well as Zoloft (sertraline)

**Try talk therapy.** When you're depressed, you may want nothing more than to be alone—but that's when you most need to be with others. Discussing your problems with supportive and caring friends, relatives, a religious advisor, or therapist helps you feel less isolated, says *Jessie Gruman, Ph.D.,* executive director of the Center for the Advancement of Health in Washington, D.C. It also provides other—often less personally critical—perspectives on your situation. Consider a support group, organized through most local hospitals. Or try your religious counselor.

*Exercise may help depression as effectively as psychotherapy or medication. Just 90 minutes a week lifts your mood.—Hinda Dubin, M.D.*

**Get moving.** Exercise is one of the best things you can do for yourself when you're depressed. It improves blood flow to the brain, thus elevating mood by triggering the release of endorphins and relieving stress, says Dr. Dubin.

Because SSRIs have fewer—as well as more benign—side effects than the other categories of antidepressants, most physicians will start you off with this kind of antidepressant, says Dr. Dubin. If the first SSRI doesn't work, the doctor will probably prescribe another before trying a different category of medication. Your doctor will take into account your medical history and symptoms when choosing an antidepressant for you. For example, Prozac may keep you awake, so if you already have trouble sleeping, a better option might be Paxil, with its more sedating effect.

While these drugs are generally effective and have fewer side effects than earlier generations of medications, they are not reaction-free, says Dr. Dubin. For instance, tricyclics can cause dry mouth, constipation, and irregular heartbeat.

MAOIs can produce food and drug interactions (avoid aged cheeses, yogurt, sour cream, beer, and wine). And SSRIs may induce mild gastrointestinal problems and sexual difficulties, such as decreased desire or inability to reach orgasm.

All antidepressants approved by the U.S. Food and Drug Administration are equally effective in general and offer a 60 to 80 percent chance of improving your symptoms. They are not equally effective in each case, however, says Dr. Dubin, and doctors can't always predict which drug is best for which patient.

If your doctor prescribes medication, don't get impatient, says Dr. Dubin. Antidepressants, while effective, are not a quick fix. Many may begin to work within two weeks, but it may take up to eight weeks before you see noticeable improvement.

Working out allows you to focus on something other than your depression and can provide a sense of control and feeling of accomplishment, as well as an improvement of self-esteem. In studies, researchers have found that jogging for 30 minutes, three times a week, can be just as effective as psychotherapy in treating depression. You don't have to jog, though—any exercise you enjoy will give you the same benefits. Even if you've been sedentary a long time, adding half an hour of activity (such as walking, gardening, or housecleaning) to your routine will help.

**Take a break.** If you're depressed because you're in a rut or going through stressful times, get lost for a few days, suggests *Annette Annechild, Ph.D.,* director of the Healing Arts Center of Georgetown in Washington, D.C. Don't think of it as running away; instead, consider it a much-needed gift to yourself to gain perspective on everyday life. You may have friends or family who can fill in at home while you're gone. If days away are out of the question, settle for an afternoon off—go to the movies, get a massage, sit in the park. Or perhaps treat yourself to a weekend free of errands, laundry, cooking, or other chores. Stock up on books, magazines, and videos. Order in, light a fire, and stay in your pajamas all weekend. If you have kids, let your husband or best friend look after them. Any change of routine—no matter how brief the experience—will give you a lift.

## MOTHER NATURE, M.D.: DEPRESSION

The herb Saint-John's-wort is as effective a treatment for mild to moderate depression as such antidepressants as Prozac. Even better, studies show it has none of the side effects of prescription medications, says *Hyla Cass, M.D.,* assistant clinical professor of psychiatry at the University of California at Los Angeles School of Medicine and author of All About St. John's Wort.

Saint-John's-wort probably acts as a selective serotonin reuptake inhibitor, says Dr. Cass. It may also enhance the brain's stimulant neurotransmitters: dopamine and norepinephrine.

Saint-John's-wort isn't addictive and has no withdrawal symptoms, says Dr. Cass. It improves sleep and dreaming, but doesn't cause drowsiness or agitation. It can also be used as an antianxiety and anti-insomnia remedy. Because Saint-John's-wort can have serious interactions with certain drugs and herbs, always check with your doctor before you take it or start any other herbal therapy.

Dr. Cass recommends a dose of 300 milligrams standardized extract (0.3-percent hypericin), two to three times daily. Saint-John's-wort is available in tablets, capsules, or tincture, depending on your preference. Though Dr. Cass has seen it work almost immediately, Saint-John's-wort usually takes several weeks for the full effect.

**Say no to junk food.** The sugary foods you may eat when you're depressed boost the feel-good brain chemical serotonin—but for a few minutes only. Once the sugar high fades, so does your elevated mood and energy, says *Shoshana Zimmerman, N.D.,* a naturopathic physician in Palo Alto, California, and co-author of *My Doctor Says I'm Fine ... So Why Do I Feel So Bad?* And seeing the pounds creep on won't do anything for your self-esteem. A diet that includes protein (such as lean meat, poultry, and fish) at least three times a day, a source of healthy fat (such as olive oil), and complex carbohydrates (such as whole grains) ensures that your brain has adequate levels of mood-boosting serotonin, energy-giving blood sugar, and depression-defeating essential fatty acids.

*Sweets may lift your spirits briefly, but a consistently healthy diet helps keep you supplied with mood-boosting serotonin.—Shoshana Zimmerman, N.D.*

Researchers at the National Institutes of Health in Bethesda, Maryland, are currently studying the link between depression and a type of fatty acid known as omega-3 fatty acid. Decreased levels of an omega-3 fatty acid called docosahexaenoic acid (DHA), have been linked directly to depression. More research is needed, says Dr. Dubin, but "the more natural and healthy foods you can bring into your life, the better." Foods high in omega-3 fatty acids include flaxseed and seafood, such as sardines, salmon, Atlantic mackerel, herring, lake trout, striped bass, tuna, Pacific halibut, channel catfish, swordfish, red snapper, sole, shrimp, and Dungeness crab.

**Change your sleeping patterns.** If you're depressed, you may have trouble falling or staying asleep, says Dr. Dubin. Conversely, you may sleep too much. If you are not getting enough slumber, you should avoid caffeine, not exercise right before bedtime, and drink a cup of herbal tea or warm milk before retiring for the night. To keep from oversleeping, set your alarm, get up, and exercise instead of lying in. If the idea of working out—indeed, the mere thought of getting out of bed—is more than you can handle, see your doctor immediately. She may want to prescribe an antidepressant that can help lift the fog and get you moving in the right direction.

**Keep a journal.** Spending 20 minutes a day writing down your emotions can be very therapeutic, says Dr. Gruman. "It's a good way to start coping with depression," she says. "It's not aggressive, it's something you can do by yourself, and it lets you see your feelings in black and white—and perhaps then make plans to do something about them."

Dr. Gruman suggests two journaling strategies: The first is known as automatic writing. Sit in a comfortable chair, take a deep breath, and just start writing. Keep it going for 20 minutes without stopping and see what comes out. "If you are having trouble putting your finger on what's bothering you, this may help you narrow the field," says Dr. Gruman. The second journaling tip, she says, is to focus a 20-minute writing session on a problem or concern that is plaguing you. Write down, in detail, what it is that worries or angers you. Then predict three scenarios for what might happen next. Which one do you like best? Why? What role might you play in making each scenario come to pass?

*Look for answers instead of living in the problem. Solutions are an antidote to feelings of helplessness and hopelessness, major components of depression.*—Helen Grusd, Ph.D.

**Switch your birth control.** Some birth control pills trigger depression, says *Elizabeth Lee Vliet, M.D.*, founder of HER Place: The Women's Center for Health Enhancement and Renewal in Tuscon, Arizona, and Dallas-Fort Worth and author of *Women, Weight, and Hormones*. Different pills contain different levels of estrogen and progestin, Dr. Vliet explains, as well as various chemical types of progestins. The higher the progestin relative to the estrogen, the more likely you are to experience such negatives as irritability and depression (along with increased appetite, weight gain, low sex drive, fatigue, and headaches). Ask your doctor about switching pills or consider another form of birth control.

**Boycott alcohol.** Alcohol is a depressant and will only bring you further down. The same applies to most recreational drugs, including marijuana, says Dr. Dubin.

**Laugh out loud.** When you really don't feel like chuckling is just when you should, says Dr. Annechild. Laughter can act as a natural antidepressant, so rent a funny video, listen to a recording of your favorite comedian, or call an amusing friend.

**Learn to relax.** The same techniques that work to reduce stress can help ease your depression, advises Dr. Dubin. Try meditation, visualization, and deep-breathing exercises. (See "Stress-Busters," page 283.)

**Change your thinking.** "We feel the way we think," says Dr. Grusd. Avoid saying toxic things to yourself, such as "I'm fat" or "I'm a failure," which only send you on a downward spiral to depression. Instead, tell yourself, "OK, I've put on some weight. What have I been eating and why? What can I do to change?" Or, "I didn't receive that promotion. Why? Do I need to go back to school or get additional training?" Dr. Grusd warns, "When you look for solutions instead of living in the problem, you don't feel as helpless and hopeless, two major components of depression."

## SEASONAL AFFECTIVE DISORDER: BANISHING THE WINTER BLUES

Feeling out of sorts on a bleak February day isn't unusual. But if you're down throughout most of the winter—and perhaps have a near-constant desire to sleep, low energy, carbohydrate cravings, poor concentration, and no sex drive—you may suffer from seasonal affective disorder, which goes by the all-too-apt acronym of SAD. Although some people also experience SAD in the summer, most go through their doldrums in the winter, when days are short and—the likely cause of the problem—there's little exposure to sunlight.

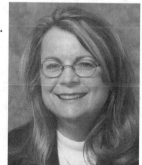

Approximately 11 million Americans suffer from SAD and 70 to 80 percent are women. Researchers don't yet know the reason that women are more affected than men, says *Sandra T. Sigmon, Ph.D.,* associate professor of psychology and director of clinical training at the University of Maine at Orono. However, there is the fact that women are more likely to ruminate, obsessing on thoughts and feelings. "Rumination keeps you focused on your

*Seasonal affective disorder, aka the winter blues, strikes four times as many women as men. Sandra T. Sigmon, Ph.D., suggests you get more light to help reset your inner clock.*

emotions and lengthens your depressive episodes," says Dr. Sigmon. She has found that women who concentrate on their SAD symptoms are apt to have longer and more serious bouts than those who don't.

Fortunately, your doctor can treat SAD simply and effectively with extra light, using a technique called phototherapy, says Dr. Sigmon. Researchers don't understand exactly how phototherapy works, but they suspect light affects the release and use of the brain chemicals serotonin and dopamine, which affect mood. Or the light may reset your biological clock, which runs more slowly in the winter.

*Even 10 minutes in the sun will lift your mood. What counts is the light that reaches your eyes.*
*—Sandra T. Sigmon, Ph.D.*

If SAD is making you sad, Dr. Sigmon suggests these light-increasing strategies.

**Get more natural sunlight.** Keep your blinds and curtains open. Decorate your home with pastel colors, such as off-white, yellow, or blue. Not only do light colors enhance your mood, but also such shades on your walls reflect any natural light that comes in.

**Up the wattage.** Use high-watt lightbulbs. Just make sure your lamps are equipped to handle the extra watts to avoid electrical fires.

**Grab some extra rays.** Whether you're at school, at work, or exercising indoors, try to position yourself near windows.

**Spend time outdoors.** Even 10 to 20 minutes a day in natural sunlight can brighten your mood. Because the antidepressant effect comes from the light waves reaching your eyes, bundling up if it's cold won't keep you from getting the benefits of the outdoor light. Go on a winter vacation—head for the islands. It may be just what the doctor ordered.

**Investigate light-box therapy.** If getting more light, both indoors and out, doesn't lift your spirits, talk to your doctor about light-box therapy. A light box is a bright-light appliance that does not include ultraviolet light, so you don't have to worry about sunburn or an increased risk of skin cancer. Exposure to a light box burning at 10,000 lux (the measure of light intensity) for 30 minutes to 2 hours a day can chase away your dark mood.

You should feel better within about a week of starting the treatment. The effects are temporary, however, so you need to use the light box daily, usually from October through April. You can buy light boxes at specialty stores, such as Sharper Image (www.sharperimage.com, 800-344-4444) or Hammacher Schlemmer (www.hammacherschlemmer.com, 800-321-1484). Or order directly from a light-box supplier, such as The SunBox Company in Gaithersburg, Maryland (www.sunboxco.com, 800-548-3968). A light box costs around $200.

Another device that works well against SAD, says Dr. Sigmon, is a dawn simulator, which is a night-light timed to begin glowing around 4 a.m. Over the ensuing hours, the light gradually brightens—just as daybreak does. A search on the Web under "dawn simulators" or "light boxes" will link you to sources—including The SunBox Company—for these appliances. Dawn simulators cost between $100 and $200.

## POST-TRAUMATIC STRESS DISORDER: RELIVING THE PAIN

After the terrorist assaults of September 11, 2001, mental-health experts predicted an epidemic of post-traumatic stress disorder (PTSD), even among people who lived thousands of miles from the attack sites and weren't personally affected by the tragedies.

Any catastrophic event—whether as intimate as a rape or as broad as the terrorist attacks—can cause an emotional hangover still felt long after the initial trauma fades. Common reactions to tragedy include depression, anxiety, sleep disorders, fear, and helplessness, which typically last for several weeks. If such feelings persist for months or even years, you may be suffering from PTSD, says *Phebe Tucker,* M.D., professor of psychiatry at the University of Oklahoma Health Sciences Center and an expert in the treatment of PTSD. Doctors used to think PTSD, originally dubbed shell shock, only affected war veterans. But researchers now know that PTSD disrupts the lives of as many as 10 percent of Americans,

*Experts used to think shell shock only affected soldiers. We now know that emotional trauma has long-lasting effects on victims of violence and abuse, says Phebe Tucker, M.D.*

about one-third more women than men. In addition to rape, common causes of PTSD in women include childhood sexual abuse and domestic violence.

A woman with PTSD may be jittery, avoid places associated with the triggering incident, replay the event over and over in her mind, and have vivid and recurring dreams, says Dr. Tucker. She may have difficulty functioning at work and in social settings, and may abuse drugs or alcohol in an attempt to self-medicate. Some women with PTSD become suicidal.

To diagnose PTSD, a therapist will question you about the trauma, as well as the symptoms you're experiencing. If you have the disorder, individual therapy may help you regain the sense of self-control and self-esteem you've lost. Family therapy may assist your loved ones to understand your condition and how it affects them. Group therapy can put you in touch with people who have gone through similar experiences.

In addition to talk therapy, such medications as Paxil (paroxetine) and Zoloft (sertraline) may relieve the depression, anxiety, or panic that often accompany PTSD. Drugs alone, however, are usually not enough.

*You don't have to cope with PTSD alone. Group therapy can put you and your family in touch with people who have had a similar experience.*

Dr. Tucker suggests these additional techniques to combat the anxiety associated with PTSD.

**Clear your environment.** Remove yourself from what is traumatizing you. For example, if you're in an abusive relationship, get out. If you don't have a family member or friend to whom you can turn and can't afford to make it on your own at first, seek assistance from a local shelter for victims of domestic violence. Or if you have witnessed a tragedy—such as the September 11 attacks—limit the amount of television you watch and the number of newspaper accounts you read about the event to avoid the sense of reliving it time and again.

**Create a support network.** This could comprise friends and family or fellow PTSD sufferers.

**Be good to yourself.** Eat well, get enough exercise and sleep, and take part in recreational activities.

**Get out.** Stay away from places that remind you of the trauma but don't hide out at home and miss opportunities to socialize. If certain situations make you uncomfortable, take a friend along.

**Avoid self-medication.** Don't use alcohol or drugs to numb out. If you have been abusing these substances, seek treatment from your physician or attend such meetings as Alcoholics Anonymous or Narcotics Anonymous.

## JEALOUSY: TAMING THE GREEN-EYED MONSTER

"There will always be someone who is younger and thinner, and has longer hair," says *Annette Annechild, Ph.D.,* director of the Healing Arts Center of Georgetown in Washington, D.C. But that's no reason to be jealous—at least not for more than a minute or so.

A twinge is normal if your husband announces that his new business partner is a former beauty-pageant winner who holds a Ph.D. in particle physics and speaks six languages. But if that initial pang turns into a constant stab in the heart, what you're actually experiencing is insecurity and low self-esteem. "When you really envy someone else, it always starts with not believing in yourself," says Dr. Annechild.

Envy is not necessarily a bad thing. It can motivate and inspire you to make changes. But when feelings of jealousy get out of hand, they do just the opposite by keeping you from focusing positively on your life.

*When you really envy someone, it always starts with not believing in yourself.—Annette Annechild, Ph.D.*

Here are some of Dr. Annechild's tips for turning envy into action.

**Admit your feelings.** First, acknowledge that you're jealous. Then ask yourself *why* you are jealous: Do I envy a colleague's promotion? Am I jealous of my best friend's relationship with her new boyfriend? Confront what's causing your feelings and then see what you can do to improve your situation. Do you need to earn additional certification to better your chances of being promoted? Should you join a club so you can meet new people and increase your chances of finding a relationship?

**Avoid assumptions.** Just because your friend got a raise doesn't mean you can't get one, too. Witnessing another person's success shouldn't keep you from achieving your own.

**Use jealousy constructively.** What you envy about someone is very often what you would admire about them if you weren't so jealous. If your friend has lost a lot of weight, congratulate her on her success and ask how she did it. Learn from others and then apply what you've gleaned to your life.

## MEMORY PROBLEMS: FORGET ABOUT THEM

Six-year-old Lia says she remembers everything from her "whole life." Her 50-year-old mom, Gail, who runs her own computer consulting company in suburban Washington, D.C., is lucky if she can recall where she left the car keys (and on some days, where she parked the car). Gail may think her memory is not as sharp as it once was because she's getting

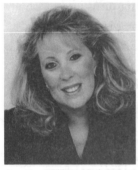

older, but that's not necessarily the case, says *Donalee Markus, Ph.D.,* founder of Designs for Strong Minds in Highland Park, Illinois. Dr. Markus creates and teaches brain exercises to strengthen memory and learning capacity. It's not age that is responsible for forgetfulness, she says, but rather a lower tolerance for doing more than one thing at the same time as we get older.

"In the normal aging process," says Dr. Markus, "memory itself remains largely intact. We may not store as much information at any given time, but what we store, we keep and can retrieve at a later time." We store less, Dr. Markus explains, not because we have a problem with recall but because our memory storage strategies change with age.

*It may seem like you're losing your memory as you age, but it's more likely that you're losing the ability to concentrate on more than one thing at a time, says Donalee Markus, Ph.D.*

When you're young, you can do many things at once and pay attention to all of them. You can pick up the phone and talk to a friend, and not forget that you have something on the stove. But as you get older, your ability to attend to multiple tasks at one time is taxed.

So as you come into the house thinking about what to make for dinner, you're not really going to pay attention to where you put your keys. When you go to get them the next day and can't find them, it's not that you've forgotten where they are, Dr. Markus explains. Rather, you didn't pay attention in the first place and so never recorded the event in your memory.

Dr. Markus suggests these strategies to strengthen your ability to keep track of numerous things at a time.

**Think positive.** Telling yourself you have a memory problem is almost a self-fulfilling prophecy. It leads to worry and keeps you from figuring out how you can avoid such difficulties in the first place. Instead, be positive and proactive.

> *To exercise your brain, try bouncing a ball with alternating hands while counting in multiples of three.*
> —*Donalee Markus, Ph.D.*

**Give your mind a workout.** Mental exercises can help increase your ability to keep your brain nimble. Practice these tasks that require you to handle several things simultaneously.

- While sitting at a table, raise your right hand and left foot at the same time. Bring them down and alternate tapping with the opposite hand and foot. See if you can maintain a fluid conversation at the same time.
- Listen to a book on tape and do a household chore, such as organize your bookcase or scan a magazine to pick out articles you want to read later.
- Watch television while you fold laundry, make a salad, or write a note to a friend.
- Bounce a ball with alternating hands and count by multiples of any given number (i.e., 3, 6, 9, etc.) with each bounce. Experiment using different numbers.
- Work a jigsaw puzzle. This activity requires you to pay attention to shape, size, and orientation of the pieces.
- Solve a crossword puzzle. Such a mind stretch encourages you to think of alternative meanings for the same words.

**Improve your imagery skills.** We remember what we see, so take a drawing class (realism, not impressionism) or check out *The New Drawing on the Right Side of Your Brain* by Betty Edwards.

**Crank up your intent to recall.** "We have to become vigilant and involved in making sure we attend to what we care about," says Dr. Markus. She cites these examples.

- Forming habits: Develop routines for what you do most frequently so that you have fewer chores to remember. If you make a point to put your keys on the coffee table when you walk through the door, it'll become a habit—and, therefore, one less thing you'll have to remind yourself to do. You have to pay attention only until the act becomes automatic.
- Arranging items: Organize your environment to keep like objects in particular places. "That way, when you get a new tool, you will know where to find it because it will be with its friends," says Dr. Markus.

**Keep less in your head.** No one remembers everything, so it's helpful to develop strategies that are essentially memory assistants. Try some of these techniques.

- Taking notes: "Don't all executives have a secretary?" asks Dr. Markus. To keep track of information, get a spiral notebook that has multiple tabbed sections; use one section for appointments, another for a to-do list. If you're the techie type, store data on a personal digital assistant.
- Planning ahead: Get in the habit of outlining your plans for the next day. Anticipating events prevents mistakes and a feeling of being rushed.
- Thinking big: Remember that large events require a lot of planning. When going on a trip, have a designated place to assemble all the items you want to pack. Make a list of essentials, even if you don't think it's necessary.

Finally, says Dr. Markus, accept that your senses will take in less information as you age: Your eyesight will be poorer, and your hearing less acute. Don't resist getting help to correct such changes. For example, bifocal contact lenses and tiny hearing aids are now available. Even having your doctor remove any earwax buildup can dramatically improve your hearing. "If you can't receive information through your senses, you won't remember it," says Dr. Markus.

## ANXIETY AND PANIC ATTACKS: YOU'RE NOT GOING TO DIE—YOU JUST THINK YOU ARE

Worrying about going to the doctor, attending a parent-teacher conference, or meeting your boyfriend's parents is not unusual. But when concern becomes full-fledged anxiety, you may find yourself jittery, sleepless, and unable to function well at home, on the job, and in your social life.

Anxiety can also seriously affect your health. In addition to experiencing a surge in stress hormones that contribute to high blood pressure and heart disease, researchers now believe a woman who suffers from anxiety tends to hold her breath. This can further affect hypertension and cardiovascular function. **Margaret Chesney, Ph.D.**, professor of medicine and epidemiology at the University of California at San Francisco, is an expert on women's health, particularly in the fields of stress and coping. Even she finds herself holding her breath when she's feeling anxious. "It's part of our cultural training," says Dr. Chesney. "We don't wear veils, but we sometimes veil our feelings."

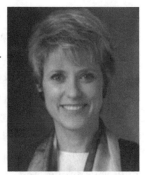

*The first prescription for battling anxiety? Take a deep breath, says Margaret Chesney, Ph.D. Then try meditation and yoga to help you stay calm.*

Dr. Chesney recommends—and practices—these tips for reducing anxiety.

**Learn to breathe.** Yoga and meditation are excellent strategies for helping inhale more oxygen. Both help relieve tension and lower blood pressure.

**Visit a safe place.** In your mind, that is. Think of a spot where you feel completely at peace. Let your mind wander there for a few minutes every day. As you experience the feeling of safety, your breathing will become deeper and more relaxed.

## YOGA FOR TENSION RELIEF: SHOULDER AND CHEST OPENER

*This technique is often recommended for meditation and stress relief, as well as to ease anxiety.*

When your chest and lungs are weak and sunken, your breathing becomes shallow, which exacerbates any tension you're feeling. The yoga pose recommended by **Cyndi Lee,** director of the OM Yoga Center in New York City, helps by creating flexibility in the muscles of the respiratory system that allow you to breathe more fully. This pose opens the chest, rib cage, throat, and heart *chakra*, or life force.

• Sit cross-legged on the floor with a cushion under your rear or perch on the front edge of a chair or stool.

• Interlace your fingers behind your back and press your palms together.

• Touch the floor or chair behind you with your thumbs and index fingers as you lift your chest toward the ceiling. Try to keep a sense of length in the back of the neck as you raise your face.

• Inhale and exhale deeply. Visualize your breath opening the spaces between each rib, your shoulder blades, and your ears.

• Hold this position for five deep breaths.

• Inhale. Sit up. Exhale and rest.

## GENERALIZED ANXIETY DISORDER

Everyone feels anxious when there's reason, but if you've been overly worried about everyday things for at least six months, your doctor may diagnose you with generalized anxiety disorder and prescribe antianxiety medications. With or without medication, self-help techniques—such as deep breathing, progressive relaxation, and meditation—can help you cope, says *Annette Annechild, Ph.D.,* director of the Healing Arts Center of Georgetown in Washington, D.C. Aerobic exercise, such as walking, jogging, swimming, and cycling, also has a calming effect.

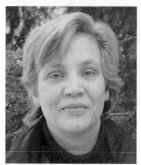

*Planning ahead can help manage anxiety. Julie K. Norem, Ph.D., wears flat-heeled shoes at speaking engagements so she won't worry about tripping in front of the audience.*

Analyze what's bothering you. "If you focus your energy on the situation and not on your anxiety, you have a much better chance of managing your stress," says *Julie K. Norem, Ph.D.,* associate professor of psychology at Wellesley College and author of *The Positive Power of Negative Thinking: Using Defensive Pessimism to Harness Anxiety and Perform at Your Peak.* Dr. Norem refers to this approach as defensive pessimism.

Are you concerned, for example, that the big conference you're planning will be a flop? Fine, accept that as a possibility. Then focus on how you can make sure it won't. Confirm travel arrangements for the speakers, check that the audiovisual equipment is working, have more press packets on hand than you think you need. Do everything you can to ensure success and then let events take their course. Dr. Norem realized the stress she felt about speech giving centered around worrying that she would trip when she walked across the stage. So now she wears flat-heeled shoes whenever she speaks in public.

## PANIC ATTACKS

As *Diane Ulicsni, C.Ht.,* can tell you firsthand, panic attacks are more than just a case of nerves. For more than a dozen years, Ulicsni suffered from chronic attacks that led her, like many with panic disorder, through a round-robin of doctors' offices and emergency rooms, convinced she was having a heart attack or nervous breakdown. Ulicsni finally found relief through hypnosis. She is now director of the Hypnosis Center in Lake Oswego, Oregon, and a board certified hypnotherapist who works with panic-disorder patients.

Three out of four people with panic disorder are women. For no apparent reason, sufferers experience repeated episodes of extreme terror, says *Jerilyn Ross, M.A., L.C.S.W.*, president of the Anxiety Disorders Association of America and director of the Ross Center for Anxiety and Related Disorders in Washington, D.C. The author of *Triumph Over Fear: A Book of Help and Hope for People with Anxiety, Panic Attacks, and Phobias,* Ross defines a panic attack as the abrupt onset of intense fear or discomfort, which peaks in approximately 10 minutes and includes at least four of the following symptoms.

- Feeling of imminent danger
- Need to escape
- Palpitations
- Sweating
- Trembling
- Shortness of breath or smothering feeling
- Feeling of choking

- Chest pain or discomfort
- Nausea or abdominal discomfort
- Dizziness or light-headedness
- Sense of unreality
- Fear of dying
- Tingling sensations
- Chills or hot flashes

Because these symptoms can be associated with a variety of medical problems—from indigestion to heart disease or stroke—it is important to call your doctor if you experience them.

There are three types of panic attacks, says Ross: the unexpected, in which the attack comes without warning and for no apparent reason; situational, in which certain experiences—such as entering a tunnel—trigger an attack; or situationally predisposed, in which you're in a situation that is likely to bring on a panic attack, but doesn't always.

A diagnosis of panic disorder is made when you suffer at least two unexpected attacks, followed by at least one month of concern over having another, says Ross. How often the episodes occur and how severe they are varies from person to person. You may suffer from repeated attacks for weeks, while someone else could have short bursts of severe attacks. Like Ulicsni, people who suffer from panic disorder often become convinced that the attacks indicate an undiagnosed illness—either physical or emotional—and make frequent trips to doctors' offices and emergency rooms in search of answers.

Ross says that people who suffer from panic attacks may modify their behavior in order to cope, such as avoiding the scene of a previous attack in hope of preventing another. If this kind of fear becomes intense enough, you may develop a frequent side effect of panic disorder called agoraphobia, which can cause you to establish a fixed route from which you can't deviate or refuse to leave your home—or your safe place—altogether.

Panic disorder tends to run in families, says Ross, and can have psychological or physiological causes, such as mitral valve prolapse, hypoglycemia (low blood sugar), inner-ear disturbances, or a hormone imbalance. Ulicsni sees many patients whose panic attacks are rooted in past events. "Anger, sadness, hurt, guilt, and fear get stored in your body," she says. Emotions may stay buried for years until a trigger causes them to bubble to the surface.

Since panic disorder is difficult to diagnose, therapy is sometimes delayed. Ross says effective treatments include psychotherapy, hypnotherapy, and antidepressant or antianxiety medications, such as BuSpar (buspirone) or Xanax (alprazolam).

## A WOMAN'S RIGHT TO THE *RIGHT* TREATMENT: SOCIAL ANXIETY DISORDER

*More than five million Americans suffer from social anxiety disorder, also known as social phobia. It's shyness with a capital S. Without proper treatment, the condition can significantly impair work or social situations throughout a woman's life.*

Social anxiety disorder is the third most common psychiatric disorder in the United States. People with this condition experience intense, persistent fear that causes them to avoid social or performance situations to the point that everyday activities are affected. Symptoms include rapid heartbeat, trembling, sweating, tense muscles, upset stomach, and blushing.

Even though it can be disruptive, most people who suffer from the condition wait more than a decade before seeking help. A study published in the *American Journal of Psychiatry* reports that the average social anxiety-disorder sufferer doesn't know where to go for help, is afraid of what others will think or say about the condition, or worries about how much treatment will cost.

**Barbara G. Markway, Ph.D.,** a clinical psychologist and expert in social anxiety disorder,

helped people with such problems for years but didn't tell anyone that she struggled with the same difficulties. Markway, author of *Painfully Shy: How to Overcome Social Anxiety and Reclaim Your Life,* was a shy, quiet child who never raised her hand in class. As a teenager, she never dated. And in college, she avoided classes where she had to speak—she even received a D in public speaking because she missed so many classes.

Markway says she decided that discussing her own social anxiety disorder would help other sufferers realize "there is hope out there." Her condition was treated with a combination of talk therapy and medication.

Some health-care professionals are more familiar with other disorders—such as panic disorder, generalized anxiety disorder, and depression—and may not ask the questions that

Even if you're receiving professional care, practicing these techniques will help you deal with the disorder.

**Be in the here and now.** Stay focused on the present and not on what you fear might happen. Ulicsni recommends this self-hypnosis technique: When panic-attack symptoms start, sit down, take several deep breaths, and look up at a chosen focal point on the ceiling. Put your hands on either side of your face. Slowly pull your hands away until you can no longer see them in your peripheral vision. This focuses your attention on something other than your symptoms and the fear of those symptoms, Ulicsni says.

Or try tapping your legs with your hands, starting with the right leg and hand and alternating back and forth. This is a variation of thought-field therapy, in which you tap acupuncture points along your body to change the

could help diagnose your problem. So it may be up to you to evaluate your condition and ask your doctor to work with you in determining if social anxiety disorder could be causing your discomfort.

Dr. Markway recommends asking yourself the following questions:

- Am I literally sick with fear at the thought of being in social or performance situations (speaking in public, participating in class, attending meetings, meeting strangers, going to parties, dating)?
- How long have I felt this way?
- How much does it affect my day-to-day life?
- Do I have other existing conditions, such as clinical depression?

If your answers reveal that social anxiety is a chronic problem that is keeping you from getting what you want out of life, you and your doctor should consider treatment.

A therapist who specializes in social anxiety will concentrate less on your past and more on coaching you to face your fears. Talk to your therapist about your goals—where you want to go and how to get there. Your therapist may

recommend such a medication as Paxil (paroxetine), the first drug approved by the U.S. Food and Drug Administration for this disorder.

Dr. Markway also recommends these self-help tips that can make your life easier:

**Have realistic expectations.** Not everyone is the life of the party. Accept yourself and don't worry about what others think of you. "There's a place in the world for people who are thoughtful and quiet," says Dr. Markway.

**Don't fight the symptoms.** If your heart is racing or you're short of breath due to a stressful situation, realize you're just experiencing anxiety. "It's uncomfortable, but it's not life-threatening," says Dr. Markway. Most of the time, other people can't detect the discomfort you're feeling. The more you struggle against the symptoms, the less you're concentrating on the task at hand.

**Face your fears.** Take small, continued steps. Go to a party. Raise an issue in a meeting. Ask a co-worker to lunch. "What's the big deal if it doesn't go as planned?" asks Dr. Markway. "Set small goals and congratulate yourself for your efforts."

energy patterns. Ulicsni says the tapping neutralizes emotional distress by breaking the loops—whether physiological, psychological, or behavioral—that cause the problem in the first place. (If you want to learn more about thought-field therapy and self-help techniques, read *Instant Emotional Healing: Acupressure for the Emotions* by Drs. Peter T. Lambrou and George J. Pratt.)

**Talk yourself through symptoms.** They may be frightening, but they won't hurt you, says Ross. Tell yourself, "I'm having a panic attack, not a heart attack. This is uncomfortable, but it will pass." Learning to halt unproductive thoughts is the objective of cognitive behavior therapy (CBT), one of the most widely used and successful therapies for panic disorder. "One benefit of CBT is that you learn to examine your feelings and separate realistic from unrealistic thoughts," Ross says. "You learn recovery skills that you can use on your own." Being involved in your recovery and having a sense of control are important parts of any treatment plan for panic disorder.

**Use positive affirmation.** Every time you make it through a panic attack, tell yourself how much better you are at coping with such episodes and how prepared you are for the next one, Ulicsni suggests.

*When you feel a panic attack coming on, look up at a point on the ceiling to focus your mind on something other than your symptoms.*—Diane Ulicsni, C.Ht.

**Don't fight the feeling.** Allow your panic to come up, advises Ulicsni. Trying to avoid it can trigger shallow and rapid breathing, as well as increased adrenaline levels as your body goes into fight-or-flight mode. These responses just intensify the discomfort you're already experiencing.

**Consult a clinical hypnotherapist.** A good hypnotherapist can teach you self-hypnosis techniques to help cope when panic attacks, says Ulicsni. Hypnosis has been recognized by the American Medical Association since 1958 as a useful form of treatment in both medicine and surgery. Ulicsni says hypnosis can amplify the effect of the mind on the body, changing the way you perceive sensations. It focuses your attention and relaxes you physically, so that you're not overwhelmed by the symptoms of a panic attack. Relaxation techniques, such as deep breathing, are also helpful.

## ANGER AND HOSTILITY: DON'T BLOW YOUR TOP

Most women are raised to be nice and polite, which translates into never being allowed to express unpleasant feelings publicly.

Years of holding in emotions can take its toll, says **Margaret Chesney, Ph.D.**, a professor of medicine and epidemiology at the University of California at San Francisco. Many women stuff their anger inside, letting it build up—until one day it just explodes. Anger isn't a bad emotion, rather a sign that something in your life probably needs to change. And keeping it bottled up can be harmful. Research has linked repressed anger to increased risk of heart disease, impaired immune systems, and cancer.

There are right and wrong ways to manage anger, says **Helen Grusd, Ph.D.**, past president of the Los Angeles County Psychological Association. These are some of her recommendations for the best ways to control your anger.

**Stop in your tracks.** If you're so incensed that you can't think straight, just come to a halt. Wait until you calm down and then address the problem.

**Walk away—mentally or physically.** When you're furious, try to remove yourself from the situation until you can cool down. If you can't get away—if you're in the middle of a meeting, for example—use visualization techniques to imagine yourself in a calmer setting.

**Face your anger.** Not letting off steam the minute you get irate doesn't mean you should ignore the feeling. Suppressing emotions leads to resentment. Admit that you're angry, but make an effort to express it in a reasonable manner.

**Put yourself in the other person's place.** Examine what made you hot under the collar in the first place. Then look for any extenuating circumstances. If your boss blows up at you for what seems to be no good reason, consider that he or she may simply be having a bad day.

**Talk it out.** Once you've had time to think about the situation, discuss it with the person who angered you. Avoid such statements as, "You made me mad," which will just put the other person on the defensive. State your case by focusing on the situation rather than the person's actions. Try starting out with, "I was angry because ..." and go from there.

**Know when you need help.** If you often overreact to people and situations that never used to bother you or lash out physically at your partner or children—or yourself—ask your doctor to refer you to a qualified mental-health professional. She can teach you anger-management techniques, as well as help get to the root of what's bothering you.

# 16 Mouth and Teeth
## Preserving a Sparkling Smile

*The signature smile of Julia Roberts or Sophia Loren lights up a room with a message of self-confidence and joy. But you don't have to be a movie star to have a stellar smile.*

It's difficult to muster up a happy grin if you have tooth or mouth pain or if your lips are sore and cracked. And women—thanks, of course, to hormones—may have more challenges with their oral health than men.

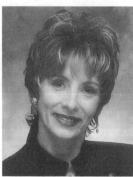

A woman's hormones increase her risk for unpleasant dental and mouth problems, says Maria Perno Goldie, R.D.H., M.S.

A woman's hormones play a tremendous role in the lifelong health of her mouth, explains **Maria Perno Goldie, R.D.H., M.S.,** of San Carlos, California, president of Seminars for Women's Health. That's because your mouth has many hormone receptors for estrogen and progesterone. Throughout a woman's lifetime, she is at risk for various dental and mouth problems—hormone- as well as nonhormone-related—that can cause discomfort, pain, and embarrassment.

According to the Centers for Disease Control and Prevention, most adult Americans have some form of dental disease. If you're among the fortunate few who don't, you can turn to the next chapter. But if you're not (and if you're a woman, you're likely not), read on about some of the dental and mouth problems you may face—and why—and what you can do about them.

# PERIODONTAL DISEASE: GETTING A GRIP ON HEALTHY GUMS

Periodontal disease is a bacterial infection that affects the gums and bones that support the teeth. *(Periodontal* literally means "around the tooth.") It's sometimes referred to as a silent disease, because many women don't realize they have it until it reaches the serious stage.

Periodontal disease begins with gingivitis—inflamed, receding gums. If untreated, gingivitis progresses to periodontitis—worsening gum recession and loss of supporting ligament and bone. Telltale symptoms of gingivitis are bleeding and red, puffy gums. "Gingivitis is the only reversible form of gum disease," says Goldie. "If you start self-care at home and receive professional care from a dental hygienist, you can probably reverse the problem 100 percent." You'll need professional cleanings and maintenance about every three months, however, until your gums return to health, she advises.

Both estrogen and progesterone play a role in gingivitis, says Goldie. That's why it's so common in pregnant women, whose hormone levels are in flux. In fact, 50 to 70 percent of women get gum disease during pregnancy. Changing hormone levels also make women more susceptible to gingivitis during puberty or when taking oral contraceptives.

If you don't treat gingivitis, you're hanging out a welcome sign for periodontitis. In this next stage of gum disease, the gum line recedes, and you gradually lose the supporting ligaments and bone around your teeth, thus loosening the teeth. Special dentists, called periodontists, typically treat this problem. Treatment involves deep cleaning to the roots to get rid of plaque. (Plaque is the gummy buildup of bacteria and food particles that accumulates

## SHOULD I SEE A DENTIST?

*Keeping a healthy smile takes professional help. See your dentist every six months for a checkup and cleaning.*

*Flora Parsa Stay, D.D.S.,* of Ventura, California, author of *The Complete Book of Dental Remedies,* says that some cases will require your dentist to recommend more frequent cleanings, depending on the condition of your teeth, gums, and bone. Dr. Stay urges women who are pregnant or have diabetes or an autoimmune condition to see their dentist every two to three months.

Any trauma to the mouth (due to a fall or accident) should be checked immediately by a dentist or, if appropriate, a dental surgeon. See your dentist if you have tooth, gum, or mouth pain, bleeding or swollen gums, difficulty chewing, or a chronic mouth abscess or ulcer. If you're having *any* pain or discomfort, call your dentist. The two of you can decide if you need to be seen.

on teeth, as well as along and below the gum line.) If the condition is severe, it may be necessary to scrape the roots of the affected teeth or remove infected tissue. Sometimes, periodontal surgery is necessary.

Periodontitis sounds bad enough, but, when left untreated, the news gets even worse. "The real issue is that periodontal disease is an *infection* that can affect the body in ways that we were not aware of five years ago," says Goldie. Research suggests a link between periodontal disease and cardiovascular disease. And periodontal disease has been shown to increase a pregnant woman's risk for a preterm, low-birthweight baby. Such oral infections as periodontitis can also play a significant role in other health conditions, such as lung disease and diabetes.

> *Your risk of gingivitis increases with hormone fluctuations, such as during puberty and pregnancy or when taking oral contraceptives.*
> —*Maria Perno Goldie, R.D.H., M.S.*

**Flora Parsa Stay, D.D.S.**, of Ventura, California, author of *The Complete Book of Dental Remedies*, sees many women in various stages of gum disease. She recommends these steps to help control symptoms of gingivitis.

**Get regular checkups.** Have your teeth cleaned and checked every two to six months by a dental hygienist, dentist, or periodontist, depending on the condition of your gums and teeth.

**Be diligent—and gentle.** Brush with a soft brush after every meal to remove food particles.

**Power it up.** If possible, use an electric toothbrush, which stimulates and cleans the gums. The best kinds have a small head with soft bristles that clean one tooth surface at a time.

*The best toothbrush is an electric model with a small head and soft bristles, says Flora Parsa Stay, D.D.S. These clean one tooth at a time.*

**Go with aloe.** To soothe your gums, rinse out your mouth with 1 cup warm water mixed with 1 tablespoon aloe-vera gel (available at drugstores). You can also apply the gel directly to the problem areas.

**Flush 'em out.** A water-irrigating device (e.g., Water Pik) is helpful for flushing plaque from hard-to-reach places.

**Pick the right paste.** Toothpaste that contains aloe vera and baking soda soothes the gums. NutriBiotic's Dental Gel features both; others, such as Kingfisher's Fluoride Free Toothpaste Aloe Vera and Kiss My Face's AloeDyne, contain only aloe vera but are still good choices.

**Forget the sweet and spicy.** Sugary foods and beverages, meats, and spicy foods irritate the gums and promote bacterial growth. Include more raw and steamed vegetables and fruits in your diet.

## FLOSS UP!

*Face it, brushing just isn't enough. You also need to floss every day to help keep your teeth and gums healthy.*

But you just don't do it, do you? Why do we find it so hard to floss? It's often because we're doing it wrong. "Flossing properly, with the type of floss that is correct for you, will help with compliance," says *Maria Perno Goldie, R.D.H., M.S.,* of San Carlos, California, president of Seminars for Women's Health. "Flossing can prevent periodontal disease, which is a risk factor for diabetes, cardiovascular disease, and respiratory disease, as well as preterm, low-birthweight babies. Since heart disease is the number-one killer of women, helping to prevent or control it should be a motivating factor." It also improves your smile and helps control bad breath.

Worried that the floss will fray or break? Floss is available with or without wax, fluoride, or whitening agents, and in a variety of thicknesses. Thin, waxed floss glides easiest between teeth without fraying. If you use a flavored floss, you get the added bonus of fresher breath. Choose a thick floss if the spaces between your teeth are large.

"Concerned that your gums will bleed? In most cases, gums bleed because they are inflamed or infected," says Goldie. "Flossing helps to reverse that condition." If you notice blood the first few times you floss, rinse with an aloe-vera mouthwash afterward to soothe your gums. And remember: Floss gently!

Here's a quick lesson in flossing, courtesy of the American Dental Hygienists' Association:
- Wind 18 inches of floss around the middle finger of each hand. Pinch the floss between the thumb and index fingers of each hand, leaving about 2 inches of floss in between.
- Gently guide the floss between your teeth. While keeping the floss taut, use your index fingers to guide the floss between the teeth, using a zigzag motion. Contour the floss around the sides of each tooth.
- Gently slide the floss against each tooth and under the gum line. Do not snap the floss as this can cause it to break or dig into your gums.
- Use a clean section of floss for every two teeth you clean.

If you have arthritis or other difficulties that affect being able to maneuver the floss between your teeth, a dental-floss holder may help. You can get one at your local pharmacy or drugstore. Ask your dentist or dental hygienist for instructions.

## TOOTHACHE: TAMING THE PAIN

"Toothaches shouldn't happen," says **Maria Perno Goldie, R.D.H., M.S.,** of San Carlos, California, president of Seminars for Women's Health. But *shouldn't* is a far cry from *don't*.

Toothache can be caused by a reaction to dental treatment, due to irritation or pressure, or by food particles caught between your teeth. Take a mild painkiller—such as acetaminophen, aspirin, or ibuprofen—to help with treatment reactions. Rinse your mouth with warm water and use dental floss to dislodge food.

> *Just like it helps teething babies, a pain-relief ointment can ease the agony of your toothache until you get to the dentist.*—Flora Parsa Stay, D.D.S.

In other cases, a toothache may be a sign that something's wrong. Toothache can be the result of gum infection, tooth decay, or a cracked tooth. You might have an impacted tooth (a tooth positioned in the jawbone in a way that prevents it from erupting properly) or an abscess (a pocket of pus caused

### KISS BAD BREATH GOOD-BYE

*How often do you do the bad breath test? You know, when you cover your nose and mouth with your hand, exhale, and smell your breath? Are you offending yourself more often than you care to admit?*

Bad breath, known as halitosis, is a universal problem. Nearly everyone experiences morning breath, the easily remedied first breath of the day, which is caused primarily by dehydration. During sleep, metabolism slows and saliva production decreases. Less saliva means that acids, bacteria, and food particles left behind—did you brush before retiring?—putrefy in the mouth. The result can be breath rank enough to scare a dog.

If bad breath is a frequent problem, identify the cause. *Flora Parsa Stay, D.D.S.,* of Ventura, California, and author of *The Complete Book of Dental Remedies,* notes that bad breath may be caused by dehydration, alcohol or tobacco use, tooth decay, gum disease, or digestive problems. Sometimes, bad breath is related to a diet lacking in fresh fruits and vegetables, whole grains, and other healthy foods; poor-fitting dentures or crowns; or old, broken, or worn-out fillings. It may also be a symptom of a medical condition, such as diabetes, cancer, kidney disease, sinus infection, or constipation. If the cause is something you can by an infection). The pain may radiate from a specific tooth, or it may feel like your entire mouth is involved. In either case, see a dentist as soon as possible before the pain—and the possible damage to your tooth—gets worse.

Until you get into the dental chair, *Flora Parsa Stay, D.D.S.,* offers these suggestions to combat the pain.

**Avoid hot or cold.** That includes drinks and foods. Also skip any hard, chewy foods (peanut brittle is definitely out).

**Baby yourself.** What do you do when a baby has teething pain? Apply an over-the-counter ointment pain reliever, such as Anbesol or Orajel. A good herbal substitute is clove or wintergreen oil. Place an oil-soaked cotton ball directly on the painful tooth for a few minutes.

**Take a pill.** Over-the-counter pain relievers, such as acetaminophen, aspirin, and ibuprofen, are helpful. Ibuprofen products, such as Advil and Motrin, also reduce inflammation. (Swallow these medications. *Never* leave aspirin or other pain pills on the gums to dissolve, as this burns the tissues.)

**Rinse well.** Wash your mouth several times a day with 1 cup warm water in which you've dissolved either 1 teaspoon salt or 1 tablespoon aloe-vera gel.

**Cool it.** For an impacted tooth, place a small piece of ice over the swollen gums for temporary relief. (This is an exception to the rule that extremes of hot or cold should never be placed on the teeth or any part of the mouth.)

change, addressing the situation may be enough to solve the problem.

Dr. Stay also has these tips to banish bad breath:

**Rinse with an effective mouthwash.** Avoid those with alcohol, which can contribute to dry mouth and, thus, bad breath. Good mouthwash choices contain parsley or aloe vera, such as Grace's Dental Essentials Natural Mouthwash.

**Brush after every meal or snack.** If you can't brush, eat such mouth-cleansing foods as carrots, celery, or an apple as part of every meal. At the very least, rinse your mouth with water after eating.

**Brush your tongue daily.** Bacteria that accumulates on the tongue can cause bad breath.

**Hydrate yourself.** Drink at least eight 8-ounce glasses of water daily. Then try adding 1 teaspoon lemon or lime juice to each glass.

**Pick parsley.** That sprig on your plate in restaurants is there for a reason. Chew on fresh parsley or take parsley tablets or capsules according to package directions.

**Choose chlorophyll.** This plant pigment is a natural deodorizer and is available in tablets and capsules. Follow package directions.

**Chew cloves or fennel.** Try two or three seeds after each meal to help eliminate bad breath.

## SENSITIVE TEETH: WINCE NO MORE

Have you ever eaten a spoonful of ice cream and had such a sharp pain in your teeth that you immediately swore you'd never break a diet again? If so, you may have sensitive teeth, which are caused by sensory nerves within the teeth reacting to various stimuli and causing pain.

Vigorous brushing can cause your gums to recede, exposing the sensitive root surfaces. "You actually remove more plaque and bacteria when you're gentle," says *Maria Perno Goldie, R.D.H., M.S.,* of San Carlos, California. And use a soft brush, never a medium or hard one.

Teeth can also become eroded by braces or partial dentures or from chewing such hard objects as toothpicks or pencils. Periodontal disease and enamel erosion from acidic foods or liquids are other causes of sensitive teeth. If you practice any poor brushing or chewing habits, then it's time to improve your daily dental regimen.

To treat your teeth right, try these recommendations.

**Use a desensitizing toothpaste.** There are many on the market from which to choose. They all contain potassium nitrate, which reduces reactivity of sensory nerves in the soft center part, or pulp, of teeth. You must faithfully brush with the toothpaste each and every day. "If you stop using it, you'll eventually lose the effect," warns Goldie. Pain usually eases after two to four weeks.

**Visit a professional.** If the sensitivity lingers or is more pronounced or painful, see your dentist. You may require a filling or crown. Or the dentist may need to apply a bonding material that acts as a surface sealing agent over the sensitive spot.

**Fortify with fluoride.** Your dentist or dental hygienist may also apply a fluoride varnish or even prescribe a fluoride rinse or gel for home use. These products work by blocking the dental tubules (minute tubes that extend from the pulp, where the sensory nerves are, toward the surface of the tooth) with fluoride and tin particles.

**Electrify your efforts.** A powered toothbrush is more effective yet more gentle and less abrasive than a regular toothbrush, says Goldie. It's also an excellent choice for people who have sensitive teeth. One of the best toothbrushes on the market is the Braun Oral-B 3D Excel, because it has so many different brushing movements. Stick to the traditional powered toothbrush and forget those disposable power toothbrushes. "There is no comparison," says Goldie, "and no data to support their use. True power toothbrushes, like the Braun, are superior and have data to prove their claims."

*If your teeth are yellow and stained, it's likely due to tobacco, coffee, or black tea.*—Flora Parsa Stay, D.D.S.

## STAINED TEETH: GET THEM SPARKLY WHITE

Within the dull colors of stained teeth lies a road map of your eating and drinking habits, as well as your vices. Coffee and black tea are two of the most common villains, says *Flora Parsa Stay, D.D.S.* They can get into the pits and grooves and onto the outer covering (enamel) of the teeth, causing dark brown stains.

If you smoke cigarettes, your teeth may sport stains ranging from yellowish brown to black. Smoking marijuana, besides being illegal, can also stain your teeth dark brown or even black. An injury can break blood vessels in the teeth, turning the affected tooth brown, gray, or black. And, of course, teeth tend to yellow as we age.

Regular professional cleanings can, in many cases, remove most of the stains caused by food or tobacco. But these days, many women prefer to turn to home bleaching kits. These products should never be used without professional supervision, warns Dr. Stay. You may have minute cracks or undetected cavities in your teeth, as well as other tooth or gum problems, that can be irritated or worsened by bleaching. So if you want to bleach your teeth at home, first discuss doing so with your dentist. If a home bleaching kit is right for you, your dentist can recommend one and then explain how to use it.

For very stubborn stains, your dentist may try one of these approaches.

• Bonding and porcelain veneers: Stubborn stains may need this approach. Bonding, often used for minor stains, is the application of acrylic resins to a tooth. A porcelain veneer is a thin cover that is bonded to the entire front of a tooth, covering unsightly stains.

• Caps: Teeth discolored by ruptured blood vessels inside the teeth must be capped, or crowned. A cap is a metal, porcelain, or plastic covering that fits over an existing tooth or portion of a tooth.

- Hydrogen peroxide or hydrochloric acid solutions: These substances can remove yellow stains due to aging or long-term tobacco use. The dentist applies the solution directly to the teeth and activates it with heat, light, or a laser. Do not use these solutions on your own—only a dentist should apply them.

*Don't use an at-home bleaching kit without first consulting your dentist. These can be harmful if your teeth have tiny cracks or cavities or if you have gum problems.*—Flora Parsa Stay, D.D.S.

## CAVITIES: DECAY ISN'T OKAY

The most common health problem in Western society is cavities, also known as dental caries or tooth decay. A cavity is a bacterial disease that can affect all parts of a tooth. Typically, it begins on the tooth surface, or enamel, where bacteria produce toxins from certain foods—especially those containing sugars and other simple carbohydrates, such as doughnuts, white bread and rice, cakes, and cookies. The toxins form plaque, which sticks to the enamel and erodes the tooth surface.

Eventually, plaque can cause the enamel to disintegrate. Then what started as a small surface cavity becomes deeper. If bacteria reach the inner layer of the tooth, or dentin, the cavity may grow inside the tooth.

Twice-a-year dental checkups are critical if you expect to keep a handle on cavities. If the dentist finds a small cavity on the surface only, you don't need any treatment. But its presence is a warning to practice good oral hygiene and dietary measures. If the damage has extended into the dentin, you'll need a filling. Then you have a choice to make.

These days, there are nearly as many types of fillings to choose from as there are lipstick colors.

- Amalgam, or silver, fillings: Composed of silver, nickel, mercury, and copper, these fillings used to be considered more durable than the composite fillings described here, too. But amalgam use is controversial among dental professionals. Some say mercury from the fillings can leak into your body over time, causing or contributing to serious problems, including fatigue, mental confusion, tremors, headache, and vision problems. Others, including the American Dental Association, say the risk is unproven and nonexistent. However, given the toxic qualities of mercury and the superior nature of composites, the composites are the better choice.

- Composite (plastic) fillings: These match the color of your teeth and are, thus, more aesthetically pleasing. Composed of plastic resin and a finely ground glasslike substance, composites, until recently, didn't stand up to wear as well as amalgams. But new advances have produced composites superior to amalgams. For example, composites expand and contract less than amalgams, which can allow cavities to form and mercury to leak.
- Porcelain inlays: Composed of ceramic materials, these inlays bond to the teeth. They are more fragile than amalgams or composites and more expensive, since they're custom-made. They can be matched to the color of your teeth, however, and resist staining.
- Gold inlays: These may be the best filling material, unless you're one of the few allergic to gold. They have a long life (20 years or more), but—because they're gold—are the most expensive option.

## DRY MOUTH: MOIST RELIEF

Dry mouth, or xerostomia, is caused by an insufficient amount of saliva. It is a common problem, in some cases coming on suddenly—just before an important speech or job interview, for instance—then disappearing.

But it can be chronic. The most common cause of dry mouth is medication. (See "Could It Be Your Medication?" on page 318). Dry mouth can also be caused by smoking, nerve damage, chemotherapy or radiation therapy of the neck and head, and by some diseases, including diabetes, Sjögren's syndrome (a disease of the salivary glands), AIDS, or Hodgkin's. Menopause can cause dry mouth because of the sharp decline in estrogen levels. (The contant fluctuation of estrogen levels may also be one reason canker sores are more prevalent in women than in men.)

Breathing through your mouth also causes dry mouth. If you do this only when your nose is stuffy due to a cold or the flu, don't worry. But if you find you're constantly breathing through your mouth because of blocked nasal passages or enlarged adenoids, talk to your doctor.

Dry mouth is more than an inconvenience. Saliva serves many purposes, such as reducing the amount of acidity in the mouth, thus warding off cavities and gum disease. Chronically inadequate saliva can dry the membranes in your mouth, leaving them prone to infection. Dry mouth is often associated with other problems, including burning tongue, bad breath, cracks in the corners of the mouth, mouth sores, and difficulty swallowing. Taste disorders can also be related to dry mouth. Saliva helps to make food more appetizing, so if you find food tastes different or not as good, you may have dry mouth.

Registered dental hygienist *Maria Perno Goldie* has these recommendations for banishing the desert from your mouth.

**Eliminate the cause.** This is the only effective long-term treatment. If you smoke, stop. If medications are causing your dry-mouth problem, ask your doctor to prescribe substitute drugs.

**Wet your whistle.** Use an over-the-counter mouth moisturizer or saliva substitute, such as Oralbalance, Oralube, or Xerolube. Also apply balm to your lips.

**Add moisture to the air.** Use a humidifier in your bedroom and, if possible, in your daytime environment.

**Stimulate saliva.** Rinse daily with a mouthwash specially designed for dry mouth, such as Biotene alcohol-free mouthwash, for temporary relief. You can also try sugarless gum or candies.

**Change products.** Use a special toothpaste—try Biotene brand—that is formulated with antibacterial enzymes to help against dry mouth.

If your dry mouth is due to a disease of the salivary glands (such as Sjögren's syndrome) or scarring from radiation therapy (particularly for head and neck cancers), your doctor or dentist may prescribe the drug Salagen (pilocarpine). It can stimulate saliva production in the remaining gland tissue. It is not for everyone because of various side effects, including over-stimulation of the sweat and intestinal glands.

*Lower levels of estrogen associated with menopause can leave your mouth dry as a desert.*

## CANKER SORES: SOOTHING A CRANKY CONDITION

The mouth is one of the first areas of the body to respond to stress. So when tiny, painful, blisterlike canker sores appear inside your mouth, your body is telling you to chill out. Also known as aphthous ulcers, these annoying sores begin life as white swellings that erupt into open sores that last three to six days. Canker sores can appear on the soft tissues of the mouth, such as the floor of the mouth (under the tongue) or the inner cheek surfaces.

Theories about the cause or triggers of canker sores include stress, smoking, food allergies, immunological conditions (such as the human immuno-deficiency virus, better known as HIV), or deficiencies in vitamin $B_{12}$, folic acid, or iron. In many cases, occurrence of canker sores may be in sync with a woman's menstrual cycle, says *Maria Perno Goldie, R.D.H., M.S.*

No one has yet found a completely effective way to rid the world—or your mouth—of canker sores. Left alone, they heal by themselves. Some dentists recommend an over-the-counter topical ointment, such as Orabase. Or your doctor may prescribe either a mouth rinse, such as a dexamethasone elixer, or corticosteroids, which can reduce pain and may speed healing.

*Flora Parsa Stay, D.D.S.,* offers these suggestions for treating canker sores.

**Soothe with oils and gels.** Aloe-vera gel can soothe pain and burning. If the sores appear on the lips, dab on vitamin E oil for relief. Either remedy can be used as needed until you experience significant relief.

**Take a nutritional supplement.** Nutritional supplements can help, especially if you have deficiencies. (A blood test or a review with a nutritionist can help you figure out what, if anything, you're lacking.) If you are prone to frequent outbreaks, take the following supplements daily. If episodes are infrequent, take these supplements at the first sign of an outbreak until the sores disappear.

- Folic acid: 400 micrograms
- Garlic: two 250-milligram capsules three times daily (Garlic is a natural antibiotic.)
- Iron: Take only with a doctor's permission.
- L-Lysine: 500 milligrams
- Vitamin $B_{12}$: 200 micrograms
- Zinc: 30 milligrams

**Avoid irritating foods.** When you have a canker sore, skip chocolate, chewing gum, lozenges, coffee, spicy foods, hot foods, and alcohol—all of which can irritate sensitive tissues.

*Canker sores and cold sores are sometimes linked to a woman's menstrual cycle.*—Maria Perno Goldie, R.D.H., M.S.

## COLD SORES: MAKE THEM DISAPPEAR

Wouldn't you know it? The night before a critical sales presentation or a date with that special someone, a cold sore suddenly appears. Can you make it disappear just as quickly?

Unfortunately, no. The good news, though, is that cold sores, like canker sores, clear up on their own—the bad news is that it takes 7 to 10 days.

Cold sores, also known as fever blisters, are infections caused by the herpes simplex virus. Once the virus takes up residence in your body, it turns into the guest from hell and never leaves. Herpes simplex usually moves in during childhood and remains dormant for years.

Common triggers that activate the virus include fever, sunburn, infection, menstruation, and stress. Therefore, some effective preventive measures include regular use of sunscreen (with a sun protection factor, or SPF, of at least 15) and avoidance or management of stress (easier said than done).

Cold sores appear as blisterlike bumps on the lips, gums, and palate. Symptoms include tingling and itching, which last for several hours, followed by pain, which lasts about two days. Then sores appear and the pain worsens. Swift treatment—as soon as you feel the tingle—is most effective.

Abreva is an over-the-counter cream that contains 10-percent docosanol. Apply it five times a day to shorten the course of a sore by about one day, while relieving pain, tingling, and burning. If the sores are in your mouth, *Flora Parsa Stay, D.D.S.,* recommends rinsing with an alcohol mouthwash (this is the *only* time she advises using commercial alcohol mouthwashes), followed by a rinse with an aloe-vera mouthwash, such as Grace's Dental Essentials Natural Mouthwash.

*Cold sores heal on their own in 7 to 10 days. Denavir, a prescription cream, requires frequent applications but clears them up in four days.*

You may want to ask your doctor about the new prescription cream Denavir (penciclovir), which can relieve cold sores in about four days. But this quicker relief comes with some inconvenience: Denavir must be applied every two hours when you're awake for four days if it's to be effective.

Some natural treatments may do the trick as well as Abreva, without the side effects of headaches and possible allergic reactions, which include rash and hives. Dr. Stay suggests these natural treatments.

**Rub on tea tree oil.** For best results, apply tea tree oil (available at health-food stores) as soon as you feel the tingle of a developing cold sore. Continue to apply it three to five times a day until the sores disappear.

**Apply herbal salve.** In a small bowl, mix 1 teaspoon each powdered thyme, myrrh, and goldenseal with 3 ounces beeswax (all available at health-food stores) and 1 teaspoon vegetable oil. Cover the bowl and put it in direct sunlight for three to four hours or in a low oven for one hour. Strain the mixture through a sieve or fine cloth and let it cool. Once the mixture is firm, apply it to sores several times daily until they disappear.

**Ease with E.** If the cold sores are on the lips and get crusty, dab on alcohol with a cotton swab two to three times a day, following up with vitamin-E oil.

**Rinse with rockrose.** Mix 1 teaspoon powdered rockrose (available at health-food stores) in 1 cup boiling water. Boil for 10 minutes. Let cool, then strain. Rinse your mouth with rockrose several times a day.

## CHAPPED LIPS: LICK THE PROBLEM

Afraid to smile because your lips may crack? Dry, chapped lips are a common problem—and not just in cold climates. Chapped lips can also be caused by overexposure to sunlight, a vitamin-B$_2$ (riboflavin) deficiency, lip biting, lip sucking, or poorly fitted dentures.

Lips are especially vulnerable to chapping and drying because their mucous membranes differ from those of the rest of your skin. Lips don't have the outer layer, called the stratum corneum, that protects skin. Nor do they have the same oil and sweat glands. The only natural source of moisture for the lips is the saliva inside the mouth. But licking your lips actually makes chapped lips worse, says *Flora Parsa Stay, D.D.S.,* since saliva contains digestive enzymes that contribute to drying.

Dr. Stay suggests the following remedies and preventive measures.

**Factor in the sun.** When you're outdoors, always apply a lip balm that contains sunblock (at least SPF 15) to your lips—and use it year-round.

**Make it gel.** Use a cotton-tipped swab to put aloe-vera gel on your lips to heal burning and drying. Apply as needed along with your sunscreen.

**Break the habit.** If you tend to bite or suck on your lips (usually a nervous habit), try chewing sugarless gum instead.

**Stay hydrated.** Dehydration can lead to dry lips. Drink at least eight 8-ounce glasses of water daily.

**Care for your kisser.** Apply ointment that contains zinc oxide to cracked lips to prevent bacteria and fungi from infiltrating and causing infection. Then apply sunscreen over the zinc oxide for optimal protection.

**Supplement your diet.** Dry lips and cracks in the corners of the mouth are a sign of a riboflavin deficiency. Take 100 milligrams riboflavin daily for several weeks. If your lips don't improve, try some of the other tips listed here.

# 17 Nails

## Hands-on Help Is Here

*Your nails reveal a great deal about your habits and personality. More importantly, their texture and color can indicate if your body is harboring disease.*

Nails are about more than looking well-groomed and picking up objects. They also support the tissues of your fingers and toes. The more active you are, the faster your nails will grow, which is why nail development is accelerated on your dominant hand and why fingernails grow quicker than toenails.

Nails are made of keratin, a hardened protein produced by skin cells. Old cells grow out and are replaced by new ones at a rate of about 1 millimeter per month. The old cells solidify to form the nails. It takes about six months to completely grow a new fingernail and approximately a year for a new toenail.

Nail development is also affected by the seasons (cold deters growth), as well as by your genes and age. As you advance in years, nails grow at a slower rate, and problems associated with poor circulation, medications, and increased nail thickness may evolve.

Hiding nail abnormalities under a thick layer of polish can just worsen some conditions. Consider what our experts have to say.

### BRITTLE NAILS: HOW TO REMOISTURIZE

Brittle nails chip, split, or break easily. The cause of such fragility is usually dehydration—but drinking more fluids won't rectify the problem. You need to moisten your nails from the *outside*.

323

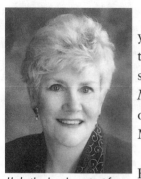

Don't be fooled, though: The more you expose your nails to water, the more likely they are to dry out. That's because moisture left on the skin and nails dehydrates as it evaporates, says *Marianne O'Donoghue, M.D.*, associate professor of dermatology at Rush-Presbyterian-St. Luke's Medical Center in Chicago.

*Hydration is as important for your nails as for your skin, says Marianne O'Donoghue, M.D. After you wash your hands, slather Vaseline or lotion on your nails to lock in moisture.*

Here's how to keep your nails healthy.

**Use a mild soap.** While it's not realistic to cut back on hand washing in hopes of stronger nails, you can minimize the drying effects of washing by steering clear of strong soaps and detergents. Instead, choose a gentle cleanser, such as Basis, Cetaphil, Dove, or Olay, suggests *Phoebe Rich, M.D.*, clinical associate professor of dermatology at the Oregon Health & Science University in Portland. And be sure to rinse well.

**Moisturize often.** While your hands are still damp from washing, slather on a rich emollient. Dr. O'Donoghue recommends Aquaphor, Neutrogena's Norwegian Formula, or a petroleum-based product, such as Vaseline, to seal in moisture.

*Ailing fingernails are not a health concern if your toenails are fine. The problem could be environmental, such as too much hand washing.*

**Wear gloves.** Detergents are formulated to cut through oil—and they'll do a number on your nails, too, by stripping away the protective surface. Remember to always wear vinyl gloves when washing dishes by hand or doing household chores that involve irritating cleansers. For extra protection, put on thin cotton gloves underneath rubber ones to act as absorbent liners. Dr. Rich warns you to never put ungloved hands into a bucket of soapy water.

**Be prudent.** Changing your fingernail polish every day is a surefire way to weaken nails. Polish removers containing acetone dehydrate your nails, depriving them of the protective layer that holds in moisture. Cutex's Quick & Gentle Felt Nail Polish Remover Pads, Mavala's Extra Mild Nail Polish Remover, and other acetone-free removers may be slightly milder. However, they still have the potential to dry out nails because they contain acetate, an ingredient similar to acetone. Even moisturizing additives, such as aloe and lanolin, don't offer much protection, since they're washed away with the remover, says Dr. Rich. So restrict your use of polish removers to once a week at most.

*Nail polish remover dehydrates your nails. Limit its use to once a week.*

*—Phoebe Rich, M.D.*

**Try biotin.** This B-complex vitamin may help thicken and strengthen your nails. One study found that more than 60 percent of participants experienced some benefits. While biotin may not work for everyone, the supplement is safe and inexpensive, so you might give it a try. Dr. Rich recommends 1,000 micrograms twice a day. Look for biotin at health-food stores and on the Internet.

## HANGNAILS: TIPS FOR HAPPIER CUTICLES

Hangnails are not really part of your nails at all. As we all unfortunately know, they're those annoying tags of cracked and ripped skin around the cuticles, the skin under the base of your nail. These painful appendages often result from cutting cuticles too aggressively.

Relief may be on its way with this advice from **Phoebe Rich, M.D.,**

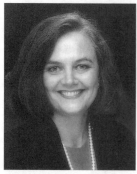

Take this cue from Phoebe Rich, M.D.: Never cut your cuticles. Instead, use a towel or soft cloth to push them back while skin is still soft after a shower.

clinical associate professor of dermatology at the Oregon Health & Science University in Portland: Never, *ever* cut your cuticles. "You don't want to get rid of cuticles. They are there for a purpose: to seal the nail and keep things out," she says. If you snip them, you open up entry points for bacteria or yeast, both of which can cause inflammation and infection.

Instead of trimming, use a towel to gently push back your cuticles after every shower, while the skin is soft. Never use any kind of instrument, especially on dry cuticles, or you'll do more harm than good, says Dr. Rich. Moisturize liberally when finished.

Heed Dr. Rich's tips, and your hangnails—as well as your dry, ragged cuticles—should disappear in several days.

**Stop chewing.** Biting only makes hangnails worse and may lead to infection.

**Have a good soak.** Twice a day, immerse your nails in about ½ cup warm water mixed with 1 tablespoon olive oil. After 10 minutes, clip any hangnails as closely as possible to the source of each tear.

**Lube up.** Finally, apply petroleum jelly—or antibacterial ointment if the site is infected—to your hangnail and cover it with a bandage.

## INGROWN TOENAILS: EASY AT-HOME FIXES

When a corner of a toenail digs into the toe, the ingrown nail causes inflammation and soreness in the surrounding skin, which can become infected.

Women who play sports that require frequent sudden stops, like tennis or basketball, can get ingrown toenails as a result of repeatedly jamming their toes into the tips of their shoes, says *Marianne O'Donoghue, M.D.,* associate professor of dermatology at Chicago's Rush-Presbyterian-St. Luke's Medical Center. But active or sedentary, anyone is fair game for this pain. If you trim your toenails incorrectly, wear snug shoes, or stand with bad posture, you're at risk.

An ingrown toenail is easy to treat at home, says **Phoebe Rich, M.D.,** clinical associate professor of dermatology at the Oregon Health & Science University in Portland. A word of caution: If you have diabetes or poor circulation, don't be a do-it-yourselfer; see your doctor instead.

Follow these recommendations from Dr. Rich to treat an ingrown toenail.

**Start with a footbath.** Soak your toes in a basin of warm, soapy water for 10 minutes, at least once a day—more often if you can manage it—to soften the nail and surrounding skin. Repeat for several days to relieve tenderness.

*Give your toes some wiggle room. Tight shoes can lead to ingrown toenails.*—Marianne O'Donoghue, M.D.

**Ease the pain.** Boil a nail file in water for 15 minutes. Let it cool. After soaking your toes, use the sterilized file to carefully lift the ingrown nail away from the inflamed skin. Insert a small piece of cotton soaked in antiseptic, such as hydrogen peroxide or iodine-containing Betadine, under the edge of the nail. (Or dab the cotton with a topical antibiotic ointment or cream, such as Bactroban or Neosporin.) The cotton will keep the nail lifted to alleviate pain-causing pressure and help the nail grow over the sore tissue. Continue this regimen each day for about a week, until the nail starts to grow correctly. If this treatment hasn't worked after two weeks, consult your doctor. The ingrown nail could become infected and require an antibiotic.

**Wear roomy shoes.** Squeezing your feet into tight shoes on a regular basis doesn't allow toenails to grow properly. Opt for shoes with a wide toe box and give your toes some wiggle room.

**Cut straight.** Next time you trim your nails, snip straight across and don't clip the corners at an angle. File down any sharp edges.

## NAIL DISCOLORATIONS: COLOR THEM HEALTHY

Under that perky polish may lurk a less desirable hue. Your nails' true tint could signal an underlying medical concern, says Marianne O'Donoghue, M.D., associate professor of dermatology at Chicago's Rush-Presbyterian-St. Luke's Medical Center. She cites these colorful examples.

- All white could point to liver disease.
- Cherry red might indicate heart irregularities.
- Paleness may be the result of anemia.
- Half white, half pink could suggest kidney disease.
- Yellow with a slight blush at the base may be a sign of diabetes.
- Black could warn of melanoma.

Pigments in nail polish can cause yellowing. To determine the actual color of your nails, stop painting them for about six weeks. Healthy nails are pinkish, shiny, and flexible. Don't worry about small white flecks. They're just signs of nail trauma—often a result of tapping nails or wearing tight shoes—and will grow out eventually.

If you think your nails are trying to tell you something, see your doctor.

## NAIL FUNGUS: CURING A COMMON PROBLEM

The first symptoms of a fungal infection are subtle: a hint of yellow or green at the edges of the affected nail, with maybe a chalky appearance under the nail. But nail fungus soon becomes hard to miss. The organisms attack the keratin that makes up the nail, causing the nail to thicken, deform, or even crumble. As the fungus eats its way through the nail to the soft tissue, dirt and debris accumulate, turning the nail an unattractive yellowish brown.

Nail fungus affects approximately 30 million Americans. It can be picked up while innocently gardening or walking barefoot in a public shower, says Marianne O'Donoghue, M.D., associate professor of dermatology at Rush-Presbyterian-St. Luke's Medical Center in Chicago.

Nail fungus is not only difficult to ignore, but also dangerous to neglect, says Dr. O'Donoghue. Fungal infections increase the risk of bacterial infections in people with impaired circulation in their feet, due to diabetes or chronic leg swelling. Resulting cracks in the skin and nails can allow bacteria to infect the tissues below or even the blood. This could lead to foot and ankle ulcers, a blood infection, or—in dire cases—foot or leg amputations.

Most people find nail fungus to be more of an unsightly inconvenience than a medical concern. Still, onychomycosis—the medical term for such an infection—won't clear up on its own and can spread to other nails. An infected nail can also become painfully ingrown. Unfortunately, topical antibiotic treatments don't get deep enough into the nail to be effective. A podiatrist can prescribe strong oral medications, but these drugs have the potential for serious bone marrow or liver toxicity and, thus, may not be appropriate for all patients. Any treatment can take up to six months to rid toes of fungus—and even then, the infection may recur up to a year later.

*A podiatrist can prescribe antibiotics, but even these can take six months to eliminate fungus. And the infection could return.—Marianne O'Donoghue, M.D.*

Here are Dr. O'Donoghue's pointers for avoiding or treating nail fungus.

**Think protection.** Wear flip-flops in communal showers and even at home if someone in your household has a fungal infection. Also, be sure to put on gloves before gardening.

**Try this polish Rx.** If over-the-counter antifungals don't help, ask your doctor about Penlac (ciclopirox), a clear solution brushed on nails affected with mild to moderate fungal infections. Penlac is mostly well-tolerated, but about 5 percent of users experience redness around the nails or burning of the skin.

**Get serious.** When all else fails, consider fighting the infection with prescription oral medication. Such drugs as Lamisil (terbinafine) and Sporanox (itraconazole) are the best weapons in the fight against nail fungus. Since some doctors won't prescribe these medications without a positive lab culture, stop using over-the-counter remedies at least two weeks before any such test to avoid getting a false negative.

# 18 Pain

## It's Time for Relief

*A woman says to her doctor, "My neck hurts when I do this." The doctor looks at her and says, "Then stop doing that."*

Pain is no laughing matter when you live with it every day. And it doesn't help that many women become frustrated when they seek medical care for chronic pain. Because family, friends, and even physicians may dismiss her complaints, a woman's pain is sometimes passed off as just a by-product of depression or anxiety.

Almost every type of pain—from common headaches to repetitive strain injuries—strikes women more often than men. Female hormones, a smaller

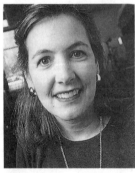

Women experience pain more frequently than men, says Julie Silver, M.D. Hormones and physiology might be to blame.

physiological build, and weaker muscles are all possible reasons for the higher susceptibility, says *Julie Silver, M.D.,* assistant professor in the department of physical medicine and rehabilitation at Harvard Medical School and medical director of the Spaulding-Framingham Outpatient Center in Framingham, Massachusetts. "Also, society may accept women giving voice to their pain more readily than it accepts men doing the same."

But that doesn't mean women get relief. For example, a national migraine study found that the overwhelming majority of those who suffer from this type of headache, which primarily affects women, do not receive the best care for the condition. In fact, half receive no treatment at all and many are misdiagnosed.

That's unfortunate, because medical advances now make it possible to control or even stop most types of pain. This chapter gives healing solutions for pain in your jaw, neck, shoulders, knees, and ankles, as well as headache, backache, and repetitive strain injury. If you have pain of any kind, there's no reason to suffer needlessly.

## WHAT IS PAIN?

Pain is debilitating—and it's *real*. Along with heat, cold, pressure, and touch, pain is one of your body's most basic sensations. You feel pain because special nerve endings throughout the body become stimulated. These nerve endings are in your skin, the covering of your bones, artery and intestinal linings, muscles, and organs. Those nerves send the "ouch" message up the spinal cord to your brain.

Your body responds to the pain much as it does to stress. Blood pressure rises and your pulse increases as blood flow shifts from your digestive tract and brain to your muscles. This prepares your body for what is known as the fight-or-flight response. In theory, this works to help your body locate the pain and take healing action. For example, when you walk on scorching pavement, the fight-or-flight response prompts you to jump away from the heat. But when you experience chronic pain, the same response can cause you to tense your muscles, resulting in even more discomfort.

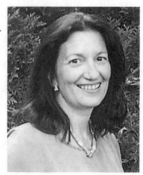

If muscle tension persists, you may continue to have pain long after the actual trigger is gone, says **Carol Kowalski, P.T.,** a physical therapist in Montague, Michigan. She says that's one reason that some types of pain are soothed by relaxation therapies, such as deep breathing, biofeedback, and meditation.

*Physical therapist Carol Kowalski recommends meditation and other relaxation therapies to soothe persistent muscle tension.*

### SHOULD I SEE A DOCTOR?
Too many women experience chronic pain needlessly. Consult a physician if any of these red flags are raised.

- You've tried to treat yourself and still have chronic pain.
- You resort to over-the-counter painkillers more than twice a week.
- Pain is the result of an accident, such as a fall.
- Pain is persistent and severe.
- Pain is accompanied by numbness, tingling, or weakness in your arms or legs.
- Pain interferes with your sleep.
- Pain disrupts your ability to enjoy life.

# BACKACHE: SURGERY IS YOUR LAST RESORT

Your lower back, called the lumbar spine, has five bones called vertebrae that are connected by six shock-absorbing disks. Muscles and ligaments support the spine's cablelike structure of nerves that connects your brain to your legs and feet. Numerous joints allow your spine to move from side to side and to twist and bend. As you age, joints in the spine can wear down, change shape, or become inflamed. If a disk ruptures, its soft interior can protrude and press on a nerve, causing pain. This is known as a herniated, slipped, or protruding disk.

To reduce swelling from acute back injuries, your doctor may prescribe a prescription nonsteroidal anti-inflammatory drug (NSAID), such as aspirin or ibuprofen. Disk problems sometimes require surgery.

Contrary to popular belief, bed rest can actually prolong back pain, whereas movement improves most cases. However, this doesn't mean you should rush

## ONE WOMAN'S STORY: CHRONIC BACK PAIN

*In April 2001, Judy Govatos, age 57, of Wilmington, Delaware, was doing what she loved most: gardening. As she pressed her foot into a shovel to dig a hole, pain shot through her lower back and she fell to her knees.*

An MRI and X-ray revealed that Judy Govatos had bulging disks in her lower spine, a condition that would take considerable time to heal. She tried various therapies over the ensuing months, and the discomfort ebbed and flowed. But often she couldn't sleep because her pain was so intense.

"At times, the pain was so bad that I couldn't exercise, which is what I had always turned to in the past to deal with stress," says Govatos. "The pain itself is so stressful. My muscles flinch to defend my body against the pain. It's a physiological response, but it sends all the muscles everywhere in my body into contraction. Then the brain sends out fight-or-flight chemicals, and I end up in a state of fear."

Govatos' reaction is common. In almost every pain condition, anxiety or depression go hand in hand with pain. As Govatos explored therapies for

managing the pain, she also met with a therapist to help her deal with her anxiety.

Here are Judy Govatos' suggestions for coping, based on her experiences:

**Keep moving.** Govatos realized that she could no longer take part in bouncy aerobics classes or dig in her garden. Yet she knew that mild exercise would help her back heal, as well as do wonders for her mood. Govatos had to find a way to work out without causing more pain. She quit aerobics classes altogether and gave up yoga and Pilates classes for six months, since all seemed to trigger back pain. Instead, she concentrated on gentle stretching and walking. When her pain became less frequent and intense, Govatos added weight lifting and aerobic exercise on "gentle" machines, such as an elliptical trainer, out to aerobics class. Normal activity and slow, gentle exercises, such as easy stretching, will help warm your back muscles and encourage circulation.

Most back pain can be treated successfully with these noninvasive techniques.

**Put out the fire.** You already know that smoking is bad for your lungs and heart, but few people think about blaming cigarettes for their backaches. Yet, when researchers from the Johns Hopkins University in Baltimore studied 53 years' worth of medical reports from 1,337 physicians, they found that patients who smoked experienced more back pain, seeking treatment for spinal degeneration more often than nonsmokers. Because nicotine from cigarettes is toxic to all body tissues, researchers theorize that smoking may cause damage to blood vessels in your back, preventing blood and oxygen from getting to the spine and back muscles. "Smoking, in general, is associated with higher pain and musculoskeletal complaints," says *Julie Silver, M.D.,*

bicycle, and treadmill. She worked out on one machine for 5 to 10 minutes and then moved on to the next. The regular exercise strengthened the muscles in her back, keeping her spinal disks aligned. "My doctor kept telling me that my back would be much worse if I was not exercising," Govatos says.

**Talk yourself through it.** On her most painful days, Govatos learned to mentally talk herself through the resulting anxiety. When she felt pain in her back, Govatos stopped fearful speculation—Will I be able to walk? What if my pain causes me to lose my job? What if I never get better?—and replaced it with more positive and realistic thinking. "I would acknowledge that, yes, I'm in pain. But I would remind myself that I'd had this pain before, that it had gone away before, that I was getting help, and that it would go away again," she says.

**Part company with the pain.** One of the most useful mental strategies Govatos learned was to keep her discomfort separate from her identity by imagining the pain as a gremlin outside her body. "I conceptualized the pain as something alien to me. So it isn't as if my entire body was in pain," she says. "It helped me see that I was not defined by my pain."

**Focus on your abilities.** For some time after Govatos began having back pain, she mourned for her old life. "I loved gardening. That was a tremendous loss," she says. "I had to accept it, let go, and then do the best I could, given the situation." So she asked her son, David, to do the digging and weeding she feared would hurt her back. "Now, I'm more my garden's manager. I still have the joy of the garden—and I get to bond with my son at the same time."

Govatos knew she had to accept some deprivations. "The greatest loss was the illusion of control," she says. "I had felt in control of my health. I exercised and ate well to be healthy, yet the pain came out of nowhere for no particular reason. Coming to terms with the pain, as well as the loss of the illusion of control, is a gradual process."

assistant professor in the department of physical medicine and rehabilitation at Harvard Medical School and medical director of the Spaulding-

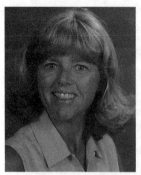

Framingham Outpatient Center in Framingham, Massachusetts. "Bone graft surgeons won't perform spinal fusions on smokers because they know the procedures won't take."

**Look on the bright side.** Stress can bring on a host of negative health changes, including back pain. A study at Ohio State University found that people are more likely to injure their backs while lifting boxes if they react stressfully to critical, nonsupportive supervisors. Research also shows that persons who are unhappy at work or home tend to have more back problems and take longer to recover from them. Stress may inflict back pain by causing you to tense your muscles, says *Letha Griffin, M.D.*, an ortho-paedic surgeon in Atlanta and team orthopaedist for Georgia State University in Athens. It may also ruin your sleep. "Sleep is when your body goes to work to repair itself," explains Dr. Griffin. When you toss and turn, those repairs go unfinished—and aches and pains set in.

*Stress can be a pain in the back, says Letha Griffin, M.D. If it keeps you awake at night, lack of sleep will interfere with your body's natural healing process, making pain even worse.*

**Lift correctly.** Women most frequently injure their backs by lifting children, laundry baskets, and other heavy items, then balancing them on their hips, says Dr. Griffin. Regardless of what you're lifting, she recommends this back-saving strategy: Align your feet directly under your shoulders for maximum support. Then bend your knees, tighten your abs, and bring the object close to your body. Use the strength of your legs to press up. If you need to turn while carrying the load, don't rotate at the waist. Instead, point your toes in the direction you want to go—keeping your weight centered over your arches—and pivot the rest of your body.

**Monitor your stress levels periodically.** Are your shoulders hunched toward your ears? Is your face all scrunched up? Is your heart racing? If you are experiencing any of these common reactions to pressure, then you are prob-ably tensing your back muscles as well. When you feel stress rising, get up and take a walk, which will help soothe and loosen tight muscles.

**Get on the ball.** Regular exercise keeps your back muscles strong and flexible. It also helps you sit, stand, and walk with good posture, thus pre-venting back strain. Dr. Griffin suggests using a fitness ball to strengthen your back. "These large balls are popular because people see them as toys or gadgets," she says. As you balance on an fitness ball, you simultaneously work numerous muscles, particularly the core muscles in your back and abdomen. These core muscles help keep your body properly aligned and ward off back pain. Look for fitness balls (also called Swiss balls and physioballs) at sporting-goods stores. Remember, though, that Dr. Griffin advises waiting until the acute pain of an attack subsides before attempting exercise with a fitness ball.

*Using a fitness ball strengthens back and abdominal muscles, which helps ward off back pain.*—Letha Griffin, M.D.

Do the following exercises with a fitness ball every other day to stretch and strengthen your back, hips, abdomen, and thighs.

- Prone scissors: Lie with your back on the floor, arms at your sides, and knees bent, with your calves balanced on top of the ball. Use your legs to pull the ball in close to your buttocks. Raise your left arm over your head as you simultaneously straighten your right leg, raising it off the ball and pointing your toes toward the ceiling. Lower your left arm and right leg, then raise your right arm and left leg in the same manner. Alternate back and forth at a slow, steady pace for one minute.
- Seated marching: Sit on the ball with your knees bent, feet flat on the floor, and arms hanging by your sides. Pull your abs in and up toward your spine as you lengthen your torso. Raise your left arm over your head, then lower it and raise your right arm. Repeat for one minute, alternating arms. If you have difficulty staying on the ball, position your feet and free arm to help you maintain your balance. Once you get the hang of the arm lifts, increase the difficulty of this exercise by simultaneously raising the opposite foot a few inches off the floor.
- Wall squats: Stand with the ball pressed between your lower back and a wall. Slowly squat as you bend your knees at a 90-degree angle. Hold the position for five seconds and slowly rise. Repeat

squats for one minute. When you are comfortable performing this exercise, challenge yourself by extending your arms over your head as you squat.

- Ball balance: Lie with your belly on the ball and your hands and feet on the floor. Raise your left arm about 2 inches off the floor as you simultaneously raise your right foot about 2 inches. Alternate opposite arms and legs for one minute.

## HEADACHE: LOOSENING THE VISE

Many doctors don't properly diagnose migraines because they incorrectly attribute the pain to tension or sinus headaches.

"There's a perception that all migraines are drag-out horrible headaches that make you vomit and send you to bed," says **Merle Diamond, M.D.,** associate director of the Diamond Headache Clinic in Chicago. "Probably

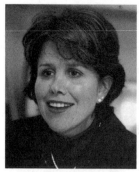

You may complain you have a hormone or menstrual headache, or a stress headache, but these are still migraines, says headache specialist Merle Diamond, M.D.

only about 30 percent of our patients vomit. And many of my patients can continue to function with a headache. They don't go straight to bed."

No one knows for sure exactly what triggers migraines. Some doctors believe they may be caused by an overreactive nervous system that inflames nerves and blood vessels in the brain. Others blame constriction and expansion of blood vessels in the head. Experts agree on one thing: Migraines *hurt*.

A migraine can last anywhere from 4 to 72 hours, often beginning as a dull pain that progresses to a throbbing headache at the temples, as well as on one side of the head at the front or back, or both. Right before their migraines set in, some sufferers see auras, which may consist of dots, wavy or jagged lines, or flashing lights; others have blind spots or tunnel vision. They may also experience nausea or sensitivity to light or sound. However, many women simply have bad headaches accompanied by no other symptoms.

Migraines are often mistakenly labeled. "If you get a headache around your menstrual period, you might call it your hormone or menstrual headache. Yes, it's related to your hormones, but it's a migraine. If you get a headache after stress, you might call it your letdown headache. It may indeed be caused by stress or by the letdown, but it's still a migraine," explains Dr. Diamond.

To find out for certain if you suffer from migraines, see a doctor who specializes in treating headaches. She'll ask about the severity, frequency, and duration of your headaches, as well as what seems to trigger them. She'll rule out other possible causes for pain, such as a sinus infection. However, despite the common misconception, sinus headaches are actually quite rare. If you don't have a thick nasal discharge, your headache is probably not sinus related; it's probably a migraine.

## A WOMAN'S RIGHT TO THE *RIGHT* TREATMENT: PAIN THERAPY

*Pain therapy has come a long way in recent years, making a visit to the doctor less frustrating than in the past.*

"Doctors like to feel successful, too," explains **Merle Diamond, M.D.,** associate director of the Diamond Headache Clinic in Chicago. When physicians had few effective pain therapies to recommend, they were more likely to dismiss the severity of patients' symptoms, she says. Now, a host of cutting-edge medications and treatments can dramatically reduce pain.

Here are some tips to ensure you get the best care:

**Allow yourself to feel justified.** Many women who suffer chronic pain are embarrassed to ask for help. Remember that all pain conditions are valid—no matter how mysterious the causes. The discomfort is *not* all in your head, and you *do* deserve to go through life free of pain. Give yourself permission to seek treatment.

**See a specialist.** Primary-care doctors can adequately treat some types of pain conditions. For example, most are now familiar with triptan prescription drugs to fight migraines. If you feel your doctor isn't providing the best care for your condition or minimizes the impact of your pain, then it's time to find someone new. For muscular conditions, ankle and knee pain, or spine-related problems, your best option is a visit to an orthopaedist or a physician who specializes in the back and spine, called a physiatrist.

**Ask questions.** Quiz your primary-care doctor about whether she feels comfortable treating your condition and how she plans to go about it. "If the doctor doesn't seem interested, then go see another doctor," recommends Dr. Diamond. "Don't give up."

**Pick the right option for you.** For any pain condition, there are myriad treatments. Ask your doctor about the choices available. "Different options work for different people. There is no single right answer that works for everyone," says Dr. Diamond. Choose a method of pain control that you know you'll be able to implement. If your physiatrist recommends 20 different exercises that will take more than an hour a day to perform and you don't have that much free time, voice your concern and seek a better option. Communicate with your doctor to get the information you need to improve your life—and alleviate your pain.

Women also often experience tension headaches, which grip the entire head, rather than one side only, making it feel as if the scalp is shrinking. They frequently occur during times of stress, anxiety, fatigue, or anger, when people subconsciously tense the muscles in their head and neck.

Here are Dr. Diamond's tips for preventing and soothing migraines and tension headaches.

**Back off on aspirin.** Many people pop over-the-counter pain relievers, such as aspirin, ibuprofen, or acetaminophen, to relieve their headaches. But if you take any of these drugs more than twice a week, your brain may begin to rely on their effects and will stop making natural pain-fighting opiates. So the medicine you take to treat a current headache may end up causing future headaches. This is known as the rebound effect. The telltale sign of painkiller addiction is a morning headache. "Your body becomes accustomed to that medicine being there," says Dr. Diamond. "So when you sleep all night without taking any additional painkiller, the medicine wears off and you wake up with a headache." If this description sounds familiar, talk to your doctor about switching from an addictive over-the-counter medication to a nonaddictive prescription medication.

*If you take aspirin too often, you may develop painkiller addiction. Frequent morning headaches are a warning sign.*—Merle Diamond, M.D.

**Ask for a prescription.** A new class of drugs called triptans is revolutionizing migraine treatment. You can take medication the moment a migraine strikes to knock out the headache within a half hour to two hours. Triptans include Amerge (naratriptan), Axert (almotriptan), Frova (frovatriptan), Imitrex (sumatriptan), Maxalt (rizatriptan), and Zomig (zolmitriptan). "These drugs don't cover up pain as over-the-counter medications do. Instead, they stop the vascular changes in the brain, turning off the headache mechanism," explains Dr. Diamond. Because there is a slight risk of heart complications, these drugs are preferable for women with no risk factors of heart disease, such as high blood cholesterol. If you suffer from migraines more than twice a week or if triptans don't work for you, talk to your doctor about such preventive medications as antidepressants, beta blockers, and antiseizure medications, which may help reduce the frequency and severity of your headaches.

**Monitor the birth control pill.** Older oral contraceptives that contained high doses of estrogen were found to intensify hormonal fluctuations, wreaking havoc on levels of a brain chemical called serotonin, which plays a role in migraines. Even today's low-dose pills are questionable. "Half the time they are helpful and actually reduce the incidence of migraines—and half the time they do not," says Dr. Diamond. Tell your gynecologist that you suffer from migraines before you start taking oral contraceptives. Be aware that birth control pills can slightly raise the risk of stroke in women who have migraines.

**Live a balanced life.** Maintaining regular sleep, exercise, and meal schedules can keep stress in check and help prevent headaches. While stress alone doesn't cause migraines, the way some women *react* to stress, such as skipping meals or getting too little sleep, may trigger migraines.

**Keep a headache diary.** To determine what triggers your migraines. as well as to help find out if your medication is working, track the following: what you eat and when, the number of hours you sleep, the medicines you take and when, when you exercise and for how long, and how stressful each day feels. Also note when you get a headache, how severe it is, and how long it lasts. After a few weeks, look for patterns in your records: Do you always get a headache soon after eating a certain food? Do headaches always hit on a particular day of the week? Once you pinpoint the causes of your headache, take the necessary steps to avoid those things or situations.

**Eliminate trigger foods from your diet.** Certain beverages and foods are known to prompt migraines. Caffeined drinks, alcohol, and chocolate top the list of culprits. Migraines may also be caused by some food additives, including yellow food coloring, MSG, and nitrates in red wine and processed meats. Some people develop headaches from tyramine, an amino acid found in aged cheeses, processed meats, peanuts, pickled foods, sourdough bread, lentils, and peas.

**Drink up.** Many headaches are related to dehydration. Much of your brain is water, so if you run a little low on this important substance, you'll get a dull headache. That's one reason that some people get migraines after exercising in the heat, when they've sweated away a lot of fluid.

**Tap into your body language.** Learn to stop tension in its tracks, and you can prevent both migraines and tension headaches. To keep muscular tension at bay, progressively tense and then relax the muscles in your body. Start at your feet, move up your legs, and proceed to your torso, arms, shoulders, neck, and face. Called progressive muscle relaxation, this tensing-and-releasing technique helps soothe muscles. "I recommend anything that makes you pay attention to your posture and breathing and state of tension in your muscles," says Dr. Diamond. Try such mind-body fitness routines as deep breathing, meditation, yoga, and Pilates.

**Prepare for stress.** If you know you are going to have a crazy day, plan ahead. "How can you find 10 minutes for yourself to take a deep breath and figure out what your body is doing? I'm a working mom, so I know it's hard to strike a balance," says Dr. Diamond, who has experienced migraines since she was a teenager. "If I can anticipate that it's going to be a rough time, I can be prepared. I make sure I have my medicine with me. I treat my headache as soon as it starts, and at the very least, I make sure to keep my sleep and exercise schedules regular."

## *Pulling on your hair can actually help reduce the pressure of a tension headache.*—Merle Diamond, M.D.

**Pull your hair out.** Well, not quite. But a neuromuscular massage technique, known as the hair pull, may help relieve tension headaches, says Dr. Diamond. Grab a hank of hair between your fingers and slowly tighten your grip, pulling slightly on your scalp where the hair is attached. Repeat along numerous spots on your head—particularly where you feel the most pressure—to stretch and release the fascia, a tight protective covering under your scalp.

**Consider biofeedback.** Some studies have reported that relaxation techniques help prevent headaches, as well as decrease their severity, frequency, and duration. One type, known as biofeedback, uses a computer to measure a patient's body temperature and muscle tension. Headache doctors trained in biofeedback can teach you how to relax, thus raising your body temperature and easing muscle tension. With guided imagery—a technique that could be called mind over migraine—you learn to relax and let go of stress by visualizing yourself in a soothing setting or situation. Try imagining yourself in a comfortable lounge chair. Notice a leaf floating down from a tree. Watch as the leaf floats to the left, then to the right. Follow it slowly making its way to the ground, where it lightly comes to rest. As you relax, migraine symptoms should ease. Other stress-reducing techniques include muscle relaxation and deep breathing. (See "Stress-Busters," page 283).

## NECK AND SHOULDER PAIN: SHRUG IT OFF

A skeleton in a science museum is held together with tiny wires. Without the wires, the head would fall off because the skull is too heavy for its seven-vertebrae neck to support. Living people don't need wires because muscles, tendons, and ligaments attach the skull to the neck and shoulder area, working in concert to hold up your head.

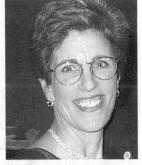

The weight of the head (about 10 to 13 pounds), sudden movement, and chronically poor posture can combine to weaken and stretch these muscles and tendons. Inflammation and pain can then result, says *Claire Wolfe, M.D.,* a clinical assistant professor of Physical Medicine and Rehabilitation at Ohio State University in Columbus.

*Soothe the aches in your neck and shoulders with massage, icing, and anti-inflammatory medication, such as ibuprofen, advises Claire Wolfe, M.D.*

"Tendon and ligament pain in the neck and shoulder can cause headaches," says Dr. Wolfe. "Pain can also mimic a pinched nerve by causing numbness and tingling in the arms. It can disrupt sleeping and daily functioning." For acute neck and shoulder pain, soothe away the ache by taking an anti-inflammatory medication, such as ibuprofen, icing the area, and lightly pressing your thumb and massaging where you feel pain.

For permanent relief from neck and shoulder pain, you must correct what initially caused the ache. These are Dr. Wolfe's recommendations for curing common problems.

**Sit up straight.** Proper posture provides support for your neck muscles. To sit and stand correctly, you need to strengthen the muscles that run between your shoulder blades. Exercises that target these muscles shouldn't hurt unless muscles are already inflamed. If you experience pain while exercising, ask your doctor for a prescription anti-inflammatory medication to reduce the swelling in your neck muscles to allow you to do rehabilitative exercises.

Dr. Wolfe recommends sitting on the edge of a bench with a light dumbbell in each hand. Lean forward from your hips, letting your arms hang down so that your hands are at midcalf level. Turn your hands so that your palms face behind you. Raise your elbows toward the ceiling as if you're rowing a boat, then return to the starting position. Repeat 10 to 15 times, three times a week. You should feel stretching in the muscles between your shoulder blades. Increase the weight of the dumbbells as you get stronger.

**Stretch it out.** Stretching can reduce muscle tension, which may lead to neck and shoulder pain. Concentrate on the muscles at the front of the neck to help you maintain proper posture. Sign up for a yoga or stretching class. Or try

## SLEEP AWAY YOUR NECK AND SHOULDER PAIN

*As you sleep, your body repairs damage caused during your waking hours. So it's no wonder chronic sleep loss is linked to many pain syndromes, including neck and shoulder discomfort.*

"In many patients, poor sleep is one of the hallmarks of neck and shoulder pain," says **Claire Wolfe, M.D.,** clinical assistant professor of Physical Medicine and Rehabilitation at Ohio State University in Columbus. Women who don't sleep well either toss and turn or simply don't get the hours of sleep that they need. "I often ask women how they feel in the morning. If they say they feel like they've been run over by a truck, then I know sleep is an issue for them."

To improve your sleep, Dr. Wolfe offers these tips:

**Get your heart rate up.** Regular aerobic exercise performed three to four times a week not only can improve sleep, but also help erase stress and improve blood flow to the neck and shoulder muscles. Aquatic aerobics is an especially good option, because the buoyancy of the water allows for more comfortable movement.

**Cut down on prebedtime drinking.** Stimulants, such as caffeinated drinks, can interfere with a good night's sleep. Avoid these for at least six hours before bedtime. While you're at it, add alcohol to the list of no-nos.

**Sleep the right way.** To position your neck properly, sleep on your back with your neck centered above your shoulders and a pillow supporting your head and neck. Sleeping on your side isn't terrible, providing you contour your pillow to provide adequate support. Avoid sleeping on your stomach, as keeping your head turned to the side all night stresses your neck muscles and causes pain.

**Consider medication.** If the previous methods don't relieve your discomfort, talk to your doctor about improving the quality of your sleep with a low-dose tricyclic antidepressant, such as Elavil (amitriptyline). "These drugs are hardly ever used to treat depression these days, but they do a wonderful job of normalizing the sleep pattern," says Dr. Wolfe. Unlike sleeping pills, these drugs have few side effects and allow you to wake refreshed, rather than having a sleeping-pill hangover.

the following neck rotations: Slowly roll your neck forward, to one side, to the back, and then to the opposite side. Do these controlled rotations five times in each direction, both clockwise and counterclockwise. Note that if you've had a whiplash injury or have compression between the vertebrae in your neck, you may not be able to tip your head back without support. So gently place your fingertips at the back of your skull as you roll your head back. If you feel pinching in your vertebrae, bring your head back up. Extend your crown upward, as if a string were pulling the top of your head up, to lengthen your neck. Then slowly lower your head as far as is comfortable.

*Good posture, stretching, and strength-building exercises can ease most cases of neck and shoulder pain.*—Claire Wolfe, M.D.

**Set up a healthy workstation.** Position your computer monitor where you won't have to move your head up, down, or to the side to see it. Your chair should be positioned so that your feet easily rest on the floor. If your feet dangle, you'll compensate for the extra space by slouching. If your chair doesn't adjust, place your feet on a footrest.

**Pay attention to your handbag.** If it's too heavy, you will walk slightly tipped to one side, inflicting neck pain. Lighten your load by removing any unnecessary items (you pack rats know who you are). Also, opt for a purse that you can wear either like a backpack or across your chest to keep the weight equal on both sides of your body.

## REPETITIVE STRAIN INJURY: WHEN YOUR HANDS NEED HELP

The cause of most repetitive strain injuries (RSIs) to the hand, wrist, elbow, and shoulder can be traced to the invention of the typewriter in the late 1800s. Because keys locked up if a user typed too quickly, manufacturers purposely designed an inefficient keyboard, with the letters *Q, W, E, R, T,* and *Y* in the upper left to slow typing speed. "Reaching these keys requires a lot of reaching and stretching as you type," explains *Julie Silver, M.D.,* assistant professor in the department of physical medicine and rehabilitation at Harvard Medical School and medical director of the Spaulding-Framingham Outpatient Center in Framingham, Massachusetts. "These extra movements probably promote injury."

Today, widespread computer usage is the primary reason for RSIs, which result from overuse of particular muscles when the same movement is performed repeatedly. Some manufacturers have tried to modify computer keyboards to make them more efficient, but consumers resist such changes. It seems we'd rather stick with what we know—even if it inflicts pain.

RSI symptoms include weakness, tingling, stiffness, and pain in the neck, shoulders, upper back, upper arms, elbows, wrists, thumbs, or fingers. The

## FIBROMYALGIA: ACHING ALL OVER, ALL THE TIME

*Doctors are only beginning to unravel why more women than men suffer from a depressing and debilitating condition known as fibromyalgia.*

If your muscles and tendons ache all the time and are tender to the touch, you might have fibromyalgia. The condition literally means "fibrous pain," or pain involving fibrous tissues. Fibromyalgia makes you feel as if you've run a marathon, even when you haven't.

This condition may be directly related to poor sleep habits. When your body doesn't enter deep sleep, known as stage four sleep, it doesn't get a chance to mend itself. Nicks in your muscles go unrepaired, leaving you perpetually sore, explains *Claire Wolfe, M.D.,* clinical assistant professor at Ohio State University in Columbus.

It is also during deep sleep that your muscles are able to truly relax. If you don't enter this phase, muscles remain tense throughout the night, says *Letha Griffin, M.D.,* an orthopaedic surgeon in Atlanta and team orthopaedist for Georgia State University.

Nonsteroidal anti-inflammatory drugs (NSAIDs), like ibuprofen, may help soothe the ache. Alternative treatments, such as acupuncture, acupressure, yoga, and massage, also show promise in easing fibromyalgia symptoms, says Dr. Griffin. But the most studied self-help strategy is exercise therapy. Aerobic exercise improves blood and oxygen flow to aching muscles, promoting healing. Exercise also helps you deal with the stress, depression, and anxiety associated with pain—and, as an added bonus, often improves your sleep.

Fibromyalgia researcher *Sue Gowans, Ph.D., P.T.,* examines various exercise programs in order to design the perfect strategy for treating fibromyalgia. In a recent study, participants gradually increased the duration and intensity of their exercise over a period of 23 weeks. By study's end, subjects reported feeling less depressed and anxious, as well as more in control of their pain. They were also able to walk longer and faster in a set amount of time.

"Some patients were fearful because they thought they would have postexercise pain, but they gradually took it upon themselves to try," says Dr. Gowans, a research associate in rehabilitative services at University Health Network at effects can be downright debilitating, with RSI sufferers often feeling too much pain to shake hands, press an elevator button, or carry a laundry basket.

You can experience an RSI in any part of your body that is moved repetitively. Tennis players often develop RSIs in their elbows and shoulders. Assembly-line workers can suffer them in whatever part of their bodies they use most. And musicians sometimes get RSIs in their fingers and hands.

The most common site for an RSI is the carpal tunnel area of the wrist and forearm. Several tendons and the median nerve run through the enclosed space in this region, explains Dr. Silver. If anything in that space swells, you feel pain in your hand, wrist, or elbow. This condition is known as carpal

Toronto General Hospital. "You absolutely need to start slow and work up. The number-one reason patients fail with exercise is because they enroll in classes available in the community, which are almost always too hard for someone with fibromyalgia. You want a class that's gentler than even ones offered to the elderly. A young Jane Fonda–type instructor is *not* what you want."

Gowans suggests exercising aerobically for 30 minutes, three times a week. Here are her tips on how to get moving without pain:

**Start and end with stretching.** Devote the first and last five minutes of your workout to gentle, mild stretching.

**Start in a pool.** Women in Dr. Gowans' study exercised in shallow water. They began by moving their arms back and forth and progressed to walking the width of the pool repeatedly. Over time, the women walked faster. By Week 6, they were able to jog in the water. Though the pool used in the study was heated to 95 degrees, Dr. Gowans says any heated pool fits the bill. Most fitness center pools are only 80 to 85 degrees, so consider sitting in a hot tub before or after your workout to soothe muscle pain.

**Advance to the land.** Once you can jog in the pool, take your workouts out of the water two days a week. Try walking for a half hour. Start slowly, then pick up the pace and work up to a jog. But don't push yourself too quickly. Those in Dr. Gowans' study weren't jogging until Week 23. And remember that if brisk walking provides enough stimulation to lift your mood, you don't have to progress to jogging at all.

**Monitor your heart rate.** One way to make sure you work up gradually is to stay below your target heart rate. To determine your target heart rate, subtract your age from 220 for your estimated maximum heart rate per minute. You want to stay between 60 and 75 percent of that—max. For example, if you are age 40, your maximum heart rate is 180 beats per minute (BPM). Sixty percent of that is 108 BPM. While exercising, take your pulse every 5 to 10 minutes to make sure you are staying between 108 and 180 BPM.

**Listen to your body.** Your muscles may ache before and even after you exercise—that's perfectly normal for fibromyalgia patients. But if the ache intensifies beyond how you usually feel, you're probably overdoing it, warns Dr. Gowans.

tunnel syndrome. Women are more prone to this syndrome than men, perhaps because their carpal tunnel space is smaller. Also, pregnancy sometimes causes these tissues to swell, creating even less space and putting more pressure on the median nerve.

*Self-help can backfire. For instance, wrist rests for the computer can press against already swollen areas, creating more pain.*—Julie Silver, M.D.

Here are Dr. Silver's tips for alleviating the pain of RSIs and preventing future attacks.

**Get a diagnosis.** Other conditions, such as osteoarthritis, can mimic an RSI. And some types of self-treatment can backfire. For example, many people use rests to hold their wrists in a neutral position at they type at the keyboard. But the rest's padding can press against the already swollen area, creating more pain. Wrist splints that are improperly fitted or worn excessively can cause your arm muscles to lose their shape, promoting weakness and, thus, perpetuating the problem. See a physician trained in rehabilitation who can customize a treatment to your needs and physiology.

**Live healthfully.** A recent study of pregnant women—who are especially prone to RSIs—cited evidence that those who smoked or drank alcohol were more likely to suffer from RSI pain than those who did neither. As noted previously, alcohol and nicotine may be toxic to tendons and muscles. Also, smoking may damage blood vessels, preventing blood and oxygen from getting to your forearms. Of course, pregnant women shouldn't be smoking or drinking anyway!

**Move around.** Many people try to soothe RSI pain by finding the most ergonomically correct positions for sitting and resting their wrists—and then try to remain that way indefinitely. Such a practice can actually make pain worse. "People get in a position where they are in perfect alignment and stay in perfect alignment all day. But your body likes to move," says Dr. Silver. "Blood likes to flow. Muscles like to contract. Sitting in the perfect position like you are in a virtual straight jacket will actually promote injury." Instead of focusing on perfect alignment, aim for comfort and ease of movement. Hold your wrists however feels good to you and change position throughout the day as needed. Also be sure to take frequent breaks—get up and walk around or stretch once every 20 minutes.

**Rearrange your office.** Many people with hand or wrist pain use one hand almost exclusively to type, manipulate a mouse, pick up the phone, and write. Relocate your mouse and phone to where you'll be forced to use your nondominant hand more often.

**Aim for comfort.** An entire industry has been built around designing office furniture and accessories for people with RSIS. Ergonomic office chairs, computer keyboards, mouse equipment, and footrests can help ease discomfort, but they are useful to you only if they conform to the unique needs of *your* body. "Companies buy 1,000 ergonomic chairs that are all the same and expect a 90-pound person and a 350-pound person to use the same chair," says Dr. Silver. "Even if the chair is adjustable, that doesn't always compensate for the different shapes and sizes of people." If you experience discomfort while using supposedly ergonomic equipment, then the equipment doesn't work for you.

> *Your checklist for an ergonomic office includes: an adjustable chair, eye-level computer monitor, and keyboard that sits below elbow level.*
>
> —Julie Silver, M.D.

Here are some general pointers for setting up an ergonomic office.

- Select a chair that is adjustable, allowing you to sit low enough that your feet rest flat on the floor. A proper chair should also support your lower back.
- Note that although experts once advised keeping the keyboard at elbow level, new research indicates that using a keyboard 4 centimeters (about 1½ inches) below elbow level puts less stress on wrists.
- Keep your monitor at eye level in front of your face, rather than to one side.

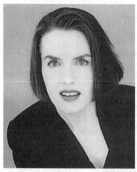

*Traditional ways of doing things might be healthier. Work by hand instead of by computer to reduce the abuse to your hands, says Deborah Quilter, a consultant on repetitive strain injury.*

**Wean yourself off your computer.** No matter how well you design your office or how much you fidget and stretch, overuse is still overuse. The best plan for easing RSI symptoms—and preventing future damage—is to rely on your computer less. "I don't use the computer if I don't absolutely have to," says *Deborah Quilter,* an RSI consultant and personal trainer in New York City and author of *The Repetitive Strain Injury Recovery Book.* "I made a decision a long time ago that my hands are more important than keeping up with the crowd. Most people are not willing to go that far, but as a consequence, they lose normal use of their hands. The body was not designed to be doing such intensive static work everyday, all day long."

Instead of using the computer, Quilter offers these suggestions.

- Phone or fax rather than e-mail.
- Don't surf the Internet for information that you can find through other forms.
- Rely on a newspaper, not the Internet, for news and checking your stock portfolio.
- Nix computer games, opting to play solitaire with real cards instead.
- Keep a paper appointment calendar and address book rather than computerized versions.
- Balance your checkbook by hand rather than using checkbook-balancing software.
- Support the post office by paying bills the old-fashioned way.

"If you can perform a task without the computer, do it," says Quilter. "It makes no sense to abuse your hands if you can use another part of your body."

**Consider injections and surgery.** If you continue to feel pain—even after rearranging your office and inserting numerous rest and stretch breaks into your routine—you may require further help. A physician can prescribe an anti-inflammatory medication to reduce pain and swelling if no over-the-counter medication is effective. Many people find relief from a cortisone shot, which reduces swelling. As a last resort, surgery can open up the carpal tunnel area, eliminating restriction on the median nerve, advises Dr. Silver.

## TEMPOROMANDIBULAR JOINT DISORDER: RELAX YOUR JAW

If your jaw pops, clicks, locks, or hurts when you open or close your mouth, you probably have temporomandibular joint disorder (TMD). Named for the jaw joint that it affects, TMD, formerly known as TMJ, can lead to pain in the ears, head, and neck.

TMD is two to five times more common in women than in men—but experts don't know why. One theory is that TMD might be linked to estrogen levels, though research is still divided on the issue.

"Researchers investigating the role of supplemental estrogen use in women have come to different conclusions," says *Dushanka Kleinman, D.D.S., M.Sc.D.*, deputy director of the National Institute of Dental and Craniofacial Research and chief dental officer of the U.S. Public Health Service in Bethesda, Maryland. "Some say their findings indicate that estrogen replacement therapy does *not* place women at increased risk for TMD. Others say these hormones *do* play a possible role in TMD pain." In other words, it could be estrogen ... or it could be something else.

If you have serious and recurring jaw pain, see a dentist to get a definitive diagnosis before trying any home remedies. Sinus flare-ups, toothaches, and even perodontal disease can cause similar symptoms—and each requires different treatment. To find a female dentist in your area, go to www.womendentists.org.

*When your jaw is relaxed, your teeth don't touch and your lips are slightly parted.*—Dushanka Kleinman, D.D.S., M.Sc.D.

Once you are diagnosed with TMD, try these self-help fixes from Dr. Kleinman.

**Warm it up.** When you experience pain, apply a moist, warm washcloth or a hot-water bottle to your jaw. Heat helps increase circulation and soothe jaw muscles.

**Take medication.** Nonsteroidal anti-inflammatory drugs, such as ibuprofen, will reduce inflammation and dull the ache.

**Consider a bite plate.** TMD pain is caused partly by the chronic tensing of jaw muscles during sleep or periods of stress. Your dentist can design a plastic mouthpiece for you to wear—particularly at night—which prevents you from unconsciously clenching your jaw. You can find similar bite plates at some drugstores, but one custom-made by a dentist will contour to the unique shape of your mouth. "In general, customized bite plates are reported to be more comfortable," advises Dr. Kleinman.

**Relax already.** The advice is so simple, yet so often ignored. Pay attention to your jaw, particularly during stressful times. When you're maneuvering in traffic, negotiating a pay raise with your boss, or waiting for your teenager to get home at night, remember to relax your jaw. In a relaxed state, your lips are slightly parted and your teeth aren't touching. You might have to remind yourself to unclench, as you probably tense your jaw more often than you think.

*Research shows that improved posture can reduce TMD pain by half. Keep your head centered over your shoulders, not jutting forward.*

**Stop slouching.** Research conducted on 60 TMD patients in Lackland, Texas, found that those who received posture training cut their TMD pain and frequency nearly in half, compared to a control group who had no such therapy and experienced little relief. People who normally stood with their heads forward of their shoulders, as if they were being pulled forward by their noses, gained the greatest relief from their improved posture. To keep your head centered above your shoulders where it belongs, try the following exercise: Place your fingertips about 1 inch behind the back of your skull. Press your head back and try to touch your skull to your fingers, as if you were a turtle retracting into your shell. Hold for a few seconds, then release. Repeat 10 to 15 times a day to train yourself to hold your head correctly.

## KNEE PAIN: STRONGER MUSCLES ARE THE SOLUTION

Knee pain is often caused by muscle imbalances that make the kneecap track improperly, thus creating friction. The usual culprits are weak inner thigh and abdominal muscles, as well as a tight iliotibial band, a thick strip of tissue that starts at your hip and runs along your outer thigh to your ankle.

The general wear and tear of life can also result in knee pain. As you age, you may develop osteoarthritis in a knee joint, as well as microtears to your meniscus, the cartilage cushion under your kneecap. Wearing high-heeled shoes eight or more hours a day makes any condition worse by putting too much pressure on your knees and back. Degenerative wear cannot be reversed, but physical therapy can help change the way you use the knee muscles in order to protect your cartilage and joints from further damage. Getting a cortisone injection in the affected knee or taking a prescription medication can also reduce inflammation and pain. A knee brace can take pressure off the joint, thus reducing pain.

Try these remedies to control and prevent knee pain.

**Strengthen the right muscles.** To eliminate the imbalances that cause knee pain, focus on strengthening your inner thigh and abdominal muscles, suggests *Anne Zeni Hoch, D.O.*, assistant professor of physical medicine, rehabilitation, and orthopaedic surgery and director of the women's sports medicine program at the Sports Medicine Center at the Medical College of Wisconsin in Milwaukee. She recommends these exercises.

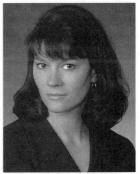

*Anne Zeni Hoch, D.O., says that exercise can help keep your kneecap aligned and reduce your knee pain.*

- Leg raise: Lie on your back with your right leg extended. Bend your left leg and place your left foot on the floor, with your toes pointing up toward the ceiling. Angle the toes on your right foot to point in a 2 o'clock position. Raise your extended right leg about 45 degrees, or about halfway up. Simultaneously, press your abdominal muscles down, flattening your lower back to the floor. Then lower your leg and repeat as often as you can without experiencing pain—stop immediately if your knee starts to hurt. Repeat with opposite leg. Once you can do 20 repetitions with each leg, increase the difficulty by adding 1-pound ankle weights.
- Roll up: Borrowed from the Pilates exercise approach, this move strengthens your abdomen. Tight abs pull your pelvis into proper alignment, which in turn also helps you properly align your legs and put less pressure on your knees. Start by lying on the floor with your legs bent and your feet flat on the floor. Stretch your arms over your

head. Expel all the air from your lungs by pressing your tummy down toward the floor. Inhale as you slowly roll up to a seated position, moving one vertebra at a time. Try to curl your abdomen into a C-shape as you roll up. Once you reach a seated position, reverse the motion by rolling back down, letting one vertebra at a time touch the floor. Repeat 5 to 10 times.

- Stand on one foot: Any injury to your lower legs also damages important nerve receptors that are responsible for keeping your balance. Damaged receptors don't provide the feedback your brain needs to keep your legs in proper alignment, making you more likely to accidentally bend or twist a knee painfully. One-foot standing drills help retrain these nerve receptors and strengthen your inner thigh and ab muscles, which in turn keep your knees aligned and soothe away pain. Stand in front of a mirror, with a chair nearby for balance if needed. Make sure that your hipbones are level and that your toes and knees point forward and don't angle in or out. Shift your weight onto your right foot and center your body over your right arch. Slowly lift your left foot off the floor, bending it behind you. As you do so, try to keep your right knee from collapsing inward. Hold for up to 20 seconds, then release and repeat six times. Do the same repetitions while standing on your left foot.

# Many people will experience a little knee pain as they age. Wearing high heels makes any condition worse by putting too much pressure on your knees and back.

Consider supplements. About half of osteoarthritis-related knee pain sufferers who take glucosamine and chondroitin experience less inflammation and pain, says Dr. Hoch. These supplements are thought to work by providing important healing nutrients to ligaments, bones, and tendons. Studies show that a daily dose of 1,500 milligrams of each is required to see results, which usually take a few months. These two supplements don't interact with prescription pain medication or have any side effects. "We know from studies that glucosamine and chondroitin are not harmful—and that's the most important thing," says Dr. Hoch. They are available at heath-food, convenience, and grocery stores. Look for a supplement that is standardized, which means that it has been proven to actually contain what the ingredient label claims. It is always a good idea to talk to your doctor before taking any kind of supplements for any kind of pain.

*The supplements glucosamine and chondroitin ease knee pain in about half of women who take them. They're free of side effects, but it can take months to see results.*

*—Anne Zeni Hoch, D.O.*

**Lose weight.** Excess poundage puts pressure on your knees and aggravates degenerative knee conditions. You can safely lose 1 pound a week by eliminating 500 calories a day. Daily exercise will burn 250 calories, roughly the number a 160-pound woman burns in one hour of water aerobics—a perfect exercise for those with knee pain, by the way. Cut out a soda a day to rid yourself of another 250 calories. Another simple tip to spur your weight loss: Eat eight or more servings of fruits and vegetables a day to help you feel full without piling on calories.

## MUSCLE PAIN: WARM UP TO RELIEF

To some extent, sore muscles are a necessary evil. In order to improve your fitness, you need to push your muscles a little beyond their comfort zone—however, then you risk tearing muscles. When these microtears become inflamed, you feel sore. But there is good news: The next time you perform the same activity, those tears will have strengthened your muscles and prepared you for the challenge.

Sometimes, muscles hurt for reasons not associated with exercise, or they just ache all the time. Both suggest a systemic condition, such as the flu or fibromyalgia. (See "Fibromyalgia: Aching All Over, All the Time," page 344.) A muscle cramp is an involuntary contraction. When your calf or foot is involved, the ache goes by the unlikely moniker of charley horse. This type of cramp can occur while exercising, as well as when you're resting. A charley horse often strikes at night. And beware: Such cramps become more common as you age.

## Take one ibuprofen or aspirin tablet before a tough workout to reduce postworkout pain.—Julie Silver, M.D.

Here's how to avoid or stop muscle pain.

**Pop a prepain pill.** If you plan to intensify an exercise session, take ibuprofen or some other nonsteroidal anti-inflammatory drug (NSAID) before revving up. One pill will help keep muscle tissue from swelling and reduce postworkout pain, says *Julie Silver, M.D.,* assistant professor in the department of physical medicine and rehabilitation at Harvard Medical School and medical director of the Spaulding-Framingham Outpatient Center in Framingham, Massachusetts.

**Take a soak.** Immediately following a workout, massage any sore areas with ice to reduce inflammation. If you still feel pain 24 hours after exercising, heat is the most effective remedy, as it improves circulation to the painful muscle, promoting quicker healing, says Dr. Silver. A 10-minute soak in a hot tub or regular bathtub will help ease the ache.

**Stretch often.** For muscle cramps, stretching may be your best option for relief. It not only helps get rid of a cramp in progress, but also can prevent future cramps by halting the muscle contractions that cause the problem. For a cramp in your foot or calf, try this stretch: Gently flex your toes toward your knees, stretching your calves, Achilles tendons, and arches of your feet. If you often get leg cramps at night, stretch before going to sleep (and remember to *always* stretch after exercising). Keep a towel near your bed. When you get a late-night cramp, loop the towel around the ball of the foot of the cramped leg and curl your toes toward you.

**Boost your antioxidants.** Molecules known as free radicals form during exercise and are partly responsible for postworkout muscle pain, explains *Liz Applegate, Ph.D.,* professor of nutrition at the University of California at Davis and author of *Eat Smart, Play Hard.* Antioxidant nutrients—such as vitamins A and C, zinc, and selenium—help neutralize free radicals. You can easily increase your intake of antioxidants by eating five to nine daily servings of fruits and vegetables—the same level recommended to ward off heart disease and cancer. Dr. Applegate also recommends a daily supplement of 400 International Units of the antioxidant vitamin E, since it's difficult to get enough of this vitamin from food alone.

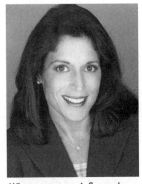

*What you eat can influence how you feel after a workout, says Liz Applegate, Ph. D. Fruits and vegetables contain antioxidants that prevent some postexercise muscle pain.*

## ANKLE PAIN: NEW TWISTS IN TREATMENT

When you sprain your ankle, the ligaments are overstretched and nerve receptors responsible for balance lose their sensitivity. Left untreated, such problems increase your risk of spraining your ankle again.

Here's how to break the cycle of pain and treat an ankle sprain properly.

**Wrap it, ice it, and prop it.** To recover quickly from a sprained ankle, you want to prevent fluid from accumulating in your ankle tissues. If you are injured away from home, keep your shoe on. It will act like a bandage to help support the ankle and contain the swelling, says *Letha Griffin, M.D.,* an orthopaedic surgeon in Atlanta and team orthopaedist for Georgia State University. If possible, keep your leg elevated until you get to where you can rest. Then take off your shoe and ice your ankle for 10 minutes with a flexible blue ice pack. These packs usually come with a protective covering that prevents the pack from making your skin too cold. If your pack doesn't have a protective covering, place a paper towel between the pack and your skin. (In a pinch, a bag of frozen vegetables makes a good substitute for the pack.) After icing, wrap the ankle snugly in a woven elastic bandage, starting at the arch of your foot and wrapping upward. You want the bandage to be snug, but not so tight that it cuts off blood circulation to your toes, advises Dr. Griffin. Prop your foot on a pillow or coffee table. Ice the ankle for 10 minutes each hour. Continue this treatment for the first 24 hours to reduce inflammation.

**Get back on it.** Doctors used to warn people to stay off a recently sprained ankle. Now, however, they encourage you to get a move on. As soon as you start using the ankle joint, you begin regaining the strength and flexibility damaged by the sprain. Stretch your injured ankle by drawing the letters of the alphabet in the air with your big toe. Rather than hopping around, try putting a little weight on your ankle every time you walk. In due course, the combination of compressing, icing, and flexing will help you increase the weight your ankle can bear. Of course, severe sprains may require some immobilization. Dr. Griffin advises that you see a doctor immediately after suffering a sprain to determine your best course of action.

*Don't pamper a sprained ankle. Move it as soon as possible. Stretch it out by drawing letters in the air with your big toe.—Letha Griffin, M.D.*

**Balance it out.** Once you can walk on your sprained ankle, balance drills will help retrain the nerve receptors in your lower leg. Start by balancing on the foot you injured. This will be difficult at first, so use a chair for balance if necessary. Once you can stand on this foot for 1 minute, try doing it with your eyes closed. Then move your head back and forth, as if shaking your head no, with your eyes still shut. Once you master that, you've probably improved your balance beyond even presprain, says Dr. Griffin.

**Choose footwear wisely.** High-heeled shoes are less stable than sneakers and make you more likely to roll your ankle when you encounter a bump in the road. If you must be a slave to fashion, Dr. Griffin suggests choosing a heel with a wide, stable, square base, rather than any of the skinnier versions.

# 19

chapter

# Pregnancy Discomforts
## A Little Mothering for Your Nine Months

*Instead of wishing away nine months of pregnancy, I'd have cherished every moment, and realized that the wonderment growing inside me was the only chance in life to assist God in a miracle.*—Erma Bombeck, "If I Had My Life to Live Over"

If you think you're having a tough time with pregnancy-related discomfort, consider the wife of Feodor Vassilyev. This 18th-century Russian woman holds the world record in the pregnancy department: 27 pregnancies that produced 16 pairs of twins, 7 sets of triplets, and 4 sets of quadruplets, for a total of 69 babies. Ouch!

Aside from comparing yourself to Mrs. Vassilyev, there is much you can do to ease your own pregnancy woes. Most importantly, take care of yourself *before* you dim the lights or break out your most alluring teddy to attempt to procreate. "Catch up on your Pap smear and vaccinations, get some basic lab work, make sure your pelvic exam is normal, and start taking vitamins with additional folic acid—and you're set," advises *Suzanne Trupin, M.D.,* professor in the department of obstetrics and gynecology at the University of Illinois College of Medicine at Urbana-Champaign. Once you suspect you're pregnant, talk with your gynecologist right away so that you and your baby can get proper care from the beginning.

During your pregnancy, the changes in your body can cause some discomfort. But there are many things you can do to prevent and treat some of the most common pregnancy-related complaints.

## MORNING SICKNESS: NEUTRALIZE THE NAUSEA

After a positive pregnancy test, morning sickness—a misnomer, since many women feel nauseated throughout the day—is often the first indication that a pregnancy is real.

"Some women get so sick, they have to be hospitalized," explains *Lisa R. Domagalski, M.D.*, clinical instructor in the department of obstetrics and gynecology at Brown Medical School in Providence, Rhode Island. "But others never vomit during their pregnancies, and we're not sure why there is such a difference." Some scientists attribute the nausea to human chorionic gonadotropin (HCG), a hormone the embryo secretes that prevents the uterus from shedding its lining and enables the embryo to implant. It could be that some women produce higher levels of HCG.

It may be cold comfort while you're in the throes of nausea, but having morning sickness is actually a good sign. Many doctors believe it indicates that the placenta and fetal membranes are developing well. A study conducted at Cornell University found that women who had morning sickness were significantly less likely to miscarry than women who didn't have morning sickness.

"There's also a theory that morning sickness is an evolutionary adaptation to keep a woman from ingesting things that could potentially harm her or her baby," says *Colleen Senterfitt, C.N.M.*, a faculty member at Yale School of Nursing in New Haven, Connecticut. However, a woman who can't keep anything down due to severe nausea and vomiting runs the risk of dehydration. With permission from your physician, you may opt to take a prescription antinausea medication, such as Phenergan (promethazine) or Tigan (trimethobenzamide). In extreme cases, a woman may need to be hospitalized to rehydrate her system, says Dr. Domagalski.

*Douse yourself with cold water to shock the nausea out of your system.*
—*Colleen Senterfitt, C.N.M.*

If you're sick and fed up, remember that you won't feel this way forever. "Morning sickness usually recedes by the end of the first trimester, at about 13 or 14 weeks," says *Thelma Patrick, Ph.D., R.N.*, research assistant professor of obstetrics, gynecology, and reproductive science at the University of Pittsburgh.

In the meantime, use these helpful hints to feel better during those first months.

**Greet the morning with crackers.** "Keep crackers next to your bed, where you can eat a few before you even get up," says *Katherine Zieman, N.D.*, an associate professor of obstetrics at the National College of Naturopathic Medicine in Portland, Oregon. "They will help you skip that initial wave of nausea." Crackers aid in preventing nausea by boosting your blood sugar.

**Eat small and often.** "A major cause of morning sickness may be hypoglycemia (low blood sugar) because the hormones that support early pregnancy tend to lower blood sugar," says *Carol Archie, M.D.*, associate clinical professor of obstetrics and gynecology at the David Geffen School of Medicine at the University of California at Los Angeles. Fight the light-headed, shaky feeling of hypoglycemia by eating a small amount every few hours. "It's been rare for me to have to hospitalize women for hyperemesis (severe nausea) if they do this," says Dr. Archie. Carry complex carbohydrates with you. Good choices include whole wheat cereal and nuts, and a peanut butter or cheese sandwich on wheat—something you can stick in your purse and nibble on.

**Take some B₆.** If nausea persists despite eating frequent small meals, Dr. Archie recommends taking 50 milligrams vitamin B₆ twice a day. Use nutritional supplements only with the supervision of your health-care provider.

**Squeeze your wrists.** Acupuncture points on your wrists are related to nausea. To get relief, apply light pressure in the center of the underside of a forearm, about 1½ inches from your wrist. "Seasickness bands, which stimulate these points, can be very helpful," says Dr. Zieman. These bands are available at boating stores, travel agencies, and some pharmacies.

**Shock your system.** "When I was pregnant, my husband and I took a boat ride, and I was really nauseated," recalls Senterfitt. "All of a sudden, the boat captain poured a bucket of seawater over my head, and it was like flipping a light switch—I felt better instantly." If you get desperate, she suggests you try this trick yourself. "Get into a place where you can get wet, such as a tub, and splash or pour a gallon of very cold water over your face and neck. I've never seen this fail."

**Follow cravings.** If saltines don't work for you, but something sweet does, head for the nearest doughnut shop. "Your body is telling you what it wants and can handle," says Senterfitt. "For the short period that nausea usually lasts, nutrition doesn't have to be your first goal."

**Sniff a lemon.** Cooking aromas, cigarette smoke, and exhaust fumes are just a few of the odors that can trigger nausea in expectant mothers. For quick relief, Senterfitt suggests slicing a fresh lemon in half and holding a piece under your nose. It will cut through the offensive odors.

**Don't drink with meals.** "Fluids dilute the small amount of helpful hydrochloric acid you have left in your stomach," explains Dr. Zieman. Hydrochloric acid destroys fermenting bacteria that might cause intestinal tract disturbances. "So drink *between* meals, not with them." If you just have to have something drink with your food, Dr. Zieman recommends drinking 1 cup warm water mixed with 1 teaspoon cider vinegar or lemon juice. Either will help break down food by increasing digestive enzymes.

**Try an Asian flavor.** Some women claim to calm their nausea with umeboshi, a pickley tasting Japanese paste used to make sushi, reports Dr. Zieman. It's definitely not a mainstream treatment, but you can try it on crackers or bread.

**Consider cardamom.** In the days before pharmaceuticals, this herb was a traditional treatment for nausea. Old wives' wisdom prescribed chewing two cardamom seeds to settle an upset tummy. Whether powdered or ground, cardamom's flavor and texture is similar to cinnamon and can be used much like it: sprinkled on cereal or toast, or mixed in eggnog, decaffeinated tea, baked goods, or casseroles. Dr. Zieman suggests adding cardamom to warm milk. Dr. Zieman says Yogi Tea brand contains helpful amounts of cardamom. According to their spokesperson, these types are safe for pregnant or nursing women: Classic India Spice Tea, Cocoa Spice Tea, Egyptian Licorice Tea, Ginger, Jamaican Roast Tea, Lemon Ginger, Raspberry Ginger, Simply Green Tea, Tropical Hibiscus Tea, and Vanilla Hazelnut Tea.

**Don't worry.** Most women fear their babies will suffer as a result of morning sickness. "Some studies show that the baby gets enough nutrition from its mother's stores and does well, even in a woman who is so sick she's in bed," says Dr. Domagalski.

## SHOULD I SEE A DOCTOR?

*When you're pregnant, visit your doctor or midwife at least once a month.*

Call your health professional between visits if you experience any of these symptoms, since they could indicate a problem:

- Bleeding that's heavier than spotting
- No movement from the baby during normally active times of the day

- Severe headaches, which could indicate toxemia (also known as preeclamsia or pregnancy-induced hypertension)
- Any severe pain, particularly in your abdominal area
- Numbness or pain that radiates down your leg

# BACKACHE: GREAT IDEAS FOR RELIEF

If you feel like someone is sticking a metal fork in your lower back in the latter stages of your pregnancy, know that it's normal. Many expectant women experience significant pain in the lower back, the area that's supporting the growing bulk in the front of the body.

The pain can begin even before you start to show. "Earlier in pregnancy, the added pressure on the front of your body can push on your sciatic nerve, causing pain in your upper legs, hips, and back," says *Thelma Patrick, Ph.D., R.N.*, research assistant professor of obstetrics, gynecology, and reproductive science at the University of Pittsburgh. As your pregnancy advances, strain on your back increases. "The curvature of your spine becomes exaggerated, sometimes creating pressure and pain," explains *Adelaide Nardone, M.D.*, an obstetrician and gynecologist in Providence, Rhode Island, and medical advisor to the Vagisil Women's Health Center.

Fortunately, there's plenty you can do to ease the pain.

**Stretch in the a.m.** The following exercises helps alleviate sciatica, an inflammation along the sciatic nerve that runs through the thigh and leg. It's best to do it in the morning, because your lower back is stiffest when you first wake up. "It may sound awkward, but lie on your back and slowly bring one knee toward your chest, even with the big belly," advises Dr. Nardone. Then repeat with the opposite leg. Rolling from side to side from the same starting position is another excerise that Dr. Nardone recommends. In the morning, do each exercise six times, holding each stretch for 10 seconds.

As your pregnancy progresses, however, lying on your back for more than a few minutes at a time may compress your superior vena cava, a primary blood vessel that drains the blood from your upper body to your heart, resulting in reduced blood flow to your uterus. So avoid lying on your back more than 10 to 15 minutes at a time. To avoid feeling dizzy or faint when you get up, roll over onto one side and gradually push yourself up to a sitting position; then pause for a few seconds before you slowly stand.

**Tone your abs.** "The abdominal muscles support the back, and the back supports the abdomen. So it helps a lot to keep your stomach muscles strong, particularly in early pregnancy," says *Suzanne Trupin, M.D.*, professor in the department of obstetrics and gynecology at the University of Illinois College of Medicine at Urbana-Champaign. Try each of the following exercises once a day to strengthen your abdominal muscles.

- Pelvic tilt: Lie on your back, with your legs bent and your feet flat; then try to push your back down to the floor, says Dr. Trupin. This exercise will help keep your body properly aligned so that it can hold the additional weight. It also may help alleviate back pain. Start with five repetitions and work up to 10 or 15.
- Cat stretch: Get on your hands and knees. Arch your back toward the ceiling, then bring it back to a flat position. Do not let your back sag, as that will strain the back and pelvis. "You'll train your back to lift the gradually increasing weight on your stomach, like using a little Nautilus machine," says *Katherine Zieman, N.D.,* a naturopathic family physician and midwife at diMedici Natural Family Clinic in Gresham, Oregon, and an associate professor of obstetrics at the National College of Naturopathic Medicine in Portland. She recommends doing this exercise once a day for 5 to 10 minutes throughout your pregnancy.

**Be a fish.** "The buoyancy of water naturally supports the extra weight of your abdomen and puts less force on the joints and ligaments in your back," says Dr. Trupin. For maximum benefit, swim at least 20 minutes every other day. As an added bonus, the coolness of the water reduces leg swelling, another by-product of pregnancy.

**Support your tummy.** Worn around the stomach, a prenatal girdle lifts the uterus slightly to take some of the pressure off the back and the ligaments in the front. "I've seen women respond tremendously to them," says *Colleen Senterfitt, C.N.M.,* certified nurse midwife and faculty member at Yale School of Nursing in New Haven, Connecticut. Maternity girdles are available in maternity shops or online.

**Elevate your legs.** "If you have backaches in the second half of pregnancy, lie with your knees elevated on a couch arm or chair seat (if it's comfortable for you). Then place a hot-water bottle under your lower back as needed," suggests *Carol Archie, M.D.,* associate clinical professor of obstetrics and gynecology at the University of California at Los Angeles.

**Boost your calcium.** Backache can be partially due to low levels of calcium. "In pregnancy, you need 600 to 1,200 milligrams calcium a day," says Dr. Zieman. Check how much calcium your prenatal vitamin contains, then add calcium-rich foods to your diet to reach the recommended amount. (For examples of calcium-rich foods, see page 28.) Use dietary supplements *only* with the approval and supervision of your health-care provider.

*Make sure you get 600 to 1,200 milligrams calcium each day while you're pregnant. Your back—and baby—will be the better for it.*
—Katherine Zieman, N.D.

**Take Tylenol.** "If you are in a lot of pain, you can probably take Tylenol with your doctor's approval," says Dr. Nardone. "It is one of the pain relievers I feel is safe in pregnancy but should be taken only when needed."

**Try oil and herbs.** *Aviva Jill Romm,* midwife, president of the American Herbalists Guild, and author of *Natural Health After Birth: The Complete Guide to Postpartum Wellness,* recommends the following alternative remedies to ease pregnancy-related backache.

- Oil massage: Ask your partner to give you a rub or go to a professional or prenatal massage therapist. Try an oil containing Saint-John's-wort.
- Herbal soak: Put a few drops each of lavender, rose, and chamomile essential oils in a hot bath to help you relax.

## INDIGESTION AND HEARTBURN: DON'T STOMACH THE PAIN

Indigestion and heartburn can get so severe during pregnancy that you may wonder if you're carrying a baby or a giant chili dog. The reason? "Women commonly get indigestion because pregnancy hormones, particularly progesterone, slow the gastrointestinal tract," says *Lisa R. Domagalski, M.D.,* clinical instructor in the department of obstetrics and gynecology at Brown Medical School in Providence, Rhode Island.

When you're pregnant, food isn't digested as quickly, acid sits in the stomach longer, and the sphincter between the stomach and esophagus relaxes, says Dr. Domagalski. This causes food to back up into the esophagus, a condition called reflux. As the baby grows and gets closer to your sphincter, the severity of your indigestion increases. "Women who get severe indigestion, or those who have had reflux or other stomach problems prior to pregnancy, may choose to go on a prescription H2 (acid) blocker, such as Axid (nizatidine) or Zantac (ranitidine)," says Dr. Domagalski. "Both are safe to use during pregnancy." Always talk with your doctor before taking any medication while pregnant.

*As your baby grows, you're more likely to have indigestion and reflux. Avoid caffeine, citrus, spicy foods, and chocolate, which make the problem worse.*—Lisa R. Domagalski, M.D.

If your heartburn and indigestion are not severe, take these steps to soothe your fiery insides.

**Watch what you eat.** Stay away from foods that you know will worsen indigestion and heartburn. "Common aggravators include caffeine, citrus, spicy foods, and chocolate," says Dr. Domagalski. Other foods known to trigger heartburn include mints, gum, onions, and tomato products, as well as fatty, greasy, and fried foods, says *Yvonne Romero, M.D.,* an esophagologist and assistant professor at the Mayo Medical School in Rochester, Minnesota. You may not have a problem with all of these foods.

**Give digestion a hand.** "Taking digestive enzymes helps during pregnancy because the enzymes in your stomach aren't working as well as usual," says *Katherine Zieman, N.D.,* a naturopathic family physician and midwife at diMedici Natural Family Clinic in Gresham, Oregon.

"Papaya enzymes help break down food faster, so the food moves through the system more efficiently and doesn't back up as much," says Dr. Zieman. You can buy papaya enzymes and other digestive enzymes at most drugstores and health-food stores. You can also eat a fresh papaya or drink a glass of papaya juice after a meal to get the same effect. Of course, don't take anything without first checking with your medical advisor.

**Wet your whistle.** "Water will keep things moving through you, which helps prevent constipation, hemorrhoids, and urinary tract infections," says *Carol Archie, M.D.,* associate clinical professor of obstetrics and gynecology at the Geffen School of Medicine at the University of California at Los Angeles. She recommends you drink 64 to 80 ounces water throughout each day.

**Take antacids.** Antacids neutralize stomach acid and provide short-term relief of heartburn symptoms. "You can take any of the over-the-counter (OTC) antacids, like Mylanta, Rolaids, Tums, and Maalox, without consulting a physician," says Dr. Domagalski. Tums has the additional benefit of providing calcium.

**Stop the burn before it starts.** H2 blockers reduce acid production and can be used to prevent heartburn or treat the symptoms when heartburn occurs. Pepcid AC (famotidine) and Zantac 75 (ranitidine) are OTC options that are considered safe for pregnant women, says Dr. Domagalski.

**Stay active after eating.** "Don't eat late at night," advises *Adelaide Nardone, M.D.,* an obstetrician and gynecologist in Providence, Rhode Island, and medical advisor to the Vagisil Women's Health Center. Once you do hit the hay, position yourself to keep acid from rising. Use several pillows to prop you up at a 30- to 45-degree angle (about halfway to sitting

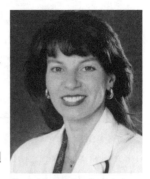

*To avoid nighttime heartburn, make sure you eat your last meal well before bedtime, says Adelaide Nardone, M.D.*

upright). Or raise the head of your bed a few inches with bricks, blocks, or heavy books.

*Eat pineapple and papaya to keep your stomach on an even keel—they contain enzymes that aid digestion.*
*—Katherine Zieman, N.D.*

**Take the natural route.** *Aviva Jill Romm,* midwife, president of the American Herbalists Guild, and author of *Natural Health After Birth: The Complete Guide to Postpartum Wellness,* recommends the following alternative remedies to ease pregnancy discomforts.

- Almonds: Chew 8 to 10 almonds until they liquefy to ease an upset tummy. Use as often as needed. These nuts contain a compound that improves the function of the sphincter between the stomach and esophagus, preventing acid from coming up and irritating the esophagus. Almonds are also a good source of protein and calcium.
- Slippery elm lozenges: These herbal lozenges act as an emollient antacid for the stomach and are safe to use as needed during pregnancy. They are available in several flavors at health-food stores.
- Yogurt: Some women find plain or flavored yogurt helpful. It is thought that yogurt contains live cultures of good bacteria that may keep the intestinal tract healthy and aid in digestion.

## INSOMNIA: GETTING A GOOD NIGHT'S SLEEP

Pregnancy creates a number of changes in your body that can jeopardize sound slumber. "It may be a myth, but insomnia during pregnancy could be nature's way to get you used to getting up at night for the baby," says *Lisa R. Domagalski, M.D.,* clinical instructor in the department of obstetrics and gynecology at Brown Medical School in Providence, Rhode Island.

Insomnia in pregnancy—as well as the vivid and sometimes frightening dreams some pregnant women have—is probably caused by hormonal fluctuations, says *Adelaide Nardone, M.D.,* an obstetrician and gynecologist in Providence, Rhode Island, and medical advisor to the Vagisil Women's Health Center. Then as your uterus grows, there is added discomfort, including difficulty positioning yourself comfortably and the frequent need to urinate.

Whatever the reason for your sleeplessness, here are some strategies that can help limit restless hours.

**Return to kindergarten.** If you're having trouble sleeping at night, get your z's whenever you can. "If you're tired during the day, take a nap, if you're in a situation where you can," suggests Dr. Domagalski. If your body tells you to hit the sack at 7 p.m., do it.

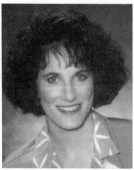

Try taking a pregnancy-safe antihistamine, such as Benadryl, to help you sleep, suggests Suzanne Trupin, M.D.

**Doze with Benadryl.** This over-the-counter (OTC) antihistamine makes people sleepy and is considered safe to take during pregnancy, says *Suzanne Trupin, M.D.,* professor in the department of obstetrics and gynecology at the University of Illinois College of Medicine at Urbana-Champaign.

**Educate yourself.** The third trimester tends to be a worrisome time for many pregnant women. "The mother may become concerned about her upcoming labor, as well as what her baby is going to look like," says *Thelma Patrick, Ph.D., R.N.,* research assistant professor of obstetrics, gynecology, and reproductive science at the University of Pittsburgh. Learn as much as you can about labor so that you know what to expect. It may also be comforting to read up on how small the chances are that your baby will have any physical abnormality.

**Warm some milk.** Grandma was right: "A glass of warm milk before bed makes you sleepy," says Dr. Trupin. Milk contains tryptophan, the same amino acid found in turkey and an important precursor to serotonin, a neurotransmitter that plays a role in sleep-wake cycles. Warming the milk simply makes it more soothing.

**Adjust accordingly.** For optimum blood flow, it's best to lie on your left side, advises Dr. Trupin, but don't panic if you awake in a different position. Add to your comfort with fluffy pillows and soft, roomy pajamas.

**Put snuggling on hold.** "As unromantic as it sounds, sometimes partners just have to sleep in separate beds if the mom is really restless," says Dr. Domagalski. "Otherwise, no one gets any sleep."

**Try natural tea and tinctures.** *Aviva Jill Romm,* midwife, president of the American Herbalists Guild, and author of *Natural Health After Birth: The Complete Guide to Postpartum Wellness,* recommends these alternative remedies to ease pregnancy discomforts.

- Herbal tea: After your first trimester, try drinking chamomile tea before bed. Steep 1 teaspoon dried chamomile in 1 cup boiling water for 10 minutes. You can also use lemon balm tea or lavender tea.
- Tinctures: Tinctures are liquid herbal extracts. Good choices for easing pregnancy-related insomnia include catnip, chamomile, lavender, lemon balm, passionflower, and skullcap. They can be used individually or in combination. Take a few drops directly or, following the manufacturer's directions, add them to water, tea, or juice.

## VARICOSE VEINS: GET A LEG UP ON RELIEF

Varicose veins—dilated veins in your legs, groin, or pelvis due to blood backing up—are common in pregnancy. Though usually not dangerous, varicose veins can be very uncomfortable, says *Lisa R. Domagalski, M.D.,* clinical instructor in the department of obstetrics and gynecology at Brown Medical School in Providence, Rhode Island.

Here's what you can do to prevent or ease the discomfort of varicose veins.

**Take some C and bioflavonoids.** "Vitamin C and especially bioflavonoids—the compounds found in plants, fruits, and vegetables that your body needs in order to process vitamin C—will help strengthen the blood vessel walls and help prevent or improve varicose veins," says *Katherine Zieman, N.D.,* a naturopathic family physician and midwife at diMedici Natural Family Clinic in Gresham, Oregon. Talk to your physician about a dosage before you use any nutritional supplement.

**Wear special stockings.** Leg girdles, also known as compression stockings, may not be comfortable, but they help prevent aching and swelling, and keep blood from collecting in distended areas of varicose veins. "They are especially helpful if you have a job where you're on your feet all day," says Dr. Domagalski. If you have a personal or family history of varicose veins, you might want to use the stockings as a preventive measure.

**Give your uterus a lift.** Increased pressure on the groin area during pregnancy can weaken valves and vessels, causing veins in the pelvic area to engorge. "Maternity girdles, which are worn around the stomach, lift the uterus off the pelvis to relieve some of that pressure," says Dr. Domagalski. They're also helpful in relieving backaches. They're available at maternity shops or online.

*Prop your feet up for a few minutes every four hours to relieve aches in your legs.*—Thelma Patrick, Ph.D., R.N.

**Cool it.** "If your veins are painful at night, use cold compresses," suggests Dr. Domagalski. Apply them as needed to help constrict veins and ease pain.

**Prop your legs.** Lie on a couch and rest your legs on the arm for 10 to 15 minutes at a time, advises **Thelma Patrick, Ph.D., R.N.**, research assistant

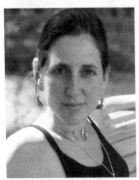

*Keep moving, advises midwife Aviva Jill Romm. You may avoid getting varicose veins if you stretch your legs at least once an hour.*

professor of obstetrics, gynecology, and reproductive science at the University of Pittsburgh. Do this about every four hours to take pressure off your veins and relieve the heavy, achy feeling. "If your veins are really engorged, prop your legs even higher," she adds.

**Walk around.** One of the best things for varicose veins is moderate exercise, says **Aviva Jill Romm,** midwife, president of the American Herbalists Guild, and author of *Natural Health After Birth: The Complete Guide to Postpartum Wellness.* Movement helps increase circulation and keeps your veins from stretching. "If you have to be in a sitting position, make sure to get up every hour to walk around and stretch your legs," says Romm.

## chapter 20

# Reproductive System
## Beyond Babies

*A male gynecologist is like an auto mechanic who never owned a car.*
—Carrie Snow, actress and comedy writer

Biologically speaking, a woman's reproductive system defines her as female. Yet it's astonishing how little American women seem to know about this vital part of themselves. In 2001, the American Infertility Association quizzed 12,382 women about their reproductive lifecycle, and only one was able to answer the entire 15-question survey correctly. It seems women need to educate themselves about their inner workings.

This chapter is a great starting point for bridging that information gap. Here, women health-care professionals tell you how to prevent and identify conditions that are uniquely female—from relatively minor irritations to life-threatening reproductive cancers—and then get the best self-care or medical treatment for whatever ails your "womanly" parts.

## VAGINITIS: ITCHING TO GET BETTER

Itching, burning, inflammation, discharge, painful sex—you likely know the signs. You've got vaginitis, the most common reason among adult American women to seek medical attention. Many types of vaginal infections have similar symptoms, but each has a different cause and requires different treatment.

"The vagina is a complex and delicate ecosystem," says *Rosemary "Mimi" Clarke Secor, M.Ed., M.S., R.N.*, who teaches at Massachusetts General Hospital and Boston College, and practices as a nurse-practitioner at the Center for Women's Health in Natick, Massachusetts. "It's dominated by 'good'

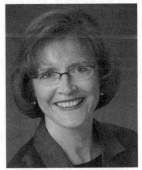

*Your vagina has lots of "good" bacteria to keep its pH balance normal, says Rosemary "Mimi" Clarke Secor, M.Ed., M.S., R.N.*

bacteria, which protect the vagina by keeping the pH balance normal—not too alkaline and not too acidic—which inhibits overgrowth of bacteria and maintains the protective mucin layer over the vaginal tissues."

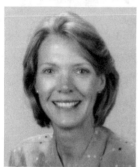

These good bacteria, called *Lactobacilli*, produce hydrogen peroxide, a natural disinfectant. It helps keep "bad" bacteria in check and enables your body to fight off sexually transmitted diseases (STDs), says **Cynthia Selleck, A.R.N.P., D.S.N.,** an associate professor in the department of family medicine at the University of South Florida in Tampa. "A variety of factors can affect normal vaginal flora and pH, including antibiotics, hormonal changes, semen, and menstrual blood," she says. "The worst culprit, by far, is douching." Such factors weaken the *Lactobacilli*, and the pH of the vagina rises when these bad bacteria get the upper hand, explains Dr. Selleck. As a result, your body has trouble fighting off infection.

*Douching, semen, or STDs can upset the pH balance in your vagina, leading to a case of vaginitis, says Cynthia Selleck, A.R.N.P., D.S.N.*

The most common types of vaginal infection include the following.

- Bacterial vaginosis (BV): This type of vaginitis, which involves an overgrowth of normal bacteria, is the most common vaginal infection in women of childbearing age. Women with BV have much more bacteria than normal. The exact cause of this proliferation is unknown, but Secor says anything that alters the normal vaginal pH can increase risk, such as douching, genital shaving, semen, multiple sex partners, or STDs.

- *Candida* (yeast, or fungal, infection): At least 75 percent of women experience this second most common type of vaginal infection at least once in their lives. The usual suspect is a strain of yeast known as *C. albicans.* A woman often has some *Candida* in her body, including her vagina; it only causes problems when there's too much of it. That can happen when something, such as an antibiotic, kills off the defenders. *C. tropicalis* and *C. glabrata* are non-*albicans* strains that cause up to a third of yeast infections, says Dr. Selleck.

- Trichomoniasis: Unlike BV or yeast, "trich" is a sexually transmitted disease, caused by a single-cell parasite known as *Trichomonas vaginalis.* Nearly five million people in the United States are infected each year with this most prevalent STD. The parasite can survive briefly on wet clothing, bath linens, and toilets, so even nonsexual contact poses some risk of infection.

- Noninfectious vaginitis: Some cases of vaginitis are caused by hormonal changes during menopause, pregnancy, or nursing. They can also be brought on by allergies or irritation from underwear, tampons, soaps, detergents, spermicidal jellies, and feminine sprays.

The plethora of over-the-counter creams and treatments for vaginitis might lead you to think the problem is relatively mild and easily treated. But that's not always the case; a vaginal infection can have nasty complications. BV and trich can affect your pregnancy, for instance.

To avoid the potential complications of vaginitis, heed these recommendations.

**Get tested.** During a case of vaginitis, 4 out of 10 women don't notice any symptoms; plus, the infection may not show up in routine Pap smear. If you think there's even the slightest possibility you have an infection, ask

## SHOULD I SEE A DOCTOR?

*A yearly visit to your gynecologist is good insurance against disease. But certain signs or symptoms should prompt a visit—scheduled or not.*

See your doctor as soon as possible if you notice any of these symptoms that suggest something may be amiss:

- Burning, itching, or irritation inside the vagina or on the skin outside the vagina
- Unusual vaginal discharge, such as gray, green, white, or blood-tinged
- Unusual or unpleasant vaginal odor
- Pain or discomfort during sexual intercourse
- Bleeding or spotting between periods
- Bleeding after menopause
- Excessive menstrual bleeding (menorrhagia), including heavy bleeding for more than a week or heavy soaking of tampons or pads, especially when accompanied by fatigue or dizziness (For more on menorrhagia, see page 249.)
- Missed or absent periods (amenorrhea)
- Lower back or pelvic pain
- Abdominal pressure
- Abnormal or rapid weight gain or loss that occurs without a change in eating or exercise habits
- Problems with urinating, such as pain or burning, frequent urination, or blood in urine
- Indigestion, abdominal bloating, constipation, or diarrhea that is constant, occurs daily, or is progressive and lingers for more than a month
- Abnormal facial or body hair (hirsutism) that appears suddenly and grows fast on typically male areas, such as the cheeks, chin, forehead, or chest
- Chronic fatigue
- Problems conceiving
- A sore that does not heal

If you have symptoms that you think relate to your reproductive organs, seek help from your gynecologist first. She'll be able to determine if you need to see a specialist.

your doctor to test you for it during your annual pelvic exam. Three simple tests—the vaginal fluid pH test, amine test, and hydrogen peroxide "bubble" test—can provide a reliable diagnosis in minutes. If you're planning to have a baby, know that the risks of vaginal infections are compounded when you're pregnant, so get tested before conceiving.

**Don't self-diagnose.** What you think is a simple yeast infection may, in fact, be a more serious condition. If you skip getting a proper diagnosis and treat yourself for what you *think* you have, you could end up even worse off, says **Barbara Sue Apgar, M.D.,** director of the Family Medicine Obstetrical and Newborn Service at University Hospital, and clinical professor of family medicine at the University of Michigan in Ann Arbor. "I've examined patients who self-treated with over-the-counter medications that were inappropriate for their particular infection," she says. "The resulting swelling and pain can make it impossible to insert a speculum." Though it's tempting to avoid the doctor's office and head straight to the pharmacy, taking time to verify the nature of your problem can save you a lot of grief.

## TREATING VAGINITIS: MAXIMIZING MEDICATIONS

Typically, doctors treat vaginitis with antibiotic or antifungal medications, such as with pills or ointments that you apply or insert into your vagina.

The prescription medication Terazol (terconazol) is the only treatment that gets rid of *all* types of yeast infections, says Dr. Selleck. Available as a cream or suppository, Terazol is used for three to seven days, depending on the dosage. Burning or itching around the vagina is a possible side effect. It may go away during treatment, but you should notify your health-care provider if the itching persists or becomes bothersome.

For BV, doctors usually prescribe one of the following medications.
- Metronidazole is available in gel form as MetroGel-Vaginal or in pill form as Flagyl, which is also prescribed for trichomoniasis.
- Cleocin (clindamycin) can be taken as a pill or may be inserted vaginally as either a cream or suppository.

Remember these guidelines when using these medications.

**Boycott the booze.** Do not drink alcohol when taking Flagyl. When you take your last dose, wait at least 72 hours before consuming alcohol, cautions **Tori Hudson, N.D.,** professor of gynecology at National College of Naturopathic Medicine in Portland, Oregon, and author of *Women's*

*Encyclopedia of Natural Medicine.* The interaction of alcohol with this drug can cause severe nausea and vomiting, headaches, and flushing.

**Consider a single dose.** Ask your doctor about the benefits of taking the stronger single dose of Flagyl, instead of the usual seven-day course. Studies show the sole dose works in 84 percent of patients, versus 95 percent for the seven-day regimen, says Dr. Hudson.

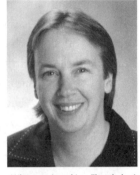

**Watch out for side effects.** Flagyl may cause nausea, headache, diarrhea or constipation, stomach pain, and loss of appetite. Seizures and tingling of the hands and feet have been reported in a few cases. Side effects for Cleocin may include vaginal or genital itching or burning, nausea, vomiting, or diarrhea. Contact your doctor if these side effects persist.

*When you're taking Flagyl, don't drink any alcohol until at least three days after your last dose, warns Tori Hudson, N.D. Flagyl's interaction with booze can cause nausea and vomiting.*

"If you have any irritation from a cream or gel that's prescribed for you, speak with your physician," says **Shaun D. Biggers, M.D.,** assistant professor of obstetrics and gynecology at the Weill Cornell Medical Center at New York Presbyterian Hospital. "It may mean that particular cream isn't a good match for you. There are alternatives, so there is no reason to use something that causes irritation."

**Take heed if you're pregnant.** Talk to your doctor about the potential hazards of the disease versus the risks of treatment for you and your unborn baby. Some health professionals caution against the use of Flagyl during pregnancy because of potential complications, such as gene mutations and birth defects. But BV also poses risks to your child. The Centers for Disease Control and Prevention advises that pregnant women with BV be treated with oral Flagyl or Cleocin. "Since the first 12 weeks of pregnancy are the most vulnerable for the child's developing organ systems, we try to avoid using Flagyl then," says Dr. Biggers.

ZAPPING A YEAST INFECTION First and foremost, don't treat a yeast infection until the condition has been confirmed by your doctor, cautions Dr. Apgar. Once you have a proper diagnosis, your doctor may suggest one of the stronger over-the-counter (OTC) preparations or may leave you to choose one on your own.

There are dozens of OTC preparations that claim to treat yeast infections. It's easy to narrow the selection, says Dr. Biggers, because only a few are actually antifungals—such as Femstat One, Gyne-Lotrimin, and Monistat—which is what you need if your itching and burning are due to yeast. "Products such as Vagisil and Yeast-Gard treat vaginal itching, but not the fungus," warns Dr. Biggers.

Your next decision is whether to get the two-day suppository or the seven-day cream. "There is no dosage length that is better than any other," assures Dr. Biggers. "All the products have been rigorously tested. Most were prescription medications before they became OTCs, so they're prescribed at a strength and length of time that are effective."

Keep in mind that any antibiotic you take to treat other infections may worsen your yeast infection and make your treatment less effective. "If your infection doesn't get better with an OTC treatment, see your gynecologist," advises Dr. Biggers. "You may need a higher level of therapy." If you're pregnant, check with your physician before using *any* OTC treatment.

## TREATING VAGINITIS THE NATURAL WAY

There are many options for treating vaginal infections naturally, rather than with medication. After diagnosis, try these tips from Dr. Hudson, a naturopath, and *Andrea Candee,* master herbalist and author of *Gentle Healing for Baby and Child.* Experiment and see which work best for you.

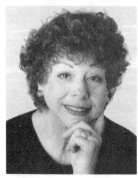

*Eat at least one clove of garlic a day to help kill off offending bacteria, advises herbalist Andrea Candee. If you're not keen on the real thing, you can substitute odor-free capsules.*

**Cut down on sugary foods.** To help prevent all types of vaginal infections, try to eliminate simple sugars that fuel microbial infections, says Candee. These include alcohol, fruits, fruit juices, and such refined carbohydrates as white bread and white rice. To keep your blood sugar on an even keel, focus your diet on such high-protein, low-fat foods as chicken, fish, and soy, as well as leafy green vegetables. "This is a good suggestion for a way of life," she adds. Cutting down on sugar may be particularly helpful in treating *Candida* infections. As you decrease sugar, Candee suggests taking a three-month course of a natural treatment, such as *Lactobacillus acidophilus* (see below).

**Take a helpful supplement.** *L. acidophilus* is a probiotic, which increases the amount of good bacteria in your vaginal ecosystem. Candee recommends taking two to three capsules, two to three times a day. Take the last dose at bedtime, so the probiotic can work without hindrance.

*Eating healthfully and choosing foods that are high in protein and low in fat and sugar can help prevent all types of vaginal infections.*—Andrea Candee

**Eat protective garlic.** The sulfur compounds in garlic kill bacteria and fungi, says Candee. If you're daunted by the prospect of eating at least one clove a day, Dr. Hudson suggests substituting odor-free capsules. Look for a product containing at least 5,000 micrograms allicin, the active ingredient in garlic that inhibits the growth of *Candida,* says Dr. Hudson. Take three 500- to 600-milligram capsules a day, in addition to any prescription or OTC medication you're taking, until your symptoms subside.

**Try a suppository.** Use a garlic suppository during the day and a *Lactobacillus* capsule as a suppository in the evening to help repopulate your vagina with good bacteria and inhibit the growth of *Candida,* suggests Dr. Hudson. To make a garlic suppository, wrap a carefully peeled clove (don't nick it) in gauze and attach a length of dental floss or cotton string for easy removal. Then insert it into your vagina and leave it in for six to eight hours. Insert a *Lactobacillus* capsule before you go to bed for it to dissolve overnight. Repeat until the infection clears.

**Rub on vitamin E.** Applied topically once or twice a day, vitamin E can reduce redness and swelling, says Dr. Hudson. Pierce a gel capsule with a pin so you can squeeze out the oil and smear it around your vagina. You should experience relief in a couple of days, says Dr. Hudson.

**Try the 98-percent effective treatment.** Boric acid creates an inhospitable environment for yeast. In a study of 100 women with chronic, resistant yeast infections for whom conventional therapies have failed, treatment with boric-acid suppositories twice a day for four weeks cured 98 percent of the subjects. Insert one 600-milligram capsule (available at most pharmacies) in the morning and one in the evening, advises Dr. Hudson. Repeat the treatment for 3 to 7 days for mild cases and up to 14 days for resistant cases.

If you're pregnant, don't use boric acid or any herbal remedy without first consulting your doctor.

**Sit in a sitz bath.** Add 2 cups Epsom salts to a tubful of warm water; soak in the water for 20 to 30 minutes, says Candee. Epsom salts help draw toxins out of your vagina and may relieve the itch as you sit in the bath.

*Taking a 20-minute sitz bath in Epsom salts can relieve the itch of a vaginal infection.*—Andrea Candee

## LOWER YOUR RISK FOR VAGINITIS

The best way to deal with vaginitis is not having to deal with it in the first place. Help prevent the problem by taking this advice from our women experts.

**Eat yogurt.** In a study of women with recurrent *Candida* infections, those who ate 8 ounces yogurt every day had one-third fewer infections than those who didn't eat yogurt at all. Yogurt that contains *L. acidophilus* helps maintain a healthy pH balance in the vagina, explains Dr. Hudson. Look for yogurts that meet the National Yogurt Association's requirements for live active cultures. In order to bear the "Live and Active Cultures" seal, yogurt must contain at least a hundred million live cells per gram.

Though douching with *L. acidophilus*–containing yogurt was once advised for vaginitis, it has since been linked to infertility and pelvic infections and is, therefore, no longer recommended, warns Dr. Hudson. In fact, douching with any type of liquid while you have vaginitis can carry organisms up into the reproductive organs, putting you at risk for pelvic infections. Douches or deodorant sprays that mask odor may also hide clues your doctor needs for diagnosis. And if you're pregnant, you should *never* douche.

**Stay dry.** Strip off a wet bathing suit or exercise clothes as soon as your workout is finished. "Moisture can cause a woman to get an external fungal infection, just like guys get jock itch," says Dr. Biggers. If an infection does strike, your doctor will probably treat it with an external antifungal cream.

**Nix synthetic underwear.** Choose cotton over man-made fabrics, since it doesn't trap moisture. Be aware that women who wear panty hose have three times more yeast infections than those who don't, says Dr. Hudson. So buy a brand that has a cotton crotch and then wear them only sparingly.

**Call on cranberries.** Cranberries contain proanthocyanidin, a substance that prevents *E. coli* bacteria from adhering to the walls of the urinary tract. An overgrowth of *E. coli* weakens your overall immune structure and provides a hospitable environment for other bacteria, viruses, and fungi to increase, including those that contribute to vaginal infections. To prevent such an overgrowth, drink a glass of unsweetened cranberry juice every day. (Sugar feeds bacteria, so sweetened cranberry juice defeats your purpose.) Or take a cranberry supplement. Candee recommends a 400-milligram pill, two to three times a day, for 10 days.

**Avoid overuse of tampons.** They can irritate the vagina and can absorb and remove good bacteria, says Secor. Instead, use unscented sanitary napkins (the scented variety can cause irritation).

**Don't shave pubic hair.** Irritated hair follicles can throw off the balance of the vagina, increasing the risk of infection and of acquiring sexually transmitted diseases, such as herpes, HPV and HIV, to name a few, says Secor.

**Don't douche—unless it's prescribed.** Women who douche have more vaginal infections than those who don't and may increase their risk of developing pelvic inflammatory disease. "Douching removes good bacteria and leaves the vagina unable to protect itself," notes Secor.

*Don't sit around in a wet bathing suit or sweaty gym clothes, since moisture can lead to an external, itchy fungal infection.—Shaun D. Biggers, M.D.*

**Stick with safe sex.** Limit your sexual partners and always use condoms. The more partners you have, the more likely you are to get trich or BV, warns Dr. Selleck. Even having condom-free sexual intercourse with one partner several times within a short time period can increase your risk of infection, since semen can disrupt the natural pH of the vagina.

**Don't play infection Ping-Pong.** A yeast infection isn't usually considered a sexually transmitted disease. But if you often get yeast infections, you and your partner could be passing yeast back and forth during unprotected sex—even if you've been treated for the infection, says Dr. Hudson. A man's body can harbor yeast without experiencing any symptoms. His semen can also affect the pH levels of your vagina. Temporarily using a condom during sex may help stop the Ping-Pong effect, but Dr. Hudson says that your best course of action is to get your partner checked and treated by a doctor, too.

## UTERINE FIBROIDS: UNRULY BENIGN TUMORS

Your stomach is so bloated that you feel—and look—pregnant. But you know you're not expecting, because you're having the worst periods ever, with cramps that feel like a hot claw digging at your insides and major bleeding. Add debilitating backaches and painful sex, and you have all the symptoms of uterine fibroid tumors.

Uterine fibroids are so common that their presence is considered normal in women ages 35 and older. Up to 80 percent of women develop these fibroids at some point, but an unlucky 20 to 50 percent really suffer their effects, says *Cynthia Morton, Ph.D.*, a geneticist at the Center for Uterine Fibroids at Brigham and Women's Hospital in Boston.

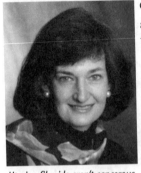

Uterine fibroids aren't cancerous tumors, but they can give you a lot of pain and trouble, says Cynthia Morton, Ph.D.

Also called leiomyomas, these benign tumors in the uterus grow from a single abnormal cell. Fibroids are *not* cancerous, but they can be very unruly in their development and growth, explains Dr. Morton. They can grow in and around the uterus. One or more can grow at the same time and range in size from as small as a pea to as large as a honeydew melon. They can be round or irregular, or hang from stalklike projections. Uterine fibroids can even twist around each other or other organs. Bottom line: They can make you miserable.

"Fibroids are the most common, least studied tumors in the world," says Dr. Morton. Researchers don't know the exact cause of them but are learning more about their biology and the factors that make some women more susceptible than others to developing them.

One factor is genetics. If your mother, sister, or aunt had fibroids, there's a good chance you will, too, says *Elizabeth A. Stewart, M.D.*, clinical director of the Center for Uterine Fibroids at Brigham and Women's Hospital in Boston. She and Dr. Morton study families throughout the world to learn more about the role genes play in fibroids.

Their research found that African-American women are about three times more likely to develop fibroids than other racial groups. "They also seem to have more severe and troublesome fibroids," probably due to genetics rather than environmental factors, says Dr. Stewart.

Hormones also play a role in development of fibroid tumors, which thrive on the female hormones estrogen and progesterone. That's one reason that fibroids often grow during pregnancy, when these hormones are in abundant supply, and shrink after menopause, when levels of both hormones decline.

The first step is a physician's diagnosis. Generally, it just takes a pelvic exam to identify the possibility of fibroids. Your health-care provider will then want to confirm the diagnosis with an ultrasound.

Once you have a diagnosis, experts recommend the following treatment options.

**Wait and see.** If your symptoms aren't severe, your best bet may be to leave well enough alone, says Dr. Stewart. Just be sure to see your gynecologist every six months for a physical exam that may pick up changes you don't notice. This is a particularly good option if you're close to or experiencing menopause, says Dr. Stewart. That's because fibroids usually shrink after menopause, as long as they're not fueled by hormone replacement therapy (HRT) or natural remedies that produce or mimic estrogen, such as isoflavone supplements, red clover, or soy products.

**Rethink hormones.** Clinical observation suggests that synthetic or natural estrogen or progesterone (in contraceptive pills or HRT) can sometimes make fibroids grow. "However, many women are able to take hormone preparations without experiencing problems," says Dr. Stewart. "If you are taking hormones and you start to have problems with fibroids, talk to your doctor about stopping the hormones and see if your symptoms improve."

**Replenish iron.** The heavy bleeding that sometimes accompanies fibroids may leave you anemic or low on iron, says Dr. Stewart. Ask your doctor if you should take an iron supplement or boost your diet with such iron-rich foods as lean meats and poultry, whole grains, beans, soy, and leafy, dark green vegetables.

**Eschew the moo.** Dairy products can stimulate your body to produce higher levels of estrogen, as well as series three prostaglandins, the hormonelike substances that contribute to inflammation and cramping. Milk may also contain bovine growth hormone (BGH), which is given to one-third of dairy cattle to promote milk production. Some research suggests that BGH may play a role in fibroid growth. If you have fibroids, consider using nondairy milks and cheese, such as soy or rice milks or soy cheese, advises *Susan Lark, M.D.,* a holistic physician and author of *Fibroid Tumors and Endometriosis.* You still need to get adequate calcium, so Dr. Lark suggests that you drink non-dairy milks that are fortified, take a supplement, or eat foods that are high in calcium and magnesium, such as leafy green vegetables.

**Clean up your diet.** Saturated fat, caffeine, sugar, alcohol, and junk foods can contribute to fibroids, since they interfere with the body's ability to metabolize forms of estrogen. And estrogen plays a role in the size and growth of fibroids, says *Tori Hudson, N.D.,* professor of gynecology at National College of Naturopathic Medicine in Portland, Oregon, and author of *Women's Encyclopedia of Natural Medicine.* These foods are also deficient in vitamin B or interfere with B-vitamin metabolism, which is necessary for your liver to regulate estrogen levels.

**Trim your body fat.** Studies show that overweight women are prone to fibroids, especially women who carry more weight around their bellies than

## ONE WOMAN'S STORY: HYSTERECTOMY

*There are many ways to deal with the symptoms of fibroid tumors. One woman explains why having a hysterectomy was the best choice for her.*

Meet Elaine Grant (not her real name): mother, defense attorney, and activist in legal causes. Grant was in her early 40s when she began having heavy bleeding and clotting related to fibroids. She sought relief in over-the-counter pain medications.

But her symptoms worsened as she aged. "I would bleed so heavily, I couldn't leave the house," recalls Grant. She eventually became anemic. And the pain was so bad, she says, "I saw stars—and I have a pretty high tolerance for pain."

Three times, Grant's doctor tried to alleviate the heavy bleeding with a dilation and cuterage procedure (commonly referred to as a D & C) in which the lining of the uterus is scraped. When that didn't work, he suggested Grant have a hysterectomy.

Since her gynecologist said the choice was up to Grant, she gave it a lot of thought, did a lot of

reading, and talked with women friends who were doctors. Grant didn't intend to have more children, so the monthly pain and debilitation, the fact that her mother had had uterine cancer, and the gnarly nature of her fibroids added up to making a hysterectomy a wise choice for her.

Grant had a total hysterectomy and oopherectomy, which removed her uterus, as well as both fallopian tubes and ovaries. To cope with having her body thrown into instant menopause, she immediately started taking hormone replacement therapy.

The result? "I feel so much better. It was such a relief to not have that pain and bleeding all the time," says Grant. While it took almost a year to fully return to her old energetic self, she says it was absolutely the right decision for her. "I would do it again—no question."

in their hips and thighs, or so-called apple-shaped. Though the reason is unclear, one theory is that fat converts such hormones as testosterone into estrogen, says Dr. Stewart.

**Keep moving.** Women who exercise vigorously tend to have few problems with fibroids. Exercise helps to regulate ovulation (irregular ovulation may make fibroids worse). It also helps keep the weight off. "And obesity can lead to higher estrogen effects on the uterus," says Dr. Hudson.

> *If you have fibroids, reduce cramping and inflammation by using soy- or rice-milk products instead of dairy.*
> —*Susan Lark, M.D.*

**Try yoga.** This tried-and-true stress-buster can help ease moderate abdominal cramps or heaviness. Dr. Lark recommends doing this exercise once a day to reduce tension, abdominal pressure, and nausea.

- Sit on the floor with your legs straight out in front or folded in the classic lotus position. Keep your spine straight throughout the exercise.
- Place your hands on your shoulders, fingers in front and thumbs in back.
- Inhale deeply as you twist your head and torso to the left.
- Exhale as you twist back to the center.
- Repeat for a total of four twists.
- Reverse direction, doing the same exercise four times to the right.

**Think twice about a hysterectomy.** Once considered the *only* treatment for fibroids, it is now the last resort for women suffering severe symptoms and complications. It's advisable for you to get a second opinion before agreeing to this surgery. If the discomfort of fibroid tumors is interfering with your daily life, see your physician, advises Dr. Stewart. There are other, less invasive, treatments that remove fibroids but leave your reproductive system intact.

## POLYCYSTIC OVARY SYNDROME: A PLETHORA OF PROBLEMS

Polycystic ovary syndrome (PCOS) is a disorder of the endocrine system, which causes a hormonal imbalance that can affect your entire body, says *Deborah Metzger, M.D., Ph.D.*, a reproductive endocrinologist and medical director of Helena Women's Health in San Jose, California.

Women with PCOS usually produce too many androgens, the so-called male hormones, which include testosterone. Androgens wreak havoc with the cycle of egg production and ovulation. Egg follicles, also called cysts, fail to release the eggs, keeping the cysts under the surface of the ovary wall. In time, the ovary fills up with a pearl necklace–like pattern of these cysts.

Even though the eggs aren't released, the uterine lining still prepares to host a fertilized egg. But women with PCOS also lack proper hormonal signals to tell the uterus to shed its lining, so the lining builds up inside the uterus, resulting in irregular menstruation and increasing the risk of endometrial cancer.

At the same time, women with PCOS tend to be less sensitive to the hormone insulin, which controls blood sugar. They become what is known as insulin resistant. Their bodies' inability to adequately respond to insulin can lead to weight gain, high blood pressure, heart disease, stroke, and diabetes. In fact, women with PCOS have five times the normal risk of diabetes, says *Susan L. Treiser, M.D., Ph.D.,* co-director and founder of IVF New Jersey, a private reproductive health clinic.

PCOS symptoms may not be life-threatening, but they are definitely disturbing. A woman with PCOS may have excess hair on her face, back, and abdomen, and, conversely, very thin hair on her head. She may also have acne, anxiety, and depression.

And PCOS is no friend to couples who want to have a baby. It's one of the primary causes of infertility in women, accounting for up to 75 percent of all cases in which ovulation doesn't occur, says Dr. Treiser.

## THE EMBARRASSING SIDE OF PCOS

*Unwanted hair and acne are symptoms of polycystic ovary syndrome that can make a woman's life miserable.*

*Susan L. Treiser, M.D., Ph.D.,* co-director and founder of IVF New Jersey, has this advice for dealing with the hair and skin problems of PCOS.

**Try medication.** Talk to your doctor about antiandrogen medications, such as Aldactone and Spironol, which both go by the generic name spironolactone. These drugs can reduce the severity of male-pattern hair growth and acne but may require up to six months to show results. Possible side effects of use include dizziness, blurred vision, and dry mouth. During the first few days of use, as the body adjusts to the medication, side effects include vomiting, loss of appetite, fatigue, sleeplessness, and nasal congestion.

**Wax or use depilatory creams.** For more permanent removal of facial and body hair, electrolysis and laser treatments are effective. Since cost is based on the number of hairs to be removed, as well as whether the hairs have been removed previously, procedures can be expensive.

PCOS tends to run in families and often strikes as young as the teen years, says *Andrea Dunaif, M.D.*, professor of medicine and chief of the division of endocrinology, metabolism, and molecular medicine at Northwestern University Medical School in Chicago. It affects up to 10 percent of all pre-menopausal women, with around five million afflicted nationwide. Even so, the syndrome often goes undiagnosed or misdiagnosed for years, since its symptoms vary and are easily confused with other conditions.

Diagnosing PCOS involves blood tests and a physical exam to rule out other health problems. Even when doctors do diagnose it correctly, there is no cure. Scientists have yet to discover the cause of the hormonal abnormalities in women with PCOS.

The best way to treat PCOS is to manage and control its symptoms. Key to treatment is improving insulin sensitivity, which will in turn help regulate ovulation, says Dr. Dunaif. Excess insulin can lead the ovaries to increase production of androgen, which interferes with the cycle of ovulation and prevents the ovaries from releasing an egg. Improving insulin sensitivity and lowering insulin levels lead to more regular ovulation, enabling women with PCOS to respond better to fertility drugs if they want to get pregnant.

If you are diagnosed with PCOS, look for a doctor who has experience treating it, usually a reproductive endocrinologist. To help your body use insulin more effectively, she may prescribe a drug, such as Glucophage (metformin), to help manage acne, infertility, and unwanted hair, as well as other PCOS symptoms.

Heed this advice for self-care and medical treatment of PCOS.

**Eat high-fiber, low-fat foods.** Dr. Treiser and her colleagues prescribe a fiber-rich diet that restricts simple carbohydrates, such as white pastas, white breads, and cake. Instead, her plan emphasizes complex carbohydrates—such as fruits, vegetables, and whole grains—as well as low-fat proteins, including beans, lean meat, poultry, fish, and eggs. "Eating these usually helps insulin-resistant patients lose weight and become more responsive to medications that treat PCOS," says Dr. Treiser.

**Lose a few pounds.** Even with PCOS, you can cut your risk of diabetes in half by dropping just 10 percent of your body weight and being more physically active, says Dr. Dunaif. If you weigh 200 pounds, for instance, losing just 20 pounds can provide huge benefits.

**Walk and lift weights.** Exercise can help reduce androgen levels, says *Marla Ahlgrimm, R.Ph.,* founder and chairman of Women's Health America, an international organization that provides information on women's health needs. Her recommendation? Walk 20 to 30 minutes a day and try weight training. "As little as 30 minutes, twice a week, can significantly increase muscle mass and lower insulin levels," suggests Dr. Treiser. Stay away from supervigorous exercise, such as marathon running, since that can actually *increase* your testosterone levels.

**Consider oral contraceptives.** If you're not trying to get pregnant, ask your doctor about using an oral contraceptive to re-establish your monthly menstrual cycle. Having regular periods is important because long-term buildup of the uterine lining can lead to unpredictable, sometimes heavy bleeding. "Over time, the abnormal lining can undergo precancerous or even cancerous changes," says Dr. Treiser.

## ENDOMETRIOSIS: A VICIOUS CYCLE OF PAIN

Listen to the voices of women who have endometriosis:

*"I had periods that would hurt so badly, I couldn't function. I was constantly fatigued (no amount of sleep was ever enough), and depressed, with headaches, muscle aches, colds, diarrhea, anemia, bladder infections, cysts, sinus infections, constant nervousness, anxiety, and tension."*

*"I've passed through scores of doctors' offices and was told I am a hypochondriac. I've been made a zombie by painkillers. I've gone through depression, pain, denial, and extreme stress."*

*"It affected every decision I made all day, every day. When you're in pain for a long time, it gets harder and harder to imagine your life without it."*

These women are not exaggerating about the misery endometriosis can bring. The condition can cause years of pain and health problems, in spite of aggressive treatment with powerful hormones and surgery.

The word *endometriosis* comes from *endometrium,* the tissue that lines the uterus and is shed each month during a normal menstrual cycle. With endometriosis, endometrial tissue is found outside the uterus, usually in the pelvic cavity around the reproductive organs. But it can also take hold elsewhere in the abdomen and intestines.

Triggered by estrogen, this wayward tissue continues to act just like uterine endometrium: building up, shedding, and bleeding each month. Since this blood has no way to leave the body, you end up with internal bleeding, inflammation, and, most notably, severe pain.

Over time, this endometrial tissue develops into nodules or growths that can cause even more intense pain and excessive bleeding, scarring on pelvic organs, intestinal obstructions, bladder function problems, ectopic pregnancies, and infertility. Other problems include painful intercourse, menstrual pain and cramps, and excessive menstrual bleeding. Some women also experience allergies, bloating, chemical sensitivities, chronic fatigue, and gastrointestinal upsets, such as constipation, diarrhea, and nausea.

One out of seven women has endometriosis. It most often affects women in their 20s to early 40s, but teenagers and even preteens can develop the condition. And because endometriosis tends to run in families, your risk is increased sevenfold if a close relative has the disease.

## CONVENTIONAL TREATMENTS FOR ENDOMETRIOSIS

"You never totally get rid of endometriosis, but there are things you can do throughout your reproductive life to ease the symptoms or temper its growth," **Shaun D. Biggers, M.D.,** assistant professor of obstetrics and gynecology at the Weill Cornell Medical Center at New York Presbyterian Hospital.

**Soothe the pain.** Take nonsteroidal anti-inflammatory drugs (NSAIDs)—such as aspirin, ibuprofen, and naproxen—as needed to reduce pain and inflammation caused by the intense uterine contractions that often accompany endometriosis, says **Susan Lark, M.D.,** a holistic physician and author of *Fibroid Tumors and Endometriosis.* NSAIDs can increase your risk for gastrointestinal bleeding and ulcers, so if you have any symptoms of stomach upset or pain, stop using the drugs immediately and consult your physician.

**Try hormonal therapy.** Since estrogen seems to stimulate the growth of endometriosis, the goal is to reduce the production of estrogen. Many women may get relief from birth control pills or gonadotropin-releasing hormone (GnRH) agonists, such as Lupron (leuprolide), says Dr. Biggers. Although it might sound counterintuitive to take hormones to reduce estrogen, the hormones in these medicines cause your body to stop producing estrogen. Be aware that depriving your body of estrogen can have potential side effects that are similar to those of menopause, including hot flashes and night sweats, and may also lead to osteoporosis.

## ARE YOU ALLERGIC TO YOUR HORMONES?

*If you have endometriosis, it's probably due to an allergy to your hormones—and a host of other things.*

"Virtually all women with endometriosis also have allergies," says **Deborah Metzger, M.D., Ph.D.,** medical director of Helena Women's Health in San Jose, California. They are often allergic to their own hormones, as well as to certain foods, chemicals, trees, grass, weeds, dust and molds, and *Candida* (fungus). Simply put, these women may have immune systems that are out of balance.

These symptoms signal that you may be allergic to your hormones:

- Your premenstrual symptoms don't respond to the usual treatments.
- Birth control pills or hormone replacement therapy results in a variety of side effects, including headaches, mind fog, muscle or joint pain, irritability, or depression.
- You feel better emotionally when you're taking a GnRH agonist, which lowers the estrogen levels in your body.

When one of Dr. Metzger's patients tests positive for a food or hormone allergy, she uses oral tolerization to desensitize the body to the allergen. This technique is based on homeopathy and has been refined by the American Academy of Environmental Medicine.

Here's how oral tolerization works: The doctor injects a small amount of the suspected allergen under your skin to provoke a reaction, which may be visible as swelling and redness at the site of the injection. After 10 minutes, you'll be asked about any sensations you are experiencing, such as nausea, headaches, mind fog, or dizziness. Then you'll take the allergen in an oral form. Every 10 minutes, you'll receive it in an increasing dilution until your symptoms disappear. The dilution that neutralizes your symptoms is the dose that you'll take each day as a drop under your tongue. After one to three years, allergic reactions are usually cured.

This process is safe and cost-effective, with no side effects, says Dr. Metzger. However, it may not be appropriate for allergies to substances, such as shellfish or peanuts, that produce an anaphylactic reaction, interfering with breathing, she says.

Oral tolerization should be conducted by an allergist or environmental specialist. Ask your primary-care physician for a recommendation.

**Consider surgery.** "We may perform surgery on a woman with endometriosis if she has intractable pelvic pain, infertility, or an endometrioma—a cyst on the ovary caused by endometriosis that can't be treated with medication," says Dr. Biggers. Surgery for endometriosis is usually done via a minimally invasive procedure called laparoscopy. The surgeon makes small incisions near the navel and lower abdomen, through which the tissue is removed. "If the condition is extensive or if there are large ovarian cysts caused by the endometriosis, we will do an open exploratory laparotomy to remove all the disease, which requires a 4- to 8-inch abdominal incision and several weeks of recovery time," says Dr. Biggers.

## NATURAL TREATMENTS FOR ENDOMETRIOSIS

Our specialists share this advice to help you manage endometrisois, as well as lower your risk of ever getting it.

**Eat right, keep fit.** Women who exercise and eat less fat and sugar tend to be thin and, thus, produce less estrogen, a primary fuel for endometriosis. Studies suggest that the high fiber and low protein associated with a vegetarian diet lead to a decrease of biologically active estrogen in the blood, says *Tori Hudson, N.D.*, professor of gynecology at National College of Naturopathic Medicine in Portland, Oregon, and author of *Women's Encyclopedia of Natural Medicine*. Also, organic foods—which don't contain the hormones and pesticides that sometimes act like estrogen in the body—can help keep estrogen levels in check. Dr. Lark recommends lowering excessive estrogen levels by eating soy, beans, peas, berries, oranges, melons, and whole grains, particularly buckwheat, oats, and rice.

**Capitalize on your Cs.** Studies show that vitamin C enhances overall immunity and decreases autoimmune progression, fatigue, capillary fragility, and tumor growth—all of which help prevent endometriosis, says Dr. Hudson. Vegetables and fruits that are high in vitamin C include broccoli, peppers, kale, tomatoes, citrus fruits, and berries. In supplement form, Dr. Hudson recommends taking 500 milligrams twice a day. Decrease the dosage if diarrhea results.

**Liven up your liver.** Certain vegetables contain compounds that enhance liver function, helping to prevent the buildup of toxins and bolster your immune system, says Dr. Hudson. These liver-strengthening veggies include onions, garlic, leeks, carrots, kale, beets, lemons, watercress, dandelion greens, artichokes, and cabbage. Eat these as often as possible to keep your liver in tiptop shape so that it can ward off toxins that may promote endometrial growth.

**Press away pain.** Dr. Lark suggests acupressure massage to ease lower back pain and cramps. Try the following exercise once a day or more when you have symptoms, working on the side of the body that has the most discomfort. (If both sides are equally painful, choose either one.) At each step, hold the position for one to three minutes.

- Sit on the floor with your back against a wall and legs straight in front of you.
- Place your right hand 1 inch above your waist on the muscle to the right side of your spine. (This muscle should feel firm and ropelike.) Your right hand should remain in this position throughout the exercise. Then

reach between your knees to place your left hand in the crease behind your right knee, bending your leg slightly as needed.

- Slide your left hand down to the center back of your right calf, just below the fullest part of the calf.
- Bend your right leg so that you can place your left hand just below your ankle bone on the outside of your right heel. Move your leg as necessary so that you can grip the front and back of your right smallest toe at the nail.

**Fight cramps with food.** Prostaglandins are hormonelike substances that act only in the immediate area from where they are produced in the body. There are three classes of prostaglandins: Series two prostaglandins cause the uterus to contract and shed its lining, and if there are too many, the result is cramps. Series one and three prostaglandins, however, decrease inflammation and can actually reduce uterine cramps. The types of food you eat influence the types of prostaglandins your body makes. Eating foods rich in essential fatty acids increases the level of series one and three prostaglandins that reduce inflammation and relax muscles, thereby reducing symptoms of endometriosis, says Dr. Lark. Choose trout, salmon, tuna, flax or pumpkin seeds, or flaxseed oil at least three times a week. Seeds and nuts, including sesame seeds, sunflower seeds, pistachios, pecans, and almonds, are particularly good choices.

You can also get your fatty acids by taking fish-oil supplements. Taking 3,000 to 4,000 milligrams standardized fish oil a day corresponds to two to three servings of fatty fish a week. To reduce the belching and flatulence that may come with taking fish-oil supplements, spread out the doses into three 1,000 milligram doses and take with meals.

*Avoid red meat to keep from making cramp-causing prostaglandins. Eat fish, nuts, and seeds to make prostaglandins that relax your muscles.—Susan Lark, M.D.*

**Eat less meat.** Foods that aggravate symptoms include such animal proteins as red meat, pork, poultry, and milk and other dairy products. They raise levels of the series two prostaglandins that trigger inflammation and muscle contractions, worsening endometriosis-related cramps. Substitute vegetable protein, soy, and almond and other nut butters, which stimulate anti-inflammatory prostaglandins that inhibit tumor growth and possibly endometrial growth, says Dr. Hudson. Dr. Lark also recommends that women with endometriosis avoid alcohol, sugar, and caffeine.

**Beat cramps with yoga.** The classic Child's Pose stretches the back and is effective for easing cramps, says Dr. Lark.

- Kneel on the floor and sit back on your heels.
- Curl your upper body forward and down, bringing your forehead to the floor. Place your hands on the floor, palms up, next to your feet.
- Stretch your spine as far over your head as possible.
- Close your eyes and hold for as long as you feel comfortable.

**Reduce stress.** Endometriosis has been called the working woman's disease because it's found more often in women who work outside the home. Work usually causes stress, which may worsen the symptoms of endometriosis. Dr. Lark suggests these stress-reducing techniques.

- Sit in a comfortable chair, holding a watch in one hand. Inhale and exhale slowly as you focus all your attention on the movement of the watch's second hand for 30 seconds. Notice how slow and calm your breathing becomes. This focus exercise helps take your attention away from your aching pelvic area and brings a sense of calm.
- Listen to quiet, calming music or recordings of nature sounds, such as ocean waves or rainfall. These sounds instill feelings of peace, decreasing stress hormones and lowering your pulse, heart rate, and blood pressure.
- Add 1 cup each sea salt and bicarbonate of soda to a tubful of warm water. Soak for 20 minutes to help reduce cramps and ease anxiety. This mixture is highly alkaline, so Dr. Lark recommends using it only once or twice a month.

# INFERTILITY: CHASING ELUSIVE MOTHERHOOD

Defining infertility is simple: If your efforts to become pregnant have been unsuccessful for a year (three to six months if you're over age 35), you're considered infertile. Finding the cause, however, is more difficult. Age, genes, environment, medical history, even your sexual technique can play a role.

Infertility is just as likely to be a result of problems with a man's sperm or testicles as with a woman's eggs or reproductive system. Or both of you may have reproductive difficulties. Overall, 50 percent of infertility is related to women, 40 percent to men, with 10 percent undetermined, reports **Carolyn Coulam, M.D.,** medical director of the Sher Institute for Reproductive Medicine in Chicago.

The following are the most common causes of infertility.

- Blocked fallopian tubes: "The majority of women with blocked tubes have them because of a previous infection or endometriosis," says **Lynn Westphal, M.D.,** assistant professor of obstetrics and gynecology at Stanford University Medical School. "An infection can lead to scar tissue all around the tubes. This scar tissue can even cause the tubes to stick to other organs, such as the intestines."
- Problems with ovulation: A woman doesn't produce enough healthy eggs.
- Low sperm count: A man has a low sperm count, meaning he produces too few sperm or sperm too weak to travel to or get into the egg.
- Nutritional deficiencies
- Lifestyle habits
- Stress

Safeguard your fertility by making smart choices early in life and continuing to make smart choices, says **Kathy Trumbull, M.D.,** assistant professor of reproductive endocrinology at the University of Illinois College of Medicine at Peoria. Here are some choices you can make to preserve your fertility.

**Practice safe sex.** Sexually transmitted diseases (STDs) often leave scarred tissue in the fallopian tubes or endometrium. This damaged tissue can prevent eggs from reaching or implanting in the uterus. "Frankly, we don't screen for STDs unless a woman is having problems with infertility," says **Shaun D. Biggers, M.D.,** assistant professor of obstetrics and gynecology at the Weill Cornell Medical Center at New York Presbyterian Hospital. So the best action you can take is to prevent an infection in the first place. That means using condoms or a diaphragm when you aren't actively trying to get pregnant because these birth-control methods reduce your risk of contracting an STD. Fertility experts don't recommend intrauterine devices (IUDs), since they can increase your risk for pelvic inflammatory disease, an infection of the upper genital tract that can lead to infertility. Also ask for an STD screening as soon as you think you may have been exposed.

**Get treated for infections.** Previous pelvic infections—including those that a woman may not even realize she's had—can cause infertility. If you are diagnosed with a pelvic infection, insist on it being treated aggressively,

# YOUR BIOLOGICAL CLOCK: AGE *DOES* MATTER

*Tick, tick, tick ... How do you know if there's still time to become a mother?*

"Women understand in a general way that they have a biological clock," says *Pamela Madsen,* executive director of the American Infertility Association. "But they usually overestimate the time remaining on their clocks by 5 to 10 years, and that makes the difference between having a baby and *not* having a baby."

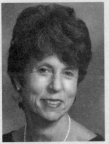

*The longer you wait to have a baby, the more obstacles you'll face in getting pregnant, says Frances Batzer, M.D.*

Statistically, a woman with normal reproductive function has a 63 percent likelihood of getting pregnant up to age 34. By the time she's 40, the likelihood drops to 36 percent; at age 45, the likelihood is down to 5 percent. Conversely, her likelihood of infertility increases with age, with an 8-percent likelihood of infertility at age 34 and 69 percent by age 45.

"Fertility is a finite gift," says *Diane Clapp,* medical information director for the national infertility organization Resolve. And too few women understand this. Instead, they feel their overall health is the best indicator of fertility. "They look great, they jog 10 miles a day, they stay fit as they get older—they don't understand why they're having trouble getting pregnant," says Madsen.

What these women don't realize is that their eggs have a shelf life. A woman is born with all the eggs she'll ever have, and they age right along with the rest of her. The older the egg, the more likely it is to have chromosomal abnormalities, be difficult to fertilize, or once fertilized, result in a miscarriage, says *Frances Batzer, M.D.,* group director at the Women's Institute for Fertility, Endocrinology & Menopause in Philadelphia.

In addition, women who delay pregnancy can face many factors that interfere with fertility, says Dr. Batzer, such as fibroids, polycystic ovary syndrome, endometriosis, and exposure to sexually transmitted diseases and environmental toxins.

So can you safely conceive and give birth to a child after age 40? Of course, but you're likely to need the help of technology to get pregnant. And the risks are far greater than when you were younger. Your chance of having a miscarriage shoots up from 11.7 percent at age 30 to more than 50 percent by age 40. And after age 35, you're more likely to deliver prematurely or have a baby with Down syndrome or other abnormalities. You're also more susceptible to high blood pressure, diabetes, fibroids, and other age-related problems that can complicate pregnancy and delivery.

If you're certain you want to have your own biological children, follow this advice from *Carolyn B. Coulam, M.D.,* medical director of the Sher Institute for Reproductive Medicine in Chicago: "I would recommend that women have families first and their careers second. The biggest risk for infertility, honestly, is age."

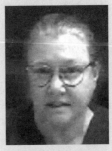

*If you want children, consider postponing your career to make having a family your priority, says Carolyn B. Coulam, M.D.*

recommends Dr. Trumbull. "I have a patient who was told when she was in her teens that she didn't need antibiotics because she was young and her body would fight off the infection. As a result, she now has terrible tubal damage and can only conceive via in vitro fertilization."

**Watch your weight.** Being 10- to 15-percent underweight or overweight can decrease your fertility. Very thin women often don't ovulate, and overweight women tend to produce excess estrogen, which upsets their hormonal balance.

*Smoking and fertility don't mix. Lighting up can harm your ovaries, negatively impact estrogen, and cause abnormalities in your eggs.*
—*Susan L. Treiser, M.D., Ph.D.*

## COPING WITH INFERTILITY

*A diagnosis of infertility may set off a torrent of emotions: guilt, anger, inadequacy, despair, or grief.*

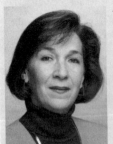

*Infertility is hurtful for both partners in a relationship. Make an effort to keep your romance alive, suggests Joann Paley Galst, Ph.D.*

"Intense anger and sadness are common, especially for the achievement-oriented couple who believe themselves capable of surmounting any obstacle if they exert enough effort," says *Joann Paley Galst, Ph.D.*, a New York City psychologist who specializes in reproductive health issues. So what are the best ways to cope with infertility?

**Do your research.** Knowledge empowers you and helps you understand what is happening medically. Read all you can, both in print and on the Web. Resolve, the national infertility organization, is an excellent resource recommended by *Alice Domar, Ph.D.*, a fertility and stress expert in Boston and author of *Conquering Infertility.*

**Follow your own path.** "What works best for any given couple is specific to that couple," says *Kathy Trumbull, M.D.*, assistant professor of reproductive endocrinology at the Illinois College of Medicine in Peoria. "Not everyone is willing to undergo in vitro fertilization, so adoption may be the best choice for some."

**Re-evaluate periodically.** It's essential that you remain open to changing your approach, advises *Diane Clapp*, medical information director for Resolve. For instance, after two years of unsuccessful infertility treatments, you're entitled to decide that your body, psyche, and bank account have had enough.

**Protect your relationship.** Men and women often cope with infertility in different

**Quit smoking.** As if you didn't already have enough reasons to quit, the American Society for Reproductive Medicine reports that tobacco smoke—even the passive kind—can harm your ovaries, interfere with your ability to produce estrogen (possibly causing early menopause), and may cause genetic abnormalities in your eggs. Men who smoke also have more sperm abnormalities, says *Susan L. Treiser, M.D., Ph.D.,* co-director of IVF New Jersey, a private reproductive health clinic.

**Curtail caffeine.** "The data on the link between caffeine and infertility isn't clear-cut," says Dr. Westphal, but women who drink a lot of caffeine may take longer to get pregnant than women who drink less or abstain. Caffeine may also increase a woman's risk for miscarriage. Studies suggest that caffeine decreases the production of prolactin, a hormone that reduces levels of estrogen and testosterone. Inappropriately low levels of prolactin are associated with infertility just as often as high levels. "I tell my patients to drink no more than two cups of caffeinated beverages a day," says Dr. Westphal.

ways, says Dr. Galst. Vital communication can break down; emotional intimacy and sexual enjoyment can disappear. "If you're not getting pregnant, understand that it's a couple thing, not a him or her thing—it takes two people to make a baby," advises **Pamela Madsen,** executive director of the American Infertility Association. "The good news about treatment is that more than 60 percent of couples walk away with a biological child."

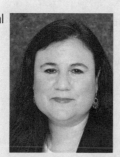

*More than 60 percent of those who get treatment are able to have a child, says Pamela Madsen of the American Infertility Association.*

To avoid the breakdown of your relationship, Dr. Galst offers these suggestions:

**Limit discussions.** Set a timer for a mutually agreed-upon time and air your feelings while your partner listens. Then set the timer again and listen while he vents.

**Show respect.** Your partner is someone you love, so listen and try to understand without criticizing or judging.

**Recapture romance.** Reminisce about fun things you used to do; create new memories with weekly dates. Take turns planning something special and leave the infertility talk at home.

**Try tenderness.** Little acts of love and kindness will help your partner feel appreciated. Massage his feet, hands, or neck with an aromatic lotion.

**Stay sensual.** Make sex fun again. Take baths or showers together. Give each other body massages. Vary the venue.

**Get help.** Consult a therapist or counselor if the strain on your relationship threatens to become too great.

**Check your medicine cabinet.** "Some medications, such as antidepressants, can affect ovulation and make menstrual cycles irregular," says Dr. Westphal. Chemotherapy drugs or radiation treatments for cancer may damage ovaries. "This side effect is usually discussed at the time of treatment," she says.

**Ease up on alcohol.** Moderate use of alcohol shouldn't affect conception, but heavy drinking can impair the ability to conceive, as well as increase the chances of miscarriage once conception takes place, says Dr. Westphal. Heavy alcohol consumption can raise your levels of prolactin—the hormone released during breast feeding—which interferes with ovulation. Extremely high prolactin levels can lead to infertility.

**Reduce stress.** "If you define stress more as depression, there's much more evidence to show that stress can contribute to infertility," says *Alice Domar, Ph.D.*, a fertility and stress expert in Boston and author of *Conquering Infertility.* One study found that a highly stressed woman was 93 percent less likely to have a baby than a woman who was not under stress. And since infertility also *causes* stress, a vicious cycle is created.

"I've done a lot of research with mind-body interventions that shows a link between decreased stress and much improved pregnancy rates," says Dr. Domar. It's the most effective intervention. These techniques usually start to take effect within a month. Try this sample exercise to lower the stress in your life.

- Choose a focus word, short phrase, or prayer that is firmly rooted in your belief system, such as *peace* or *one.*
- Sit in a comfortable position in a quiet room and close your eyes.
- Relax your muscles, consciously progressing from feet to calves, thighs, and stomach up to shoulders, head, and neck. Breathe naturally and slowly. Silently repeat your focus word or phrase each time you exhale.
- Keep a positive attitude. Don't worry about how well you're doing. If other thoughts wander into your mind, gently put them aside and return to your focus repetition.

Continue this exercise for 10 to 20 minutes. When finished, don't stand immediately but sit in silence for a minute or two, allowing other thoughts to slowly return. Then open your eyes and sit for another minute before rising.

Perform this calming exercise once or twice a day, preferably before breakfast and dinner.

**Join a group.** Spending time with women who share similar frustrations can be extremely helpful. The National Infertility Association offers Resolve support groups in every state (www.resolve.org, 617-623-0744).

**Take the pressure off.** Infertility can affect every aspect of a woman's life, from her job to her relationship with friends to her sex life. So it's normal to feel awful, to resent every pregnant woman you see, or to fight with your husband, says Dr. Domar. Don't add to your stress by being ashamed of your emotions. (To help you and your partner overcome negative emotions, see "Coping with Infertility," page 392.)

**Avoid dangerous stress-relievers.** These no-nos include alcohol and cigarettes, both of which only make it harder for you to conceive.

## TROUBLE CONCEIVING: WHAT YOU CAN DO

If you're having difficulty getting pregnant, our experts suggest you try these steps before seeking professional help.

**Track your ovulation.** You're most likely to conceive when you're ovulating, as well as a day or two afterward. Most women ovulate on Day 14 of their cycle, but numerous factors can throw you off. Try the following to determine your exact time of ovulation.

- Take your temperature: Record your basal temperature for three to four months. (You can buy a basal body thermometer at most drugstores.) Take your temperature at the same time each morning before you get out of bed. Your temperature will be slightly lower before ovulation and will rise just after ovulation.

- Use an ovulation home testing kit: You can get one at the drugstore. Use it around Day 11 of your menstrual cycle to determine when your ovaries are about to release an egg. "For most women, these tests are reliable, although they're not really useful in increasing pregnancy rates," says Dr. Westphal. "However, if a woman is having irregular cycles and she and her partner are having trouble timing intercourse because they're working or traveling, these tests can help." Follow the manufacturer's directions.

- Tune in to your body: Some women say they feel a "ping" when they ovulate and the egg is released, says Dr. Westphal. Others report a twinge in the lower abdomen where the ovaries are located, an increase in mucus or difference in mucous texture, or tenderness in their breasts.

**Avoid sperm-killing lubricants.** Nix the K-Y Brand Jelly, Lubrifax, Surgilube, Vaseline, and oils, since all create an inhospitable climate for sperm. Instead, Dr. Westphal recommends you use a water-soluble lubricant, such as Astroglide, which is not toxic to sperm.

**Don't douche.** "I usually recommend that women not douche even when they're *not* trying to conceive," says Dr. Wesphal. Douching changes the pH balance of your vagina, making you more vulnerable to infection.

*If you're trying to get pregnant, create a hospitable environment for sperm by using only water-soluble lubricants.*—Lynn Westphal, M.D.

**Give sperm a boost.** For about 20 to 30 minutes after intercourse, lie flat on your back, with your legs and hips propped up with a pillow to help sperm travel to your cervix and beyond. "It certainly can't hurt, and it may be helpful in some women," says Dr. Westphal.

**Keep your guy cool.** Make sure your partner avoids tight underwear and prolonged stays in the sauna or a hot tub, since excess heat can kill sperm.

**Don't wait too long.** Developing technologies will be able to help some—but not all—women become pregnant later in life. "The ovaries age along with the rest of us, and women simply cannot have children over their entire lives," says Dr. Westphal.

### TIME TO TURN TO THE EXPERTS

If you've tried unsuccessfully to conceive for a year (six months if you're older than age 35), consult a reproductive endocrinologist, a doctor with special training in infertility issues. Identifying the cause of infertility can require detective work—the testing alone may take several months. And the older you are, the less you can afford to lose valuable fertility time.

A fertility specialist starts by taking your family history and then performs tests. You'll have blood tests to determine ovarian and hormonal function and an X-ray to see if your fallopian tubes are open and the uterine cavity looks normal. Your partner will have a semen analysis, says Dr. Treiser. The results will help determine your treatment options.

There are numerous options from which to choose.

- Fertility drugs: The most effective fertility drugs available are gonado-tropins, which are designed to act like natural hormones to help you ovulate, says Dr. Westphal. Gonadotropins are expensive, administered by injection, and carry a risk of multiple fetuses. These drugs include the human menopausal gonadotropin Humegon, Pergonal, and Repronex (or generic menotropins) and the follicle-stimulating hormones Follistim and Gonal-F (or generic follitropin). An alternative treatment is an oral fertility medication, such as Clomid and Serophene (clomiphene), which suppresses hormones that interfere with ovulation. "These drugs are not as effective as the gonadotropins, but they work for younger women or women who don't ovulate regularly," says Dr. Westphal.

- Artificial insemination: This procedure, performed in your doctor's office, places sperm directly in your cervix or uterus. "Artificial insem-ination is very common," says Dr. Westphal. "It's great in certain cir-cumstances, especially for a woman who doesn't have a partner, whose partner doesn't make sperm, or whose partner's sperm count is low."

- In vitro fertilization (IVF): The first step of this procedure is usually for you to take drugs to stimulate your ovaries into producing multiple viable eggs. Your doctor then removes those eggs during an in-office or outpatient surgical procedure and mixes them with your partner's sperm in the labo-ratory. The fertilized egg or eggs are allowed to grow for two to five days before the doctor transfers the embryo(s) into your uterus. "IVF is the most effective fertility procedure. In the best cases, each attempt is about 50- to 60-percent effective," says Dr. Westphal. "However, it has a low chance of success in women who are older or who have poor quality eggs."

## REPRODUCTIVE CANCERS: FIGHTING BACK

Approximately every seven minutes in the United States, a woman is diag-nosed with a gynecologic cancer. Uterine cancer is the most common form; cervical cancer is the most preventable and easiest to detect. Ovarian cancer is the most difficult to diagnose and, thus, the deadliest.

However, a diagnosis of *any* reproductive cancer is not a death sentence. Research is constantly devising new tools, therapies, and resources to assist with these life-threatening diseases. Education is the key to reducing your risk and increasing your survival. Here are some basics you need to know.

## UTERINE (ENDOMETRIAL) CANCER

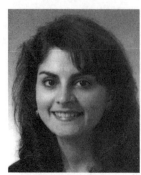

"Uterine cancer is treatable and curable with early detection," says *Mary L. Gemignani, M.D.*, assistant professor of breast and gynecologic oncology in the department of surgery at Memorial Sloan-Kettering Cancer Center in New York City. About 75 percent of women with this type of cancer are diagnosed before the cancer spreads beyond the uterus. Most are cured with treatment, which usually includes a hystero-oophorectomy, the surgical removal of the uterus and ovaries. If the cancer has spread, or metastasized, your doctor may advise radiation therapy.

*See your doctor right away if you have unusual bleeding, warns Mary L. Gemignani, M.D. It could be a warning sign of uterine cancer, which is curable if detected early.*

Uterine cancer begins in the lining of the uterus, called the endometrium. In 9 out of 10 cases, the warning sign is postmenopausal spotting or even heavier bleeding. In premenopausal women, the key may be heavy bleeding between periods or heavy periods. If you have a change in your normal menstrual cycle, see your doctor.

There is no specific screening for uterine cancer, although a few cases are detected with Pap tests. In most cases, a woman who is having symptoms is diagnosed after a pelvic exam and endometrial biopsy, says Dr. Gemignani.

To help prevent uterine cancer—or, at least, detect it early—follow these recommendations from *Carolyn Muller, M.D.*, assistant professor of obstetrics and gynecology in the division of gynecologic oncology at the University of Texas Southwest Medical Center in Dallas.

**Stay slim.** Obesity increases a woman's risk of uterine cancer by two to five times, depending on how overweight she is, according to the American Cancer Society.

**Rely on the Pill.** A woman who takes oral contraceptives for at least five years during her lifetime runs a lower risk of getting endometrial cancer, probably because the Pill prevents ovulation. This protection continues for about a decade after you stop taking the Pill.

**Know your medical risks.** If you're aware that your medical and menstrual history put you at high risk for this disease, work with your doctor to schedule more frequent screenings. You are at higher risk for uterine cancer if any of the following are true for you.

- You started having periods before age 12.
- You went through menopause after age 50.
- You have diabetes.
- You have high blood pressure.
- You are obese.
- You have never been pregnant.
- You have a history of infertility.
- You have had breast cancer or used tamoxifen to treat it.

## CERVICAL CANCER

"The most important thing women should know about cervical cancer is that Pap smear screenings reduce the rate of cervical cancer deaths by 85 percent," says **Bobbie Gostout, M.D.**, assistant professor in the division of gynecological surgery at the Mayo Clinic in Rochester, Minnesota. That's because a Pap smear can detect development of abnormal cells in your cervix—a condition known as dysplasia—*before* those abnormalities evolve into cancer. Left untreated, dysplasia can lead to cancer in a significant proportion of women, especially if the condition is severe. "Dysplasia typically has no outward signs or symptoms," explains Dr. Gostout. "So, without a Pap smear, neither a woman nor her doctor will know anything is wrong."

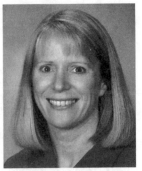

*See your doctor regularly for a Pap smear—it's your best chance of detecting the earliest warning signs of cervical cancer, says Bobbie Gostout, M.D.*

The most common sign of early cervical cancer is abnormal bleeding. See your doctor if you experience bleeding between periods or after sexual intercourse. She will examine your cervix and take a sample of cells that will be sent to a lab for a Pap smear.

If your Pap smear shows some dysplasia, your options vary. "Some cervical dysplasia doesn't require any treatment," says Dr. Gostout. Your doctor may want to examine your cervix with a binocular-like instrument, called a colposcope, in a painless procedure known as colposcopy. If your doctor sees abnormal areas during the colposcopy, she can remove them using one of the following methods.

- Freezing therapy (also known as cryosurgery): In this in-office procedure, your doctor uses a probe cooled by liquid nitrogen to freeze and, thus, kill abnormal cells.

- Laser surgery: Your doctor can perform this surgery right in her office, focusing a beam of high-energy light to vaporize abnormal cells.
- Loop electrosurgical excision procedure (LEEP): After administering a local anesthetic, your doctor will pass an electrical current through a thin wire loop and use it to scoop out the abnormal cells. The process takes about 10 minutes and can be done in your doctor's office.

All enable you to retain your fertility and usually have good outcomes. You will need to have follow-up exams to make sure the dysplasia doesn't return. If it does, you can have the treatments again.

If the cancer has spread, however, treatment options are more complex, usually including hysterectomy, radiation therapy, chemotherapy, or some combination.

The best methods for preventing cervical cancer are practicing healthy habits that keep cells from becoming abnormal, including routinely getting Pap smears, and detecting any deviant cells *before* they have a chance to become cancerous and spread.

> Don't *panic if your Pap smear shows some abnormal cells—they may revert to normal without treatment. But* do *get follow-up Pap smears to monitor those cells.*—Bobbie Gostout, M.D.

These practices can help you reduce your risk for cervical cancer.

**Get an annual exam.** A pelvic exam isn't the most enjoyable way to pass some time, but it's not the most awful experience in the world either—so there's no real reason, or valid excuse, for not having it done. Remember the old saying, Better safe than sorry. If your Pap smear detects any abnormal cells, you'll need to have a follow-up exam at least every six months until you've had two years of normal Pap smears, advises Dr. Gostout. "Most mild abnormalities go away on their own," she says. "But repeat Pap smears are the only way for a woman to be sure her body is healing."

**Reduce your exposure.** Nearly all cervical cancers are caused by the human papillomavirus (HPV), which is spread through sexual contact. Your risk is related to your total number of sexual contacts: The more partners, the higher your risk. The risk is concentrated in the 10 to 15 years after your first sexual experience with a new partner (assuming that partner doesn't have other partners at the same time). "All women who have had sexual intercourse are at some risk for dysplasia and cervix cancer," says Dr. Gostout. "But no one knows for sure how long the virus can be dormant before causing dysplasia or cancer."

Researchers are testing several vaccines that may help prevent an HPV infection from developing. In November 2002, the *New England Journal of Medicine* reported that a study found early testing of an experimental vaccine is 100-percent effective against HPV. With nearly 50 percent of young adults showing evidence of HPV exposure—although most don't have any clinical symptoms—a vaccine might offer the only real hope for real protection, aside from sexual abstinence, that is.

**Quit smoking.** Tobacco use seems to promote cervical cancer in two ways, says Dr. Gostout: Cancer-causing chemicals in cigarette smoke tend to concentrate in cervical mucus and result in damage to your DNA. And smoking suppresses your immune system, which makes it easy for HPV to gain access to and remain active in your body, says Dr. Gostout.

**Eat your fruits and veggies.** A diet rich in fruits and vegetables may help reduce the risk of cervical cancer. One study tested the affects of diet on 53 women with cervical dysplasia. Half the test subjects ate a diet high in fruits and vegetables; the other half ate little of the healthy stuff. After six months, the group who'd eaten lots of fruits and vegetables showed improvements in their condition.

## OVARIAN CANCER

Ovarian cancer struck 23,400 women in 2001, making it the fifth leading cause of cancer-related deaths in women. Dr. Gemignani explains that the difficulty in diagnosing ovarian cancer—it can't always be detected by a pelvic exam—is part of what makes it so dangerous. By the time it is found, usually on the surface of an ovary, the cancer has often progressed to an advanced stage.

Until a reliable and accurate screening test to detect ovarian cancer exists, the National Ovarian Cancer Coalition suggests you follow this advice.

- Get an annual pelvic exam, starting at age 18.
- Get an annual rectovaginal exam, starting at age 35. To perform this test, your doctor inserts one finger in your rectum and one in your

vagina, then uses the other hand to feel your abdomen for abnormal swelling and detect tenderness.

- If you have a strong family history of breast or ovarian cancer, you are at increased risk for ovarian cancer and should have these additional screenings. Your doctor may also suggest them based on your vaginal exam.
  - Transvaginal sonography: Your doctor performs this ultrasound procedure by placing a small probe in the vagina. It can help find masses in the ovary.
  - CA-125 blood test: This test identifies levels of a tumor marker that tends to increase in women with ovarian cancer. However, it cannot be considered a definitive test, since some noncancerous conditions of the ovaries also increase CA-125 levels. Conversely, some ovarian cancers may not be associated with elevated CA-125 levels. CA-125 can also be elevated in premenopausal women who have reproductive problems, such as endometriosis or fibroids, says Dr. Gemignani.

If cancer is present, treatment may include surgery accompanied with chemotherapy or radiation, or even both, depending on the stage of the disease. If the cancer is advanced, a total abdominal hysterectomy and removal of the ovaries may be required. In some cases, the affected ovary may be the only one removed, leaving a healthy ovary in place to preserve fertility.

Defend yourself against ovarian cancer with these weapons.

**Know your family history.** You can inherit an increased risk for premenopausal ovarian cancer from either your mother's or father's side of the family—especially if there's a history of breast, ovarian, endometrial, colon, or prostrate cancer. If you are a woman of Eastern European (Ashkenazi) Jewish descent, you are at greater risk if your mother or sister has or had ovarian cancer. You are also at higher risk if you are of Northern European or Northern American heritage. You are also at increased risk if you have unexplained infertility, no personal history of pregnancies or history of using birth control, or personal history of breast, endometrial, or colon cancer.

**Pop the Pill.** The American Cancer Society reports that women who do not take birth control pills are almost three times more likely to develop ovarian cancer than women who do. And the longer women take the Pill, the greater the benefit of lowered risk. Pills with a relatively high level of progestin offer the greatest level of protection.

# 21 Respiratory System
## Breathing Better Again

*Breathe in. Breathe out. Breathe in.*
*Breathe out. You do that thousands*
*of times a day without giving it a*
*thought—unless something goes wrong.*
*If you can't draw an easy breath, you*
*suddenly can't think of anything else.*

Abnormal breathing can affect your ability to work, exercise, socialize, even sleep. Just ask one of the more than 30 million Americans living with lung disease—all are acutely aware of their condition. For many, it becomes the defining fact of their lives.

From a mechanical viewpoint, your lungs are gas-exchange depots. Oxygen is the energy every cell requires for life. Every time you inhale, your lungs snatch oxygen from the air and send it into the bloodstream to be distributed throughout the body. When you exhale, your body disposes of carbon dioxide, the waste material of living.

Any condition that hinders breathing threatens your life. "It impedes body function on the most basic level," says *Sally Wenzel, M.D.,* a specialist in chronic obstructive lung disease at the National Jewish Medical and Research Center in Denver. Lung disease in general refers to conditions caused by infection, such as pneumonia or tuberculosis; it can also refer to chronic lung infections, including asthma and chronic obstructive lung disease. And of course, there's lung cancer. Lung disease is the third largest killer in the United States, responsible for one in seven deaths each year. Yet many women don't even consider it a major health threat.

That's a mistake, says Dr. Wenzel, because the sad truth is that lung disease is often incurable and incapacitating. But the good news is that proper disease management enables most patients to live full and active lives.

## ASTHMA: LIKE BREATHING THROUGH A STRAW

Place your mouth on one end of a drinking straw, then breathe through it. That's what it feels like to try to breathe during an asthma attack

Nearly 25 million Americans are living with asthma. Despite advances in treatment, the disease still claims about five thousand lives each year. Many people with asthma say it restricts their activities, preventing them from participating in even mild physical exertion.

Asthma is a chronic inflammatory condition that affects the airways of your lungs. When these airways are stimulated, they become inflamed, which causes them to swell and become narrowed. If you have asthma, you may have some inflammation at all times. Or your airways may stay inflamed for weeks following an episode, or asthma attack. Sometimes, the airways can also become obstructed by muscles that tighten around them, a condition known as a bronchospasm. In some people, excess mucus collects, which also clogs your airways. The result is the gasping wheeze associated with asthma. Sudden changes in air temperature, a respiratory infection, or an allergic reaction to airborne substances can trigger an episode. Exercise, stress, and exposure to cigarette smoke can have the same result.

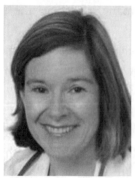

Your asthma can change over time and may require different care, says Mary Kay Wolfson, M.D.

Although there is no cure, asthma can be managed successfully so that you can lead a normal life, says **Mary Kay Wolfson, M.D.,** an asthma specialist in New Orleans. But don't fool yourself that asthma can just go away, even if you're not having any symptoms. "Asthma is a chronic condition that requires continuous care," she says. "It can change over the years, and you may need different types of treatment. But just because you're not experiencing episodes of labored breathing doesn't mean you're cured."

Most people who have asthma start having episodes in childhood. It is a hereditary disease, but a genetic predisposition doesn't guarantee that you'll develop it. Environmental conditions tip the scales, says **Sally Wenzel, M.D.,** a specialist in chronic obstructive lung disease at the National Jewish Medical Center in Denver. Research finds that a child has a greater risk of developing asthma if the mother smoked during pregnancy or while the child was younger than age 2. Asthma can be triggered in active kids by severe air pollution or cockroach infestation (cockroach droppings are powerful lung irritants).

If asthma is taking your breath away, you may feel powerless to prevent the wheezing, coughing, or gasping. But there's actually a great deal you can do to control the attacks.

**Avoid irritants.** Asthma symptoms are caused by lung irritants called triggers. You need to know what your triggers are and how to limit your exposure to them, says *Mary Beth Fasano, M.D.*, an asthma and allergy specialist at Wake Forest University Baptist Medical Center in Winston-Salem. Triggers vary widely among people with asthma, but common ones include dust, pollens, mold, pet dander, tobacco smoke, traffic fumes, perfume, cold air, and wind. Ask your doctor to perform allergy tests to determine your unique sensitivities, recommends Dr. Fasano.

*Wear a filter mask over your nose and mouth when you dust. Use a damp cloth or an electrostatic disposable wipe to remove dust, not just move it around.*—Mary Beth Fasano, M.D.

**Restrict the time you spend outdoors.** If pollen is one of your triggers, stay inside from 5 to 10 a.m.—the peak pollen hours—and on windy days when pollen levels are highest. Also keep the windows closed in your home during that time. Wear a filter mask when mowing the lawn—or better yet, get someone to cut it for you. When in the car, keep the windows closed and use the air conditioner on the recirculate setting. Pollen or other irritants can stick to your hair and clothing, so shower and change your clothes after you've been outside for any significant length of time.

**Do away with dust.** No matter how clean you keep your house, millions of microscopic dust mites live there. You're not allergic to the mites themselves, but to a protein in their waste. Over the course of a mite's short life, this critter can produce 200 times its body weight in waste. "That means simply dusting probably isn't enough. You have to get the dust mites where they live—deep inside sofas, chairs, bedding, and carpets," says Dr. Fasano. Don't buy upholstered furniture that can harbor dust. Choose wood, metal, vinyl, or leather, since they are less likely to harbor dust mites. Similarly, if you can, opt for hardwood, tile, or linoleum flooring, rather than carpeting.

Of course, you'll still want to dust, too. Wear a filter mask over your nose and mouth as you clean. Keep in mind that dry-dusting just moves dust around. Use a damp cloth or mop or an electrostatic disposable wipe, which removes dust, advises Dr. Fasano. Some electrostatic products include the Exstatic Dust Mop, Pledge Grab-It Duster, and Swiffer.

**Target your bedroom.** Studies show that dust mites inhabit bedrooms more than anywhere else in the average home. Why? Because that's where you are most likely to find their favorite food: your spent skin cells. The average adult can lose about 1.5 grams of skin each day, enough to feed about one million of the little critters. Putting allergen-impermeable covers on your mattress and pillows is the most important step you can take to reduce your exposure to dust mites, says Dr. Fasano. These vinyl or plastic covers keep dust mites from setting up housekeeping and block your exposure to their waste. They are available at department stores, but companies that specialize in allergy prevention may offer a better selection. Wash your bedding once a week in hot water (it should be at least 130 degrees) to kill dust mites living on your sheets, blankets, and pillowcases.

**Vacuum at least twice a week.** If you're sensitive to dust and can't replace your rugs, then you'll need to clean them well, since carpeting is a haven for dust. If you don't have a vacuum cleaner that is designed to reduce allergens, consider investing in one. Dr. Fasano recommends using a vacuum that has a high-efficiency particulate attracting (HEPA) filter and microfilter bags that do not allow dust, pollen, and other allergens to escape back into your

## SHOULD I SEE A DOCTOR?

*Patients sometimes forget that their asthma can be a serious, life-threatening condition.*

It's critical for people with asthma to know when to seek emergency help, says *Mary Beth Fasano, M.D.,* an asthma and allergy specialist at Wake Forest University Baptist Medical Center in Winston-Salem. See your doctor immediately if you experience any of these symptoms:

- You have difficulty walking or talking because of your asthma.
- Your lips or fingernails turn blue or gray.
- Your heart or pulse rate is very fast.

- You are still breathing hard or fast after using a quick-relief bronchodilator, which enables you to inhale medicine directly into your lungs.
- Your peak-flow meter readings drop below 50 percent of your personal best reading.

These are warning signs of an extreme asthma attack that could be fatal if not treated promptly, says Dr. Fasano. If you can't get to your doctor in less than 20 minutes, go to a hospital emergency room.

environment. Many antiallergy vacuum products are available, ranging in price from about $200 to more than $2,000. "The name manufacturers, such as Hoover and Eureka, make good antiallergy vacuums that are readily available at discount department stores," notes Dr Fasano.

**Buy a filter.** If you live in an urban area with industrial and transportation pollution, consider getting a HEPA filter for your home's air system, suggests Dr. Fasano. These special filters are designed to cut down on the amount of pollen, mold, and dust moving through your home and into your lungs, thus reducing the chance of an asthmatic reaction. A disposable filter, such as Filtrete or Purity Max, lasts about three months and costs from $10 to $25. Permanent electrostatic filters need to be washed monthly and can cost from $50 to $200.

**Be sensible about scents.** Give up heavy perfumes and don't let salesclerks spray you with cologne. "Scents of any kind can throw a sensitive, twitchy lung into an asthmatic spasm," explains Dr. Fasano. She recommends avoiding scented room sprays and using fragrance-free laundry and cleaning products.

**Be OTC cautious.** Some over-the-counter (OTC) pain relievers can trigger an asthma attack. Check with your physician before taking acetaminophen, aspirin, ibuprofen, or naproxen sodium, says Dr. Wolfson. Research into the link between asthma and pain relievers is ongoing, but evidence shows up to 19 percent of people with asthma may have this sensitivity.

*Take the daily medicine your doctor prescribes, even if you haven't had an asthma attack in a while.*

—*Mary Kay Wolfson, M.D.*

**Take your meds.** Some types of medication can help reduce inflammation and prevent the narrowing of airways so that you avoid asthma attacks. Other types help stop an asthma attack after it starts. Both kinds are important.

Anti-inflammatories reduce swelling and mucous production, thus making the airways less sensitive to triggers. Your doctor may prescribe an anti-inflammatory that you use as an inhaler, such as Azmacort (triamcinolone) and Flovent (fluticasone). Or you may take pills, such as Accolate (zafirlukast) and Singulair (montelukast). Bronchodilators open the airways by relaxing bronchial muscles.

Unfortunately, some people stop taking medication when they haven't experienced symptoms for some time. It's important to understand which drugs you should take every day to *prevent* attacks and which ones you only use to *relieve* attacks. Medications will thwart asthma symptoms if you take them properly, says Dr. Wolfson. An effective treatment plan should provide the following, with little or no side effects: enable you to breath normally most of the time, perform normal activities and exercise, and prevent asthma attacks.

Dr. Wolfson has these words of encouragement for asthma sufferers: "With proper medication, medical supervision, and commonsense precautions, you can control your asthma, rather than have your asthma control you."

## COPD: COMMON BUT POTENTIALLY DEADLY

A physical change in lung tissue can create a barrier that prevents air from getting in and out of your body. This condition is called chronic obstructive pulmonary disease (COPD). It is also referred to as chronic obstructive lung disease, or COLD. COPD includes such diseases as chronic bronchitis and emphysema. Most people with COPD have both.

Approximately 16 million Americans struggle with some form of COPD. About 14 million have chronic bronchitis and 2 million have emphysema, although the two frequently occur together. According to the American Lung Association (ALA), women experience chronic bronchitis more often than men, and more men are likely to have emphysema. Both forms of COPD cause permanent lung damage.

Recurring lung infections and exposure to industrial pollutants can be the culprits in some cases of COPD. But the ALA reports that smoking is responsible for up to 90 percent of these diseases. So if you want to really reduce your risk of developing this condition, shun tobacco and avoid secondhand smoke whenever possible, advises *Sally Wenzel, M.D.*, a COPD specialist at the National Jewish Medical and Research Center in Denver.

Not to be confused with acute bronchitis—which is due to a viral or bacterial infection—chronic bronchitis is caused by repeated exposure to irritants, such as tobacco smoke or airborne chemicals. With chronic bronchitis, the lining of the bronchial tubes are chronically inflamed and swollen. The inflammation causes excess production of mucus, which makes it harder for you to breathe. This eventually causes mucus to build up, blocking the flow of air. The first sign of chronic bronchitis is usually a cough with mucus production. The condition may start in the winter, then the problem may become continuous. As the disease worsens, you may feel short of breath.

With emphysema, tiny air sacs in the lungs lose their ability to stretch and recoil. As the lungs lose their snap, they are less able to send oxygen into the bloodstream or rid the body of carbon dioxide. As the disease progresses, every breath becomes a struggle. Having emphysema typically means you have shortness of breath, coughing, and a limited ability to exercise, says Dr. Wenzel. An accurate diagnosis requires pulmonary-function tests, where you forcefully breathe into a tube to measure airflow capacity.

*Smoking causes 90 percent of chronic obstructive pulmonary disease. If you want to breathe to a ripe old age, give up tobacco now.—Sally Wenzel, M.D.*

As either emphysema or chronic bronchitis progresses, quality of life diminishes. In a national survey of COPD patients, more than half reported that the condition limited their ability to work. Nearly 50 percent of survey participants said they get short of breath while washing, dressing, or doing light housework. One in three said they have trouble breathing while talking; almost one in four said COPD made them invalids.

What begins as minimal shortness of breath eventually requires most COPD patients to use supplemental oxygen, says Dr. Wenzel. Many are forced to rely on mechanical respiratory assistance, such as in-home oxygen tanks.

There is no cure for COPD, but Dr. Wenzel recommends these steps to maintain or improve the quality of your life.

**Get oxygen.** You need to get enough oxygen into your blood, says Dr. Wenzel. If your doctor suggests oxygen therapy, which may involve toting around a portable oxygen cylinder, don't resist. "Most women don't like to walk around with oxygen prongs in their nose—it offends their vanity. But getting enough oxygen is the number-one thing you can do to prolong your life when you have COPD," says Dr. Wenzel. Sometimes, oxygen therapy is also recommended while you're resting. Even if you don't feel short of breath, having a higher oxygen level at rest can help reduce strain on your heart.

**Live in a smoke-free zone.** The best way to prevent COPD—or keep it from worsening—is to not smoke or be around people who do. If you smoke, stop now. If you live or work with smokers, don't allow them to smoke around you. "This is not negotiable," says Dr. Wenzel. "Tobacco smoke is absolutely the worst thing for people with COPD. Avoiding exposure must be your top priority."

**Avoid pollution.** In our industrial society, doing this is like trying to escape sunlight, but steer clear of exposure whenever you can. Stay inside on days that have very high pollution levels, usually during the summer when weather conditions trap airborne chemicals from factories and automobiles. Use high-efficiency filters in your home's ventilation system to keep the air inside as

## PNEUMONIA: AN OUNCE OF PREVENTION, A POUND OF CURE

*Pneumonia was the leading cause of death in the United States until antibiotics revolutionized its treatment. But it remains a serious condition, especially for people with lung disease.*

Pneumonia is a serious infection or inflammation of the lungs that causes your air sacs to fill with fluid, making it difficult for them to send oxygen to your blood. And your body's cells can't work properly if there's not enough oxygen in your bloodstream, explains *Sally Wenzel, M.D.,* a pulmonologist at the National Jewish Medical and Research Center in Denver. Oxygen starvation on the cellular level combines with spreading infection to make pneumonia potentially fatal, particularly among those people who already have lung disease.

Pneumonia isn't a single condition. Rather, it can have more than 30 different causes, ranging from bacterial infections to fungus. Almost half the cases are caused by viruses that attack the upper respiratory track.

Because pneumonia is a common complication of influenza, getting a flu shot every fall is a sensible measure to prevent the disease, says Dr. Wenzel. There is also a one-time vaccine for a type of bacterial pneumonia called pneumococcal pneumonia. Dr. Wenzel recommends this vaccination for those at high-risk of developing pneumonia, including nursing-home residents and people with chronic respiratory illnesses, such as emphysema or asthma.

Many times, pneumonia comes on the heels of a respiratory infection, such as a cold or the flu. So if you get one of these, see your doctor about any breathing problems that linger for more than a few days. Take the full course of medicine your doctor prescribes and don't push yourself to do too much too soon. "If you have a viral infection and let yourself get rundown, you greatly increase your chances of developing pneumonia," says Dr. Wenzel.

Finally, don't forget the tried-and-true preventive: good health habits. Eating a balanced diet, as well as getting plenty of rest and regular exercise, will improve your resistance to all respiratory illness, advises Dr. Wenzel.

clean as possible. If you work where trace chemicals may be in the air, such as in an assembly line or paint shop, ask for another assignment—otherwise, you may end up having to take disability retirement, says Dr. Wenzel.

**Drink up.** Make sure you get at least eight 8-ounce glasses of liquid every day. Taking in plenty of fluids helps keep your lung secretions thin, making it easier to clear your airways. Water is best, but any nonalcoholic beverage will do, says Dr. Wenzel.

**Breathe moist air.** Using a humidifier to increase air moisture in your home helps prevent your lung secretions from becoming too thick, says Dr. Wenzel.

*Put vanity aside if your doctor recommends supplemental oxygen. Prongs in your nose are easier to live with than the need to gasp for every breath.*—Sally *Wenzel, M.D.*

**Stay active.** Staying fit maintains your strength, prevents the disease from worsening, and keeps weight off—all of which make it easier for you to breathe. Even though it's difficult to exercise when you're having trouble breathing, try to maintain an active lifestyle as much as possible, advises Dr. Wenzel. She recommends exercising at least 30 minutes a day, five days a week. "Ideally, you should incorporate equal amounts of cardiovascular work and weight-bearing exercise," says Dr. Wenzel. If you can't manage a half hour at a time, try adding what she calls "fit bits"—5 to 10 minutes of walking or lifting hand weights throughout the day. Remember that the goal is to build up your overall strength, not to exhaust yourself.

**Eat more fruits.** Here's potentially good news: A handful of strawberries every day may keep COPD at bay, especially if the fruit is dipped in chocolate. A recent British study looking into the effect of diet on lung function found that people who had a higher daily intake of vitamin C and magnesium (that's where the chocolate comes in) performed better in one test of lung function. More research is needed to determine the exact impact of diet on COPD, but many studies suggest that eating more fruits and vegetables, which are rich in antioxidants, can be protective. Smokers, who have more oxidative damage, may particularly benefit from eating more fresh fruits and vegetables.

**Don't forget your meds.** It's essential that you follow directions for the medication you've been prescribed to treat COPD. The most commonly prescribed medications are bronchodilators, which relax the muscles in the bronchial tubes, allowing air to freely flow in and out. Some bronchodilators are inhaled; others are taken in pill or liquid form. Corticosteroids are sometimes used to treat COPD, but they don't work as well against this lung disease as they do with asthma, says Dr. Wenzel.

**Get immunized.** If you're prone to respiratory congestion, which weakens your lungs over time, you may be more susceptible to COPD. Dr. Wenzel advises you to get a flu shot every year and to get the one-time pneumonia vaccination. Infections can often make COPD symptoms worse, requiring emergency office visits or hospitalization.

**Use protein supplements as a last resort.** Some doctors advocate taking high-calorie, high-protein nutritional supplementation to prevent malnutrition in people with COPD. "Unless you're having trouble eating because trapped air makes your lungs press on your stomach, there's no need for nutritional supplements," says Dr. Wenzel. She advocates eating a balanced, nutrient-rich diet. Real food is better for your body and isn't as likely to cause weight gain, which can put added stress on your lungs.

## LUNG CANCER: THE HIDDEN SCOURGE

Would you be surprised to know that lung cancer—rather than breast cancer—is the leading cause of cancer deaths in women? Well, it's true, says oncologist *Helen Ross, M.D.,* of Earle A. Chiles Research Institute and the Providence Cancer Center in Portland, Oregon. The U.S. Surgeon General has declared lung cancer epidemic among American women.

The cause of this alarming trend is easily identified: More than 85 percent of lung cancers are attributable to cigarette smoking. (Many of the more than four thousand chemicals in cigarette smoke are proven cancer-causing substances, called carcinogens.) Smoking cigars or pipes also increases the risk of lung cancer. The American Lung Association (ALA) reports that a female smoker older than age 35 is 12 times more likely to die prematurely from lung cancer than a female nonsmoker.

Nearly half of new lung cancer diagnoses are in women, says *Linda Garland, M.D.,* a lung cancer specialist at the Arizona Cancer Center in Tucson. She blames this rise among women on niche marketing by cigarette companies, who advertise smoking as the chic thing to do. "What a destructive message to give women, especially impressionable young women and girls," she says. Despite all we know about the dangers of tobacco, smoking rates are still rising among women, particularly among young ones. Twenty percent of eighth-grade girls and up to 33 percent of female high school seniors smoke.

*Teenage girls smoke to look cool. But female smokers are 12 times more likely to die of lung cancer than female nonsmokers. This is not cool.*

—*Linda Garland, M.D.*

The habit is all the more dangerous because women metabolize carcinogens in tobacco differently than men, which causes greater harm, says Dr. Ross. Even if a woman doesn't smoke, she is at risk for lung cancer from secondhand smoke, radon, air pollution, and occupational exposures, warns Dr. Garland.

Lung cancer is difficult to diagnose because of its usually nonspecific symptoms, such as a persistent cough, or because its symptoms become severe only when the disease is in the advanced stages. In addition, this form of cancer occurs most often in women who already have lung problems, so warning signs can be attributed to other diseases. Dr. Garland reports that about only 15 percent of all lung cancers are diagnosed early enough to be cured. "The problem is that lung cancer can grow unnoticed to a fairly large size," she says. "There isn't a lot of nerve tissue in the lungs, so you don't feel pain in the early stages." But the cancer can spread to other parts of the body. It tends to move into the bones, she explains, where it causes a great deal of pain. Or it can spread into the brain, triggering seizures.

If you have a cough that doesn't clear up, shortness of breath, blood in your sputum, chest pains, or aches and pains in your bones, go to your doctor for a complete physical examination as soon as possible, advises Dr. Ross. Your doctor may test sputum for cancer cells, order chest X-rays, or look inside your airways with a broncoscope. In order to know definitively if and where there is a tumor, your doctor may order other special tests, such as magnetic resonance imaging (MRI), positron emission tomography (PET), or computed tomography (CT) scan, explains Dr. Ross.

Do everything you can to reduce your risk of getting lung cancer. If you do develop it, go with the most advanced treatments. This is what experts advise.

**Toss the cigarettes.** "This can't be repeated enough," says Dr. Garland. Your risk for lung cancer drops dramatically over the first 10 years after you quit smoking. The body has a remarkable ability to repair itself if you stop the exposure, even though a former smoker's risk will never be as low as that of a nonsmoker. And since women are now living longer, even those who quit smoking decades ago sometimes develop lung cancer. Dr. Garland says she recently treated an 82-year-old woman who gave up smoking 40 years ago, yet still got the disease. "Nonetheless, quitting is the right thing to do," she says.

**Test for radon.** The second-leading cause of lung cancer is exposure to radon, an invisible and odorless gas given off naturally by soil and rocks. The U.S. Environmental Protection Agency (EPA) estimates that 1 in 15 American homes has elevated levels of radon. "If you live in an area where radon levels have been high (by EPA standards), then you can get your home tested," says Dr. Garland. Test kits are available at most hardware stores for less than $20. Select a kit with a label that states it meets EPA requirements. The EPA recommends that you take immediate action if your test reveals radon levels of 4 picocuries per liter of air. You can reduce radon levels through a variety of home repairs, including sealing cracks in the foundation, floors, or walls. But the EPA warns that sealing and caulking alone isn't enough. In most cases, to reduce radon, you'll need a subslab depressurization system, which uses pipes and fans to remove radon gas from beneath your home's foundation and vent it above the roof, keeping it from entering the building. Call your state's radon office to find a radon-reduction contractor.

**Get the best care.** If you are diagnosed with lung cancer, seek treatment from specialists who are up on the most recent techniques, advises Dr. Ross. First, get a complete evaluation so that your doctor can determine the cancer's stage. Using this information, your doctor will formulate a treatment plan. There are three standard treatments for cancer: surgery, radiation, and chemotherapy. How and when each is used depends on your situation, says Dr. Ross. Although lung cancer death rates remain high, progress is being made in many areas of care. Stage III lung cancer, which is unlikely to be cured surgically, had about a 5-percent, five-year survival rate until recently, reports Dr. Ross. Now patients who are otherwise healthy can benefit from new lung cancer therapies that combine radiation and chemotherapy, and can result in a long-term survival rate of up to 40 percent.

# 22 Sexuality

chapter

## Facing the Physical Problems of Love

*Many women still suffer sexual problems in silence, too embarrassed to reach out. If only they realized how common these difficulties are.*

For many women, tales of what happens—or doesn't happen—in the bedroom go no further. For them, sex just isn't discussed in detail. Some women won't even talk about sex with their partners, let alone their doctors. They feel alone and confused about their sexual difficulties.

Sadly, these women have plenty of company. In a 1998 survey, psychologists ranked sexual problems fourth among top family challenges. Research shows that about 30 percent of American women consistently lack sexual desire. Even more women report orgasm problems. "Not being able to reach orgasm during intercourse is normal—as many as two-thirds of women can't do that at some point in their lives," says sex therapist *Barbara Bartlik, M.D.,* a psychiatrist at New York-Presbyterian Hospital's Weill Cornell Medical Center in New York City. "To make that the goal is unrealistic for many women." So you're not alone if you lack libido, don't climax, or have pain during intercourse.

But solace isn't found in numbers. You want, need, and deserve solutions. This chapter offers the latest and best advice for overcoming your sexual troubles so that you can have the most fulfilling sex life possible.

## LACKLUSTER SEX: MAKING THE EARTH MOVE AGAIN

When a healthy appetite for sex is gobbled up by the routine of everyday life, you might not even miss it. Maybe your partner doesn't, either. But then you begin to wonder: Is this normal? Is this healthy?

It could be, assuming you and your mate are honestly content with the occasional tryst or even all-out celibacy, says **Barbara Bartlik, M.D.,** sex therapist and psychiatrist at New York-Presbyterian Hospital's Weill Cornell Medical Center in New York City. Problems arise when one person in a relationship craves sex more often than the other. You may think your partner is satisfied with the status quo, but he may not be admitting—or even aware of—bubbling resentment or deep-seated feelings of rejection. Such situations can lead to quarrels, affairs, or divorce.

Physical intimacy plays a powerful role in creating an emotional bond between partners in a relationship. "The inability to fully enjoy sex can make you feel inadequate, anxious, and depressed," says Dr. Bartlik.

Having sex seldom or not at all can also adversely affect your physical health, says **Winnifred B. Cutler, Ph.D.,** a reproductive biologist and founder of the Athena Institute, a biomedical research center in Chester Springs, Pennsylvania. One of her studies revealed that young women who had sex sporadically—such as a hot weekend followed by 10 days of celibacy—had reduced estrogen levels similar to those of older women, thus putting them at risk for osteoporosis and other health problems. However, decreased sexual activity may be a sign of low estrogen levels, rather than the cause.

*Frequent sex is good for your health. A woman's body is designed for steady loving, not for feast or famine.*
—*Winnifred B. Cutler, Ph.D.*

On the other hand, regular weekly sex is known to be associated with a regular menstrual cycle, normal estrogen levels and bone density, and a milder, later menopause. "Our bodies appear to be designed for steady loving, not for feast or famine," says Dr. Cutler.

That need for regular loving is why our bodies excrete chemical substances, called pheromones, to attract the opposite sex. Dr. Cutler, who is the co-discoverer of pheromones in humans, says her research suggests that simply having a man—and his pheromones—around can be a plus for a woman's health. In one study, Dr. Cutler swabbed male pheromones onto the upper lips of women who had abnormal or irregular menstrual cycles. After 14 weeks of treatment, the women's periods became more regular—in fact, within three days of the optimal 29.5-day cycle. "Men's pheromones somehow affect our hormones, especially estrogen," she concludes.

Sex is such an integral part of our lives that the average woman with a healthy libido reportedly has about six sexual thoughts or feelings a day. The average male has more (of course): as many as 11 a day. If these numbers seem high to you, keep in mind that the totals include everything from a daydream to a fleeting tingle triggered by an attractive passerby. If you worry that you'd score below average, relax. Dr. Bartlik points out that we're not always aware of these thoughts or feelings.

Libido is just part of the story. In her book, *Love Cycles: The Science of Intimacy*, Dr. Cutler explains that sexual desire has three components: libido, arousal, and willingness. Libido is that elusive connection between body and brain that leads us to actively seek sex. Willingness and arousal are the more tangible psychological and physical pieces of the puzzle. To figure out where your lack of desire originates, you have to examine all three components.

## PUMP UP YOUR PHEROMONES

*Having a hard time getting the object of your desire to notice you? You may benefit from extra pheromones.*

Pheromones are subtle aromas that humans secrete to attract and communicate sexually with the opposite sex.

"They lure someone to you more powerfully than—or at least as powerfully as—appearance," says biologist **Winnifred B. Cutler, Ph.D.,** who co-discovered pheromones in humans.

Research shows that pheromone production diminishes with age, especially after menopause or a hysterectomy. So Dr. Cutler created a product called Athena Pheromone, an unscented fragrance additive that is a chemical copy of naturally occurring substances. There are separate formulas for women and men.

A few small studies tested the product and concluded that it actually works. J. Clark Bundren, M.D., a gynecologist and reproductive endocrinologist at the University of Oklahoma at Tulsa, studied women who had undergone hysterectomies and had then noticed a drop in their partners' sexual interest in them. Dr. Bunden found that with regular applications of the pheromone substitute, these women reported increased attention from their once-ambivalent mates.

There's no guarantee that Dr. Cutler's faux pheromones will work for you. But if you're interested, you can order the fragrance online at www.athenainstitute.com.

## LOW LIBIDO: ANTIAGING TIPS FOR ADDED DESIRE

Estrogen plays a significant role in female arousal. Since estrogen levels drop as a woman enters menopause, arousal can be impacted. Physiological changes, such as thinning of the vaginal tissues and lack of lubrication, can cause you to feel less amorous and can make intercourse painful, even impossible.

Take these steps to help you get back in the mood.

**Restore moisture.** "If your only symptom is vaginal dryness, try a lubricant," suggests *Jane L. Murray, M.D.,* of the Sastun Center of Integrative Health Care in Mission, Kansas. She recommends Astroglide, available at drugstores.

**Help yourself to herbs.** Black cohosh is nature's alternative to hormone replacement therapy (HRT). For hot flashes and mood swings associated with menopause, Dr. Murray suggests taking 40 milligrams standardized black cohosh twice a day. Another herb that may cool your hot flashes is evening primrose oil. Take one to two 500-milligram capsules two or three times a day as needed. Both black cohosh and evening primrose oil are available at health-food stores. "Experiment to see what works best for you," says Dr. Murray. Always consult your doctor before trying any herbal treatment.

**Consider hormone therapy.** HRT is a combination of estrogen and progestin (a form of progesterone) that restores vaginal tissue and enables your body to lubricate naturally. For women who have had hysterectomies, estrogen replacement therapy (ERT) alone can restore normal moisture.

**Try a cream.** If you're not interested in HRT, you can get lower doses of estrogen from a vaginally applied cream, such as Estriol. Because a prescription cream improves tissue health with less effect on blood levels of estrogen, this method probably carries less risk for breast cancer.

**Go "natural."** Some women experience better results with so-called natural hormones than with HRT, says Dr. Murray. Don't be fooled: Natural progesterone and estrogen are still man-made prescription drugs. But unlike synthetic hormones produced by pharmaceutical companies, these natural hormones have the same chemical structure as those produced by your body. And they are custom-made for your individual needs by specially trained compounding pharmacists. These medications should deliver a more natural balance of the three types of estrogen: estradiol, estrone, and estriol. The downside is that natural hormones are not approved by the U.S. Food and Drug Administration, and there has been little scientific research on their benefits and risks. Check with your doctor for more information.

## TESTOSTERONE: THE TURN-ON TRIGGER

A woman's real hormone of desire is the one you probably would never guess: testosterone. Many women don't realize they produce this so-called male hormone. "Without testosterone, you'd have no capacity to get turned on," says *Susan Rako, M.D.*, a Boston-based psychiatrist and author of *The Hormone of Desire: The Truth About Testosterone, Sexuality, and Menopause*. Dr. Rako is among the many doctors who consider testosterone to be the foundation of female sexuality. Testosterone receptors in your nipples, clitoris, and vagina make these areas particularly sensitive to sexual stimulation, she says.

Testosterone levels usually peak in your early 20s, then begin to decline. By menopause, your testosterone production is about half what it once was. The resulting deficiency can lead to a loss of sexual desire, says Dr. Rako.

*Supplemental testosterone may help revive your interest in sex. And don't worry: It won't make you look or sound like a man.—Susan Rako, M.D.*

Yet the medical community has been slow to prescribe replacement therapy for women who are testosterone deficient. This is probably due to the mistaken belief that raising testosterone levels will increase body and facial hair, deepen the voice, cause acne, and enlarge the clitoris. "As long as women

## AM I TESTOSTERONE DEFICIENT?

*We hear a lot about a woman's need for estrogen. But a healthy female body also requires testosterone.*

While estrogen may prevent genital atrophy, testosterone prevents "libido atrophy," says *Susan Rako, M.D.*, author of *The Hormone of Desire: The Truth About Testosterone, Sexuality, and Menopause*. A lack of testosterone can lead to flatness of mood or loss of mental sharpness. Talk to your doctor about testosterone therapy if you experience some or all of these problems:

* Loss of sexual desire
* Difficulty reaching orgasm

* Loss of sensation in the clitoris and nipples
* Thinning and loss of pubic hair
* Loss of vitality and diminished sense of well-being
* Reduction in muscle tone
* Dulling and brittleness of scalp hair
* Dry skin
* Thinning and dryness in the vaginal wall, especially if hormone replacement therapy has failed to help (For more on this condition, see page 246.)

take dosages of testosterone within the appropriate low range, there is no danger of side effects," assures Dr. Rako. She emphasizes that use of a testosterone supplement should always be closely supervised to avoid overdosing.

Supplemental testosterone is marketed in various forms, including one coupled with estrogen called Estratest. But these products contain far more testosterone than most women need, says Dr. Rako. She recommends lower doses, available only through compounding pharmacies. The suggested starting dose for an oral supplement is 0.4 milligrams methyltestosterone. If you don't notice any change after a couple of weeks, talk to your doctor about increasing the dose. But if you feel agitated, have trouble sleeping, or are ravenously hungry, you may be taking too much and should reduce the dose.

If you prefer to use a topical product, Dr. Rako recommends a cream called testosterone propionate for use on the skin or genitals, provided you take care not to use too much. And she stresses that no woman who has any chance of getting pregnant should ever take supplemental testosterone because it can be risky to the developing fetus.

## AROUSAL: BREAKING DOWN THE BARRIERS

Not every woman who reaches menopause notices a dip in desire. Likewise, plenty of young, fertile women with healthy hormone levels have no interest in sex. Inhibited sexual desire—the clinical term for low libido—is a complex problem, with both physical and psychological causes.

Certain medications, for example, can dull the senses and inhibit desire, says Dr. Bartlik. Particularly notorious are the antidepressants Paxil (paroxetine) and Prozac (fluoxetine). Ironically, these drugs are designed to treat depression, a condition that is also a major contributor to loss of sexual interest. They work by impacting serotonin levels but frequently also end up dampening sexual desire.

If an antidepressant is extinguishing your sex drive, ask your doctor about switching to a different medication. Wellbutrin (bupropion) is an antidepressant that appears to improve sexual appetite by increasing levels of dopamine, a neurotransmitter linked to libido. A study in the *Journal of Sex and Marital Therapy* found that Wellbutrin enhanced desire in women who were not depressed and had no clear reason for their lack of sexual interest.

Psychological causes of low libido include marital problems, trauma from rape or incest, and religious, familial, or cultural inhibitions. Guilt, shame, anxiety, and poor self-esteem can also inhibit sexual desire or arousal, says Dr. Bartlik.

*If you're too busy for sex, maybe you need to let the housework slide. Spend that time making love instead.*
—Jane DiVita Woody, Ph.D.

To recharge your interest in sex, here's where to look for help.

**Talk to your doctor.** To determine the cause of your dysfunction, your physician should ask many questions about your sexual experiences, past and present: How long has this been going on? Is your disinterest chronic? Or does it come and go? Have you had this problem with other partners? What do *you* think the cause might be?

Talking about the problem with an objective listener may bring out intuitive hunches as to the source of the problem. The doctor should perform a physical examination to rule out sexually transmitted diseases, as well as check for vaginal dryness, thinning of the vaginal walls, loss of skin resilience, or episiotomy scarring. All of these could result in painful intercourse or signal a hormonal change that could lessen desire. She may also order tests to gauge blood hormone levels or look for signs of diabetes or cardiovascular disease. Arousal depends upon blood flow to the genitals, so hardening of the arteries can impede circulation to the sex organs. It's important to find a health-care provider with whom you can speak comfortably and frankly. Your primary-care physician is a good choice if you trust that he or she is skilled enough to fully explore all possibilities. Or you might be better off seeing a gynecologist or urologist. There are also psychiatrists and other doctors who specialize in sexual problems. Ask your primary doctor for a referral.

**Work with a therapist.** Many sex therapists believe disorders are rooted in learned patterns and values. For example, some women are uncomfortable acknowledging their sexual excitement. They may cling to old-fashioned views that a sexual woman is a bad mother or that nice girls don't like sex. A therapist can help retrain thinking that prevents sexual pleasure, says *Jane DiVita Woody, Ph.D.,*

*Are your inhibitions keeping you from enjoying physical intimacy? Working with a therapist may help you discover the joys of sex, says Jane DiVita Woody, Ph.D.*

licensed marriage therapist, professor of social work at the University of Nebraska at Omaha, and author of *Treating Sexual Distress*. Look for a counselor or therapist certified by the American Association of Sex Educators, Counselors, and Therapists at www.aasect.org.

**Change your priorities.** A lack of time for sex is one of the most common problems cited in couples therapy. The solution? Shift your priorities. You have to make time for sex, says Dr. Woody. Every day, list every single thing you need to do, including showering and preparing meals. If you find you're trying to squeeze too much into each day, let something slide. Maybe you can slack off on the housework or skip a TV program. Let dinner cook in a slow-cooker (such as a Crock-Pot) while you're at work. Identify time-stealers, such as lengthy telephone calls, poor planning, or saying yes to too many people. Taking control of your daily life will help you regain peace and balance. Then you can relax and get in the mood for lovemaking again.

**Return to romance.** Set the stage to rediscover intimacy with your partner. Plan a romantic weekend getaway. At home, create a seductive mood with flowers, candles, oils, and music.

**Let your mind wander.** Several times a day, take a few minutes to think erotic thoughts. Share your fantasies with your partner to intensify intimacy.

**Be adventurous.** Spice up your lovemaking with sex toys or such foods as whipped cream, honey, or chocolate sauce. Always tell your partner if you are uncomfortable with anything he or she is doing.

> *A couple of sexy telephone chats with your mate during the day can have you rarin' to go by evening.*
> —*Barbara Bartlik, M.D.*

**Express yourself.** About twice a day, have a conversation with your partner about something sexual or titillating. You can communicate in person, via e-mail, or on the telephone. Talk doesn't always have to lead to action, but if these sexy chats keep you aroused throughout the day, you're more apt to be in the mood when you and your partner get together, notes Dr. Bartlik.

**Be willing.** A lot of women say they don't think about sex often, but enjoy it when it happens. So even if you're not especially in the mood, take the lead and keep a neutral, open mind. See if this puts you in a receptive frame of mind, advises Dr. Bartlik. If your partner initiates sex, let yourself go with it. It usually doesn't take more than a few minutes before your body kicks in and you are interested. You may rise to the occasion and surprise yourself.

## ORGASM: THE DELIGHT YOU DESERVE

For some women, the problem isn't a matter of not wanting sex, but rather the problem is getting the pleasure they deserve from sex. They just can't climax, or reach orgasm.

The medical definition of the female orgasm sounds anything but exciting: an involuntary muscular contraction that happens in response to rhythmic pressure on the nerves of the clitoris, vagina, or cervix. But any woman who has experienced orgasm can attest to the incredibly powerful reality.

Most women are orgasmic when sufficiently aroused, says *Barbara Bartlik, M.D.,* sex therapist and psychiatrist at New York-Presbyterian Hospital's Weill Cornell Medical Center in New York City. Common reasons women don't reach climax include poor lubrication, a vagina that doesn't swell, and a lack of tightening in the necessary vaginal muscles. If these conditions needed for orgasm don't come together, a woman simply can't achieve "the big O," even if she's feeling erotic.

This can leave you extremely frustrated, especially if there's emotional pressure from your partner. But worrying about whether you'll be able to reach orgasm only creates anxiety, which can cause blood vessels to constrict and actually diminish arousal. Focus instead on sensuality. Let your partner's touch and kisses enhance your awareness of your lips, eyelids, back, butt, ears, feet, and inner thighs. Fantasize about the most arousing thoughts you can imagine, whether or not they involve your partner. Surprisingly, most people in long-term relationships think about someone other than their partner at moments of high arousal. Play these fantasies in your mind's eye as though they were X-rated movies. If you lose your momentum, just rewind your mental video and start again from a higher level of arousal, says Dr. Bartlik.

If you're still searching for the elusive G-spot, forget about it. Most experts agree that this orgasm button doesn't really exist. Terence Hines,

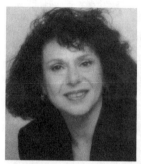

Aline Zoldbrod, Ph.D., offers this recipe for great sex: Relax, be comfortable, and experience pleasure. And don't worry about whether you reach orgasm.

author of *The G-Spot: A Modern Gynecologic Myth,* calls it "a sort of gynecological UFO: much searched for, much discussed, but unverifiable by objective means."

"Orgasm actually isn't necessary for sex to be intensely erotic or significant—neither is intercourse," says **Aline Zoldbrod, Ph.D.,** a Lexington, Massachusetts, psychologist and certified sex therapist, and author of *SexSmart: How Your Childhood Shaped Your Sexual Life and What to Do About It.* Sexuality includes anything that arouses: a gaze, dream, conversation, or thought, as well as flirting, dancing, and hugging.

Perhaps the best approach to having terrific sex is to learn to let go. Dr. Zoldbrod says being comfortable enough to enter a so-called sexual trance is a requirement for deep pleasure with a partner. For many women, that's easier said than done.

"Our childhood family patterns shape us sexually as adults," she says. "How we were touched, disciplined, and socialized determine how healthy our sex lives become." You must experience certain milestones of development to achieve sexual confidence: being loved and touched, receiving empathy, learning to trust and be soothed by the person you trust, and developing a good body image. Figuring out which of your needs weren't met while growing up can help you pinpoint the roots of your intimacy issues and bring you closer to a solution.

But the inability to orgasm isn't always psychological. Inhibited sexual desire—caused by a testosterone deficiency, depression, hormone imbalance, medical problem, or medications—can also make reaching orgasm difficult. Have a complete examination to rule out physical problems. Often, something can be done medically to improve the situation.

If you're not getting the gratification you deserve from sex, ask yourself some questions: Is this a recent problem? If so, what has changed? Have I started a new medication? Am I getting the stimulation I need? Explore all the possibilities.

These suggestions can help you find a new path to pleasure.

**Break down barriers.** For some women, the lack of sexual desire stems from a conservative or religious upbringing. They usually need a therapist who can help them break down these barriers and adopt a positive attitude toward sex. With "homework" assignments and encouragement from the therapist, you can learn to approach sex as something that isn't bad or naughty, says Dr. Bartlik.

**Watch erotica.** For many women, the typical men's pornography is a turnoff. But erotic movies that are written, directed, and filmed by women have a pace and content that is often more appealing, depicting how people really make love in private. Dr. Bartlik suggests Candida Royalle's *Femme* series, available at www.adameve.com.

**Exercise vigorously.** Twenty minutes of aerobic exercise releases endorphins, the feel-good brain chemicals that help get you in the mood for sex. Exercise also increases blood flow to the pelvic area and genitals, improving sensation, lubrication, and intensity of orgasm. In fact, some women report having orgasms while exercising. Now *there's* a good reason to get moving.

## Exercises that strengthen your vaginal muscles can heighten arousal for both you and your partner.

**Just do it.** Regular sex fosters better blood flow, which keeps your arteries and genital tissue in good shape. It also reduces stress, improves self-esteem, boosts your hormones, and lifts your mood. Plus, practice makes perfect: The more you do it, the better the odds are that you'll find the position or stimulation that's right for you.

**Tighten up.** You can intensify orgasm by strengthening your pelvic-floor muscles with Kegel exercises. Developed by Arnold Kegel, M.D., as an alternative to surgery to correct urinary incontinence, these exercises are now often used in sex therapy. Strong pelvic-floor muscles allow you to grasp the penis better, heightening arousal for both you and your partner. To tighten these muscles, practice stopping your urine in midstream. Those muscles you feel tightening inside are the ones you need to strengthen. To perform Kegel exercises, contract your vagina and hold for two to three seconds; repeat 10 times. Repeat sets of 10 at least five times a day. As these muscles get stronger, hold each squeeze 8 to 10 seconds.

**Please yourself.** There's no better way than masturbation to figure out what stimulates you. Explore your own body so you can later guide your partner.

# PAINFUL SEX: REGAINING PAIN-FREE PLEASURE

Sex is supposed to be a wonderful expression of adult intimacy, full of joy and pleasure. But, for some women, sex hurts.

Dyspareunia, the medical term for painful intercourse, is a serious problem that affects up to 30 percent of adult women, says *Deborah Metzger, M.D., Ph.D.,* associate clinical professor in the department of obstetrics and gynecology at Stanford University School of Medicine and medical director at Helena Women's Health in San Jose, California. For many of them, the pain, which can be deep inside the vagina or outside, may occur occasionally or may happen each time a woman attempts intercourse. It might feel like a sharp, shooting pain, or burning sensation, or like your partner is hitting against something very tender. It may occur during intercourse or for hours after, ache dully, or be so severe that it is impossible to have intercourse.

But 85 percent of women who experience painful intercourse can be cured once the cause is discovered, says Dr. Metzger. The challenge is to pinpoint the source of the pain.

## ALLERGIES: WHEN YOUR IMMUNE SYSTEM AFFECTS YOUR SEX LIFE

Pain associated with intercourse can be a symptom of an imbalance within the body, caused by nutrition, bowel health, stress, or antibiotics, says Dr. Metzger. One of the most common causes of pain during sex, she says, is something many women and doctors don't think to check: allergies. An allergy to yeast, certain foods, environmental factors, or even your own hormones can result in inflammation throughout the body. Painful inflammation can affect the tiny glands around the urethra (the canal that carries urine from the bladder to the outside of the body) and glands outside the hymen ring (the skin that partially closes the vaginal opening).

Therefore, Dr. Metzger examines a woman's immune system before she designs a treatment plan for pelvic pain. She assesses levels of stress, hormones, nutrition, bowel health, fatigue, and depression, and looks for symptoms of food allergies. "If you treat the whole body, you can get relief," she says.

Dr. Metzger tells patients to try these remedies for allergies and subsequent relief of painful intercourse.

**Cut the sugar.** In a 1993 study conducted at St. Jude Children's Research Hospital in Memphis, mice with weakened immune systems who were fed sugar had 200 times more yeast in their gastrointestinal tract than mice with similar immune systems who ate no sugar. Yeast, which thrives on sugar, is a common allergy in women. Eat less sugar to prevent or clear up a profusion of yeast in the bowels. Dr. Metzger suggests the Sugar Busters! diet as a model.

**Feed on friendly bacteria.** *Lactobacillus acidophilus* helps maintain the vaginal ecosystem, preventing the overproduction of yeast and unfriendly bacteria. The lactic acid it produces acts like a natural antibiotic and competes with other organisms to utilize sugar. Follow manufacturer's directions on the packaging when you buy *L. acidophilus* as tablets, capsules, or suppositories in a health-food store.

> *Cut sugar from your diet to reduce the yeast in your body, which may contribute to pelvic pain.*
> —*Deborah Metzger, M.D., Ph.D*

**Swallow herbal relief.** Caprylic acid, garlic, grapeseed extract, oregano, and uva ursi all help decrease yeast overgrowth by boosting intestinal health, aiding in sugar metabolism, or strengthening the immune system. Look for each in pill form as supplements at health-food stores. Dr. Metzger suggests that you choose any two—say, uva ursi and grapeseed extract or garlic and oregano—and take the supplements for one to three months. Follow dosage recommendations on the supplement labels. (You can't get the dosage you need from using the herbs in cooking.)

If you have a lot of yeast in your bowel when you start taking the supplements, you could experience symptoms of die-off, says Dr. Metzger. This is an allergic reaction to the toxins released by the yeast that are being killed by the potent herbal products. A die-off reaction is actually good news, because it indicates that the supplements are having the desired effect, says Dr. Metzger. The aching, bloating, and nausea you may experience is usually brief. But if the side effects are severe, stop taking the supplements for two or three days, advises Dr. Metzger, then restart them at a lower dose. Over two to four weeks, you can gradually increase how much you take until you reach the recommended dose.

**Terminate your triggers.** An elimination diet can identify hidden food allergies that may be causing anything from fatigue and sore throats to migraines, abdominal pain, anxiety, or painful intercourse. To follow such a diet, you must completely avoid such common allergens as dairy products, eggs, wheat, corn, and refined sugars for two weeks, while sticking strictly to fruits, vegetables, whole grains, chicken, turkey, fish, and lean meats. Then reintroduce the suspect foods, one at a time, to see if you have a reaction. An allergic reaction can occur immediately after you eat the offending food, but it is more likely to take 12 to 72 hours. An allergist can help you follow an elimination diet correctly and avoid any dangerous allergic reactions.

**Consider an antifungal.** If all else fails, your doctor can prescribe a pill to help get rid of a yeast infection. Nizoral (ketoconazole) and Sporanox (itraconazole) are brands that can have potentially dangerous side effects, says *Alice Chang, M.D.,* an instructor at Harvard Medical School. She says the safest brand is Diflucan (fluconazole). But some types of yeast are resistant to Diflucan, says Dr. Metzger. Your health-care provider can order lab tests to determine which antifungal medication will be most effective for the type of yeast you have, she says. Nystatin is commonly prescribed because it is not absorbed in the body; rather, it stays in the gut and kills the yeast on contact.

## OTHER CAUSES OF PAINFUL SEX: WHAT YOU CAN DO

Painful sex isn't always related to the immune system or allergies. Discomfort can also be caused by vaginal infections or irritations, scar tissue, a hernia, nerve damage, spasms of the pelvic floor muscles, varicose veins on the ovaries, or endometriosis. When any of these conditions is severe, surgery may be required to alleviate the pain.

If sex is a physical torment, heed this advice.

**Don't suffer in silence.** "Many times, women don't deal with a sexual problem. They assume it'll just go away," says *Jane DiVita Woody, Ph.D.,* licensed marriage therapist and author of *Treating Sexual Distress.* Don't continue to have sex if it's uncomfortable in any way. Take immediate steps to figure out the cause of the problem. Otherwise, your next intimate experience may be even worse. When you anticipate pain, your anxiety increases, your body tenses, and your discomfort is magnified. "The body has a memory," says Dr. Woody. Pain can lead you to stop desiring sex altogether.

**Keep a sex diary.** Document when and where it hurts, as well as how you feel toward your partner when sex is painful. By writing down these feelings, you can identify patterns that may help you or your doctor diagnose the source. Ask yourself these questions: Have I felt this way all along? What's different? Have I had pleasurable sex with my partner before? Do I wish to avoid sex but do it anyway? Is there some underlying resentment or anger? Have I recently been depressed, anxious, or sick?

If your mind is somehow preventing you from becoming aroused, your body may not be lubricating itself properly. This could be the reason intercourse is uncomfortable, explains Dr. Woody. If you think the cause might be emotional or psychological, find a certified sex therapist to help you work through the problem.

> *Tell your lover about the pain you feel during sex and make sure he knows it's not his fault.*
>
> *—Jane DiVita Woody, Ph.D.*

**Get a physical exam.** If you've recently begun experiencing pain, you might have a vaginal infection or sexually transmitted disease, such as genital warts or herpes, says Dr. Metzger. Get tested to rule out these concerns.

**Share it with your partner.** As difficult as the discussion may be, you must have an honest conversation with your partner so he understands how you feel. Talking will help keep him from feeling rejected and you from feeling obliged to have intercourse. Be sure he knows you're not pointing an accusing finger. Rather than saying, "You hurt me when, . . . " it's better to explain, "I hurt when. . . ." Don't bring up the subject during sex, though, recommends Dr. Woody. It's hard to have a rational conversation in that context.

**Try lubricants.** Lack of moisture can be attributed to menopause, dehydrating medications, or insufficient arousal. And when you're dry, intercourse can be agony, particularly at the entrance of the vagina, says Dr. Woody. Your best bet is to get your body to promote its own lubrication, recommends *Winnifred B. Cutler, Ph.D.,* a reproductive biologist and founder of the Athena Institute, a biomedical research center in Chester Springs, Pennsylvania. The solution may be as simple as slowing down and spending more time on foreplay. But if you really need help, a lubricant can reduce abrasiveness. Try such products as Astroglide or ID Personal Lubricant. *Barbara Bartlik, M.D.,* a sex therapist and psychiatrist at New York-Presbyterian Hospital's Weill Cornell Medical Center in New York City, recommends K-Y liquid, rather than the traditional gel.

## SEXUALLY TRANSMITTED DISEASES: UNINVITE THEM

Sexually transmitted diseases (STDs) are more common than most women realize. In the United States, 5 of the top 10 reported infections are STDs, with approximately 15 million new cases diagnosed a year. In some age groups, up to one in every four women has genital herpes. Yet a 1998 survey by the Kaiser Family Foundation found that almost 70 percent of women think the number of people infected with STDs is 1 in 10 or fewer. Lack of information was reported to be even higher among teens.

That same survey showed that two-thirds of single women and men don't always use a condom during sex. This false sense of security may be one of the reasons why the United States has the highest rate of STDs of any industrialized nation.

STDs don't discriminate: They affect women and men of all backgrounds and economic levels. However, there is still a social stigma attached to the subject that stifles frank discussion of this widespread problem.

A woman's body is particularly vulnerable to STDs, says *Jeanne Marrazzo, M.D.*, medical director of the Seattle STD/HIV Prevention and Training Center, and an assistant professor of medicine at the University of Washington at Seattle. The warm, moist membranes of the vagina and urethra provide an ideal environment for infectious organisms. As vaginal walls thin and become dryer with age, a woman may get tiny abrasions in the vagina during sex, which provide easy access for infection. A sexually active female teen is at even more risk, since her cervix is more susceptible to some infections. Two-thirds of new cases of STDs occur in people under age 25.

A man often knows right away that he is infected with an STD. Sores on his penis or a visible discharge broadcast the message loud and clear. But a woman's early symptoms are usually far more subtle, perhaps even undetectable. This may be why the effects of STDs are typically more severe in women because they don't know to seek treatment until serious problems develop. Dr. Marrazzo warns that the long-term consequences of an untreated STD can include infertility, a tubal pregnancy, and cervical cancer. Even when an infected woman has no symptoms, it is possible to pass the disease on to an unprotected sexual partner or, with some STDs, to a newborn baby.

There are two types of STDs: bacterial and viral. Between the two types, there are more than 20 identified conditions. Bacterial STDs, such as chlamydia, trichomoniasis, gonorrhea, and syphilis, can be successfully cured with medication. Viral STDs are incurable. You can use medicine to treat the symptoms of most viral STDs, including genital herpes, human papillomavirus (HPV), hepatitis B, and human immunodeficiency virus (HIV). Once your body is infected, though, these viruses remain there, and symptoms can recur throughout your life.

## PROTECTING YOURSELF FROM STDs

The best way to prevent getting an STD is to practice safe sex. It's also a good idea to insist that you and a partner get tested for STDs before you have sex with each other. For more information about STDs, visit the Centers for Disease Control and Prevention Web site at www.cdc.gov/health/std.htm.

Play it safe with these defensive maneuvers.

**Always use a condom.** Condoms are effective against STDs, but only if you use them consistently. If your partner is reluctant to wear a condom, consider using the female condom, Reality, available at drugstores or online at www.femalehealth.com.

Dr. Marrazzo says condoms protect women against herpes, but only up to a point. Lesions can pop up in any area of the groin not covered by a condom. Abstain from sex when you or your partner feels the early warning signs of an impending herpes outbreak or if the virus is active and lesions are visible. (See the box at right.)

There is a long list of excuses for not using a condom. Perhaps there isn't one on hand at the crucial moment. Or you may think that your lover is too young, too old, or too nice to be HIV-positive. Don't let naive assumptions lead you to infection.

**Get tested.** You cannot assume that your annual pelvic exam will include tests for any and every STD. Most health-care providers screen for chlamydia and gonorrhea during a routine pelvic exam. All pregnant women are screened for syphilis. If you think you might have been exposed to any STD, you need to ask your doctor for that specific test—it's the only way to know for sure that you'll be screened, advises Dr. Marrazzo.

### CAN YOU SPOT A POTENTIAL PARTNER'S STD?

*Sexually transmitted diseases spread quickly because they are so difficult to recognize.*

These are some signs you should look for when getting involved with a new partner:

* Swollen lymph nodes near the groin, especially after a recent bout of flulike symptoms that can include fever and chills
* Rashes, sores, bumps, or blisters near the mouth or genitals
* Foul-smelling discharge from the genitals

# During oral sex, use a condom or or dental dam to protect yourself from STDS.—*Jeanne Marrazzo, M.D.*

**Accept no substitutes.** Don't use Vaseline, baby oil, Crisco, or other oil-based lubricants. They can break down the latex in condoms, rendering them less effective. For safer sex, stick with true sexual lubricants, such as Astroglide or K-Y Liquid, says Dr. Marrazzo.

**Keep your mouth clean.** If you engage in oral sex, avoid getting semen in your mouth. Ask your partner to wear a condom or withdraw before ejaculation. When oral sex is performed on a woman, a dental dam helps protect against STDs. You can purchase dental dams online at www.condomania.com. Or you can use a piece of food-grade plastic wrap, says Dr. Marrazzo.

**Trust in vaccines.** Hepatitis B virus (HBV) infects about 200,000 Americans every year, despite the availability of a preventive vaccine. In 1991, the Immunization Action Coalition recommended that all infants be vaccinated against hepatitis B. Those at high risk for hepatitis B include anyone exposed to the blood of potential carriers. The National Center for Infectious Diseases at the Centers for Disease Control and Prevention suggests asking your doctor about getting a vaccination if you fall into any of these high-risk categories.

- People who have sex with an HBV-infected partner
- People who live in the same household with someone who has a lifelong HBV infection
- People who have multiple sexual partners
- Men who are homosexual
- People who use intravenous drugs
- Health-care workers who may come into contact with human blood
- People who get tattoos or piercings
- People who travel to developing countries in the Amazon Basin of South America, Southeast Asia, Africa, the Middle East, or the Pacific Islands, as well as people whose parents were born in those areas
- People who have hemophilia

There may soon also be a vaccine for genital herpes. Researchers are testing Simplirix, a new vaccine that appears to help protect women from the infection. The catch is that Simplirix doesn't work in men, and it only works in women who have never been infected with the type of herpes virus that causes cold sores.

## LIFE AFTER INFECTION

If you or your partner already has an STD, follow this advice to stay as healthy as possible.

**Be honest.** Tell any new partner about your STD before you become sexually intimate. If you keep it a secret and transmission does occur, any trust built up in the relationship will be destroyed, warns Dr. Marrazzo. Easier said than done, though. It can be especially difficult to discuss an STD with a new partner. Dr. Marrazzo offers these tips for handling such a conversation.

- Talk in a quiet one-on-one setting at a time when both of you are sober and in a relatively good mood. Always have the discussion before having any type of sex. It's much harder to bring up the issue after the deed is done.
- Read up on your particular STD so you can answer your partner's questions with confidence.
- Suggest that your partner talk to a doctor or other health-care provider. Offer him or her this book or other educational materials about STDs.
- Expect your partner to react strongly when first learning of your STD. You may face shock, denial, anger, revulsion, or pity. Try to be patient.
- Don't blame yourself if a potential lover loses interest after hearing about your STD. If a partner decides to opt out, there probably wasn't much to the relationship in the first place. And don't let the fear of receiving a negative response prevent you from telling future partners.

**Be careful.** If your partner has an STD, take precautions to protect yourself.

**Be assertive.** Insist on the use of a condom any time there is genital contact. Even if no symptoms or visible signs of infection are present, you are still at risk. Abstain from intercourse when you or your partner has any visible ulcers, warts, or discharge.

**Be aware.** Watch for these symptoms of STD infections in women.

- Bleeding not related to menstruation
- Genital ulcers or sore lymph nodes in the groin
- Pelvic pain during intercourse
- Abdominal pain accompanied with fever
- Abnormal vaginal discharge
- Vaginal burning, itching, and odor

If you notice any of these problems, see a doctor as soon as possible, advises Dr. Marrazzo.

# 23 Skin

● ● ● ● ● ● ● ● ● ● ● ● ● ● ● ● ● ● ● ● ● ● ● ● ● ● ● ● ● ● ● ● ● ● ● ● ● ● ●

chapter

## Restoring Your Natural Shine

*Your skin covers every inch of your body, accounting for about 16 percent of your total weight.*

If you ever tried to count the myriad of skincare products available, you might conclude that American women are obsessed with their skin. It seems every woman's skin is too dry, too oily, too wrinkled, or too susceptible to breakouts or rashes. So women overscrub, overpick, overtan, or just plain overload their skin with pore-clogging cosmetics and creams. If you're not careful, the result can be a vicious cycle of dermatological problems.

Your skin—all 21 square feet of it—protects your insides from the outside world. It prevents water loss, guards against wounds and harmful rays, produces essential vitamin D when exposed to sunlight, and regulates body temperature through the sweat glands. It is also your first line of defense against infection.

So there are many important reasons to keep your skin healthy. And the best prescription for an exceptional epidermis is prevention. In this chapter, our female experts guide you to the potions and actions that can help you avoid or—overcome—common skin problems.

### ACNE: OUTBREAKS AT ANY STAGE OF LIFE

Think your skin isn't acting its age? Well, unfortunately, you don't always outgrow the tendency toward blemishes. You can get a pimple on your 88th birthday, says *Kathy Fields, M.D.,* clinical instructor of dermatology at the University of California at San Francisco.

Granted, most females deal with acne's onslaught in high school, a wacky time of wacky hormones. But acne's two primary contributing factors—heredity and hormones—don't disappear with a diploma. The main culprit is androgen, a male hormone that stimulates oil production. Androgen surges usually level off in your 20s, but you can continue to experience them even decades later. And at certain times in your life—or times of the month—you produce a stickier type of oil that doesn't exit your pores easily, says Dr. Fields.

*If you think sunlight is good for your skin, think again. Exposure actually makes acne worse.*—Lisa Donofrio, M.D.

Don't buy into the myth that sunshine is good for your complexion. Extensive sun exposure actually worsens acne by making pores more likely to become clogged with oil and dead skin cells, says *Lisa Donofrio, M.D.,* assistant clinical professor of dermatology at Yale University School of Medicine in New Haven, Connecticut. Stress also plays a role in some acne cases.

### PREVENTING AND TREATING PIMPLES

There's no cure for acne, but the condition can be tamed. Some women opt to strike at the hormonal source by taking birth control pills that manage their hormone levels, notes Dr. Fields.

In 1997, the U.S. Food and Drug Administration approved the oral contraceptive Ortho Tri-Cyclen for the treatment of acne, after successful study results. (Some other brands of birth control pills have the same effect.) No one is suggesting that you go on birth control just to clear up your complexion. But if you're already taking another oral contraceptive, talk to your doctor about the benefits of switching to Ortho Tri-Cyclen, suggests Dr. Donofrio. But following a good skin-care regimen is still your best defense against breakouts.

A pimple erupts when oil stuck in a pore provides a breeding ground for bacteria, which feed off the oil. Avoid such an infection with this three-part strategy: Unclog pores, reduce oil, and kill bacteria. Follow these steps faithfully each day. "Skin care is like brushing your teeth," advises Dr. Fields. "You don't wait until you see a cavity to begin preventive measures."

**SHED EVERYTHING** Exfoliation is the sloughing off of the skin's uppermost layer, which is comprised mostly of dead cells. This practice opens up pores to allow oil to pass through easily and minimizes the appearance of pores by unclogging the debris that stretches them, says Dr. Fields. Exfoliating removes the accumulation of old cells and waxy oils that look like dirt in your pores, which is the characteristic of blackheads.

There are two ways to exfoliate: physically (with a scrub) or chemically (with an acid-based product). Then you have to decide if and how you should moisturize. To get the best results, follow this expert advice.

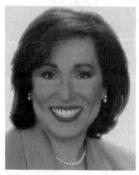

Moisturizing is a no-no if you have oily skin, warns cosmetics maven Paula Begoun. It can make you look greasy and contributes to breakouts of acne. Only women with dry skin really need to moisturize.

**Go easy with exfoliants.** Scrubs containing rough ingredients, such as large apricot kernels, can damage your skin. To protect your face, choose a product with small particles, such as Decléor's Micro-Exfoliating Face Gel, recommends Dr. Fields—and be sure to rub gently.

**Buff with baking soda.** This kitchen staple makes a mild exfoliate, according to *Paula Begoun,* author of *Don't Go to the Cosmetics Counter Without Me.* In the palm of your hand, mix a little baking soda with just enough water to make a paste. Use your fingertips to apply in a circular motion for about 30 seconds, then rinse. Caution: Don't try this self-help remedy if you're using a retinoid-containing product, such as Retin-A (tretinoin), since baking soda will negate the medication's effectiveness.

**Avoid pore strips.** Dr. Donofrio discourages the use of so-called pore-cleansing strips that you wet, apply to your face, and pull off when dry. These products can injure or tear skin, as well as cause those annoying thin red spider veins to surface. Their ingredients also irritate the skin over time, causing more breakouts.

**Clean up with acid.** Apply a thin layer of a 2-percent salicylic acid product, such as Clean & Clear's Invisible Blemish Treatment. Dr. Fields says the acid penetrates your skin to unclog pores. You can apply makeup over it without rinsing.

**Get a prescription.** Retin-A is not only excellent at fighting wrinkles, but also prevents pores from being clogged with oil. "It treats adult acne more effectively than any over-the-counter medication," says Dr. Donofrio.

> *Mix baking soda with a little water to make an excellent exfoliating agent.*
> —*Paula Begoun*

**Rethink moisturizer.** If you have oily skin, stop moisturizing. "It's a myth that everyone needs moisturizer," says Begoun. The oil on your skin is already doing the job of locking in moisture. Add more and you'll just look greasy—plus, you'll be more likely to suffer a breakout. Even oil-free moisturizers can make skin look shiny and clog pores. It's even possible that

## POPPING THE PIMPLE MYTHS

*Conventional wisdom is sometimes anything but wise. What do you really know about acne?*

**Myth:** Makeup causes acne.
**Truth:** Adult acne is primarily caused by hormones, heredity, and stress. However, heavy makeup *can* aggravate or contribute to an existing problem. For example, pressed powder usually contains mineral oil, which could definitely clog pores if used in conjunction with a heavy moisturizer or an oily foundation, or both. Play it safe and stick with oil-free, water-based foundations that are noncomedogenic—meaning they don't clog pores—and choose loose powder over pressed. Select a concealer with salicylic acid.

**Myth:** A poor diet can cause acne.
**Truth:** Although some people still insist that chocolate and caffeine upset their skin, no scientific data exists to validate such a link. It takes about two weeks for a pimple to rear its ugly head, so you can't blame last night's French fries for this morning's zit. Even a nutritionist's dream diet won't protect you from breakouts.

overmoisturizing can prevent your skin from repairing itself. Begoun is a 20-year cosmetics veteran who believes that moisturizers are the most misunderstood and abused skin products around. Only women with dry skin need to moisturize, she says. If you have normal to slightly dry skin, look for lotions labeled lightweight. Or try serums, which are water-based gels that soak into the skin quickly without leaving much moisture behind.

Here are some other tips for clearing away excess oil.

- Clay masks: Clay deep-cleans by drawing out impurities. It also slightly dries oily skin to prevent breakouts. Spread the product on

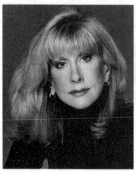

Each week use a clay mask to dry oily skin just enough to prevent breakouts, recommends beauty author Diane Irons.

your face and let it dry for about 15 minutes, then follow manufacturer's directions for removal. Use a mask just once a week to avoid overdrying your face. Palmetto's Jasmine Green Tea Clay Mask is recommended by *Diane Irons,* author of *911 Beauty Secrets* and *14-Day Beauty Boot Camp.*

- Milk of Magnesia: It may not be designed for facial use, but this laxative product absorbs more oil than clay—and, as an added bonus, soothes skin and reduces irritation. Swab the liquid onto your face with a cotton ball. Let it dry for no more than 15 minutes, then rinse. Dr. Donofrio recommends using this treatment every day or once a week, depending on how oily your skin is.

- Blotting papers: Today's face-blotting sheets are superior to the powdered rice tissues of yesteryear. Both Clean & Clear and Xpressions make soft papers that sop up significantly more pore-clogging oil than old types. If you have oily skin, you can blot your face several times a day with an absorbent sheet—without smudging your makeup.

- Rubbing alcohol: This is the only no-no on the list. True, rubbing alcohol removes oil, but it also irritates and dries out skin—which only prompts your body to secrete more oil, says Dr. Fields.

**KILL BACTERIA** The key to clear skin is treating your whole face. Applying a potent product, such as 10-percent benzoyl peroxide, onto a pimple may eliminate bacteria, but it'll also overdry and burn that area, warns Dr. Fields.

Go gentle on your face with a mild 2.5-percent benzoyl peroxide, available in drugstores. Reserve aggressive treatments—such as 10-percent benzoyl peroxide, discussed above—for your back and chest where the skin is thicker.

Benzoyl peroxide isn't your only option for reducing or eliminating bacteria. Three-percent hydrogen peroxide is an inexpensive and effective treatment, says Begoun. Apply with a cotton ball, avoiding your eyebrows and hairline, since peroxide can have a lightening effect on hair.

## AGING SKIN: BLAME IT ON THE RAYS

If you doubt the enormous role the sun plays in aging your skin, you should see the startling proof from a study conducted by Darrick Antell, M.D., who photographed the faces of identical twins between ages 45 and 75. Some subjects had spent years baking in the sun—as well as smoking—while others had taken great care to wear sunscreen and live a healthful lifestyle. The contrasts were dramatic, illustrated by one twin who appeared 10 to 15 years older than her genetically identical—yet more health-conscious—sister.

The somewhat surprising conclusion to be drawn is that heredity actually has little to do with how you age visibly. Rather, almost all wrinkles, lines, and discolorations are the by-products of overexposure to harmful ultraviolet (UV) rays. The UVs break down collagen and elastin, the skin's underlying support structures. As these proteins collapse and flatten out, grooves or wrinkles appear.

*Invest in ordinary sunscreen. It will do your skin more good than any fancy antiaging potion.*—Kathy Fields, M.D.

Of course, aging is a complicated process that involves numerous factors. For example, your skin becomes thicker and less pliant as you age. Also, women lose fat cells in the bottommost layer of the skin, known as the dermis, which gives older skin a transparent appearance. Less facial fat results in less fullness and more sagging as you age, says *Paula Begoun,* author of *Don't Go to the Cosmetics Counter Without Me.* (And before you ask: No, facial exercises won't help.)

The best advice for slowing this process? Completely avoid the sun. But that approach is hardly realistic. The best antiaging lotion you can buy? That would be good ol' sunscreen, says *Kathy Fields, M.D.,* clinical instructor of dermatology at the University of California at San Francisco. (For information on choosing the right sunscreen, see "The Truth About Sunscreens," page 450.)

## THE INSIDE SCOOP ON ANTIAGING CREAMS

Chances are, you already have wrinkles and age spots. Will anything really improve the look of them? Do antiaging creams offer actual promise?

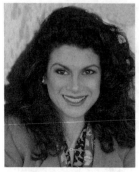

Here's the bad news: No skin-care product can erase your wrinkles. But there's good news, too. Dr. Fields says that one topical ingredient—retinoic acid, the active ingredient in vitamin A—has been proven to reduce such lines. You're probably more familiar with this acid's prescription forms, Retin-A and Renova, or the generic tretinoin. Tretinoin is the only product approved by the U.S. Food and Drug Administration to fight wrinkles.

*Kathy Fields, M.D. advises: Ask a dermatologist to prescribe the wrinkle-reducing formula that best suits your skin type.*

Research proves that its use can reverse some effects of sun damage. However, it's not a miracle cure, and it can cause skin irritation. While any doctor can prescribe retinoic-acid products, a dermatologist will know which formulation and concentration is right for your skin. For example, Retin-A may be too drying for mature skin; therefore, Renova, a creamier medication, may be a better option. Women with sensitive skin may be instructed to apply Retin-A only once a week at first, then slowly work up to a once-a-day regimen, says Dr. Fields.

Most health-insurance policies won't cover the cost of Retin-A unless you're under age 25 and have acne. But at about $65 for a 45-gram tube, it won't set you back much more than many department-store creams.

Not everyone wants to have to get a prescription, so what about all those so-called age-defying products on store shelves? Ignore the hype, recommends Dr. Fields, because most offer little to no real results. The government doesn't regulate cosmetic products, so companies are able to make any claims they desire—without having to substantiate anything. Sometimes, the only reason a product seems to work is because it hydrates.

Simply relieving dryness can plump out skin and slightly hide wrinkles, says Dr. Fields.

Check out what you can expect from some of the most commonly used cosmetic ingredients.

*Prescription Retin-A is your best weapon in the battle against wrinkles. But no miracle cream exists that will completely erase wrinkles.*

**ALPHA HYDROXY ACIDS** Of all the commercial elements, alpha hydroxy acids (AHAs) have the most research to back up their claims of efficacy. AHAs include glycolic, citric, and lactic acids, found naturally in sugar cane, citrus fruits, and sour milk, respectively. They stimulate cell turnover and increase exfoliation. Glycolic acid is best able to penetrate the skin because it has the smallest molecules, says Begoun.

## FAKE THAT SUN-KISSED GLOW
*An artificial tan can look like the real thing.*

Sunless tanning lotions and sprays have improved dramatically over the past couple of decades. That means no more orange disasters.

Are you worried about the safety of self-tanners? Don't be. The active ingredient is a colorless, completely safe sugar called dihydroxy-acetone (DHA). It interacts with skin proteins to produce a darker pigment. However, keep in mind that even sunless tanners give you little, if any, defense against ultraviolet (UV) rays, since DHA is essentially a skin stain. You'll still need to apply a true sunscreen when you're exposed to any sunlight.

To get even and natural-looking coverage, start by exfoliating and shaving so that your skin is clean and smooth. Apply the tanner generously but use less around your hairline or on dry areas. Wash your hands thoroughly with soap afterward. Let the tanner dry for 15 to 20 minutes. Don't swim or bathe for at least three hours afterward. When choosing a product, remember that, in general, lotions go on easier and are less streaky than spray-on oils.

Some lotions contain a disappearing color indicator so that you can see where you've applied it—the cream starts out brown when you first put it on and then turns clear within minutes. Another way you can get a warm glow is by using light-reflecting moisturizers with a sheer, rosy tint.

Nevertheless, you'd be challenged to find an AHA product that actually works. Many manufacturers intentionally raise pH levels to avoid skin irritation, and this practice ends up neutralizing the AHAs. Some of the most effective products are sold through dermatologists and spas. Drugstore brands may help exfoliate, but this fades only the slightest of lines over time.

If you have delicate skin, start with an AHA concentration of around 5 percent and gradually work up to 8 or 10 percent. Since AHAs can make your skin more sensitive to sun exposure, Dr. Fields recommends wearing sunscreen in conjunction with such a product or looking for one that contains a sun protection factor (SPF), such as Formula 405's AHA Facial Day Cream SPF 15. If your skin doesn't tolerate these acids well, switch to a product featuring a gentler fruit enzyme, such as bromelain (pineapple enzyme) or papain (papaya enzyme). Enzymes kick-start the rebuilding of collagen and elastin, as well as digest dead cells to help unclog pores, says *Lori Gregory,* technical director for the cosmeceutical company BioMedic.

BETA HYDROXY ACIDS Also known as salicylic acid, beta hydroxy acids (BHAs) may plump out fine lines by exfoliating and renewing cells. They are preferable for acne-prone or sensitive skin because they penetrate more effectively through oil and are less irritating than AHAs. BHAs are a relative of aspirin, so they also have a slight anti-inflammatory effect on acne, says Begoun. Be aware that BHAs can make your skin more reactive to the sun's rays, so protect yourself accordingly.

*Vitamin C is touted as an effective antioxidant. But there is no evidence that it can make wrinkles disappear.*
—*Kathy Fields, M.D.*

VITAMIN C Well-known as a potent antioxidant, vitamin C is controversial as an antiaging product. You've probably heard a lot lately about free radicals, the tiny molecules generated when your body converts oxygen into energy. When too many free radicals accumulate—usually as a result of excessive sunlight and air pollution—they kill off cells, damage tissues, and lead to disease, explains Begoun. Research shows that such antioxidants as vitamins A, C, and E taken in pill form can stop the free-radical chain reaction in your body. But it's not clear how much antioxidants help the skin.

There's no doubt that vitamin C can neutralize damaging free radicals. But because of the difficulty of keeping vitamin-C molecules stable, or active, few companies have developed formulas that truly allow this vitamin to work its wonders. Even vitamin-C blends that have proven effective in lab studies can be quickly rendered inactive upon exposure to light and air, says Dr. Fields.

So look for products housed in airtight, dark containers. Studies suggest that the type of vitamin C most likely to penetrate skin and stay active is L-ascorbic acid in a 10- to 20-percent concentration. Dr. Fields says that

## THE BEST LIGHTENER FOR AGE SPOTS

*These discolorations don't have to get between you and a porcelain complexion. There are plenty of ways to rid yourself of them.*

Age spots aren't actually caused by aging, but rather by the sun. Your body responds to sun exposure by producing a skin-darkening pigment called melanin. Thus, think of these spots as reminders of tans that have long since faded, says *Deborah Sarnoff, M.D.,* clinical assistant professor of dermatology at New York University School of Medicine and author of *Instant Beauty: Getting Gorgeous on Your Lunch Break.*

The best at-home practice is to exfoliate with an alpha hydroxy acid and to lighten darkened skin with a bleaching cream. There are numerous lightening creams based on plant extracts—such as kojic acid, mulberry, and licorice—but they are inferior to any featuring hydroquinone, a bleaching agent that actually slows melanin production.

You can buy 2-percent hydroquinone creams at drugstores. For better results, a dermatologist can prescrie Lustra, a 4-percent hydroquinone cream that contains glycolic acid to improve penetration. Dab it on discolorations twice a day.

Patience is an essential ingredient in treating age spots with any product, as it can take months to see results. If any discoloration hasn't faded after six months, it's probably never going to disappear. That's when it's time to see a dermatologist.

You doctor can use a laser to remove an age spot. Better yet, she can freeze it in a relatively painless, quick procedure that involves swabbing on liquid nitrogen to burn off abnormal cells. Be sure to wear sunscreen afterwards, as the treated site will be more vulnerable to the sun, says Dr. Sarnoff.

A final note: Don't confuse age spots with a condition known as pregnancy mask. The latter is a change in pigmentation that results from hormonal surges during or after pregnancy, or while taking birth control pills or hormone replacement therapy. These spots usually go away on their own, says Dr. Sarnoff. If they don't and your medication is determined to be the culprit, talk to your doctor about getting a new prescription.

this can be found in such upscale brands as Cellex-C (www.cellex-c.com, 800-235-5392) and SkinCeuticals (www.skinceuticals.com, 800-811-1660). But expect to pay a hefty $42 to $135 per package. Some dermatologists insist that you'll see some benefit from inexpensive brands, such as Avon's Anew Clearly C 10% Vitamin C Serum (www.avonzone.com) for around a more reasonable $20. Keep in mind, however, that no good evidence exists to support *any* vitamin-C product as a wrinkle fighter, warns Dr. Fields. For now, the best you can hope for is to keep such lines and creases at bay.

RETINOIDS  Researchers don't know if over-the-counter versions of retinoic acid offer much promise. One study found that a 0.25-percent concentration of retinol—the most popular member of the retinoid family—has the same exfoliating, skin-strengthening effect as 0.025-percent Retin-A. But many products offer only a 0.1-percent concentration of retinol, which probably does little good. In addition, Begoun points out that retinol must be converted to its effective ingredient, tretinoin, to be effective in the skin. How easily the skin achieves this is debatable.

Choose a vitamin-A cream that contains retinol, rather than retinyl palmitate or provitamin A, which are even more difficult to convert into tretinoin in the skin. Begoun suggests L'Oréal's Plénitude Line Eraser.

*Beware: Most antiaging products are more hype than hope.*—Kathy Fields, M.D.

NEWCOMERS  The list of ingredients being touted as the latest in wrinkle cures seems to grow longer every day. You may have heard the hype about green tea, grapeseed extract, Coenzyme Q10, alpha lipoic acid, Kinerase, soybean extract, and copper. But there's not enough evidence that any are effective, says Dr. Fields. While a particular extract may work wonders in a petri dish, it is then questionable as to whether the ingredient remains chemically stable in a lotion or serum. Can it penetrate the skin? Once inside the skin, will it still be active?

Although there are no definitive answers as yet, that doesn't mean you shouldn't try these products. Dr. Fields says they can't hurt and may very well help.

# THE LUNCH-HOUR FACE-LIFT

*Fast and effective cosmetic procedures are winning widespread popularity.*

The results gained from these relatively new treatments lie somewhere between a good face cream and a full-blown face-lift. They're quick enough to get you back on the job within about an hour without a telltale red face. With the exception of Botox treatments, the procedures will help conceal only the finest of lines. To keep that fresh look, you'll need to repeat your chosen treatment anywhere from two to four times a year.

These are some of the trendy treatments available:

- **Botox:** Tiny amounts of this lethal poison are injected into certain facial muscles to temporarily paralyze them, giving the appearance of ironing out wrinkles. Results are dramatic and can last up to six months, says *Deborah Sarnoff, M.D.,* clinical assistant professor of dermatology at New York University School of Medicine and author of *Instant Beauty: Getting Gorgeous on Your Lunch Break.* However, there is a slight chance that your eyelid could droop temporarily if an injection is made too close to the muscle that controls it. Expect to pay up to $450 per area, such as your forehead, or $1,000 for your whole face each time you have it done.

- **Chemical peels:** This involves swabbing a light glycolic acid (a type of alpha hydroxy acid) or salicylic acid (beta hydroxy acid) onto your face. The acid is left on for a few minutes, causing mild stinging but not the severe redness normally associated with a standard peel. Several treatments will peel away fine lines and superficial wrinkles, says Dr. Sarnoff. Expect to pay up to $250 per application.

- **Fat injections:** Also called fat rebalancing, this procedure involves suctioning fat from one area, such as the jowls or buttocks, and injecting it where fullness is desired, such as the cheeks. Expect to pay $500 to $1,000 for each plumping.

- **Collagen injections:** Collagen is a general term that applies to connective tissue. A form of bovine (cow) or human collagen is injected beneath the skin with a fine needle to fill out wrinkle lines for six weeks to four months. All collagen products contain a local anesthetic, so the area is quickly numbed for the injection; the numbness lasts a few hours. If your doctor uses bovine tissue, you'll need a test four weeks before the procedure to rule out an allergic reation. Price will vary, depending on the extent of the treatments. Expect to pay $500 to $1,500.

- **Laser resurfacing:** Most standard laser peels leave you red-faced for weeks to months. Nonablative lasers won't, though, making them a good option for lunch-hour visits. These peels zap away only the most superficial layer of skin. Expect to pay $500 at each visit.

- **Microdermabrasion:** A handheld device shoots microscopic crystals onto the skin surface for a gentle polishing effect. This treatment is good for people who are sensitive to chemical peels and offers similar results, says Dr. Sarnoff. You'll pay about $250 per touch-up.

## BURNS, CUTS, AND BITES: FIRST AID FOR YOUR SKIN

Your skin is exposed to injury from abrasions, poisonous plants, and flying pests looking to make a meal of you. Therefore, you should know how to properly treat cuts, scrapes, rashes, insect bites, and other common skin complaints. Perhaps you can't make a wound disappear overnight, but you can help ease any pain and speed the healing process.

### BANISHING BURNS

Burns that blister may be serious enough to require a doctor's attention, especially if the burn is on your face, neck, hands, feet, or genitals. You should also see your health-care provider if the burned area is larger than about the size of your palm. Any burn caused by electricity or steam should be evaluated by a physician as quickly as possible. Infection and scarring may result if such serious burns are not treated properly.

Home treatment is safe and effective for minor burns, which usually result in little more than redness, a little swelling, and mild pain.

*Use lavender oil to clean a burn and promote healing.*—Joni Keim Loughran

For routine mishaps, our experts recommend these self-care remedies.

**Raid the freezer.** Ice constricts blood vessels, thus reducing swelling. If you don't have an ice pack handy, grab a bag of frozen vegetables or wrap some ice cubes in a thin towel. Apply to a burn for five minutes, then expose the area to warm running water to soothe the pain, says *Jeanette Jacknin, M.D.,* author of *Smart Medicine for Your Skin.*

**Milk it.** Soak burns in whole milk for 15 minutes. Milk is even better for cooling burns than water because it doesn't pull moisture out of the skin. Also, its fat leaves behind a protective emollient over the burn, says *Diane Irons,* author of *911 Beauty Secrets* and *14-Day Beauty Boot Camp.*

**Enjoy the benefits of lavender.** "It's *the* essential oil for burns," says *Joni Keim Loughran,* essential oil specialist and author of *Natural Skin Care.* Lavender kills germs, fights infections, and speeds cell rejuvenation. Swab pure lavender essential oil directly onto the burn. Loughran recommends the Oshadhi brand, available at health-food stores.

## COPING WITH CUTS AND SCRAPES

If you have an unfortunate encounter with a power tool, you might want to run, not walk, to the nearest emergency room. But for minor wounds, consider these approaches.

**Fight germs.** Wash and dry your injury. To prevent infection, you should immediately apply a topical antibiotic, such as Bacitracin or Polysporin, says *Audrey Gottlieb Kunin, M.D.,* associate clinical instructor in the department of dermatology at the University of Kansas Medical School and president of DERMAdoctor.com. "I avoid recommending any topical antibiotic product that contains neomycin, such as Neosporin, since so many people have an allergic reaction to it." Cover the cut with a bandage.

**Pour on the honey.** This tasty sweetener makes a terrific topical antibiotic. It suffocates and fends off bacteria, which prevents infection and promotes healing. The enzymes in honey may even encourage skin growth. Wash the wound well with mild soap, apply pasteurized honey, and cover with a bandage, recommends Irons.

**Avoid chafing.** Rub cornstarch onto your hands before you perform any task that might lead to friction blisters—such as raking. Cornstarch provides a silky-smooth layer that can protect skin from irritating rubbing, says *Dee Anna Glaser, M.D.,* associate professor of dermatology at St. Louis University School of Medicine in Missouri.

**Repair a paper cut.** Two or three times a day, apply an antibiotic ointment that does not contain neomycin, such as Bacitracin or Polysporin, recommends Dr. Kunin. As needed, you can also apply a bland moisturizing cream—one without such acidic ingredients as glycolic or urea that could sting—to prevent dryness. At night, apply Epilyt, an oily lotion that softens the edges of the cut, allowing them to bond and heal.

### SHOULD I SEE A DOCTOR?

*Be sure to examine your skin regularly. Preventive skin care can ward off many common conditions.*

If you answer yes to any of the following statements, schedule a visit with a dermatologist:
- Have you noticed a change in a mole or a sudden new growth that hasn't gone away for weeks?
- Do you have rashes, hives, or dry patches?
- Do you have acne that is chronic or cystic, meaning you have large, inflamed, pus-filled sacs deep under the surface of your skin? Such lesions are painful and can leave scars.

## BATTLING BRUISES

Bruising can signal vitamin deficiencies or blood-cell irregularities. If you notice that you bruise frequently or easily, see your health-care provider. But to treat everyday bumps, remember these tips.

**Apply special K.** Known for helping make spider veins disappear, vitamin-K creams also work on bruises. Pierce a soft vitamin-K capsule with a pin and squeeze the contents directly onto the bruise. Or try a commercial cream, such as Dermal K, available at beauty salons, drugstores, health-food stores, or www.dermal-k.com. Taking 65 micrograms vitamin K daily helps your liver form substances that promote blood clotting, says Dr. Jacknin. Vitamin K also strengthens capillaries and heals weakened tissues.

**Use arnica.** For centuries, natural-healing practitioners have relied on this plant remedy to aid the body's recovery process. Look for liquid arnica at health-food stores. In a bowl, dilute 1 tablespoon arnica tincture in 1 pint cool water. Soak a compress in the solution, then apply it to the bruised area for a few minutes several times a day, recommends Dr. Jacknin. Or take the homeopathic form of arnica, a 30C supplement, daily for a few days, following the dosage recommendations on the label. Always be sure to consult your health-care professional before taking any kind of supplement.

**Check out helichrysum.** "This healing essential oil is unsurpassed for bruises," says Loughran. Apply this oil, also known as immortelle, directly to the site or dilute 6 drops essential oil in 1 teaspoon vegetable oil. Swab it on right after the injury, and a bruise will barely form.

**Take your Cs.** Excessive and chronic bruising could be due to a deficiency of vitamin C, which is essential to the healing process and fortification of the immune system. The bioflavonoids in vitamin C are critical for strengthening capillary walls, says Loughran. To reduce your risk of bruising, Dr. Jacknin recommends taking 300 milligrams vitamin C with bioflavonoids twice a day. To treat an existing injury, she suggests you can apply a topical 10-percent, vitamin-C serum directly onto a bruise.

## SOOTHING BITES AND STINGS

The itch of an insect bite can be misery. The marketplace has plenty of commercial insect repellents and anti-itch potions that will help. If you want a home remedy, try these for relief.

**Add onion.** The enzymes in onions help break down prostaglandins, the chemicals your body releases to signal pain. Onions also contain quercetin, which reduces inflammation. Cut a raw onion in half and rub a piece directly over the affected area, says Loughran.

**Get the venom out.** Because it's a solvent, rubbing alcohol removes any material left by the sting or bite. Swab it on with a cotton ball. As the rubbing alcohol dries, it cools and comforts the tender area, explains Irons.

*Keep rubbing alcohol and baking soda on hand to treat painful insect bites. In a pinch, you can rub an onion slice on a sting to reduce pain and inflammation.*

**Try baking soda.** Loughran explains that the alkaline in baking soda relieves pain by neutralizing the acid in insect venom. Dr. Jacknin advises mixing 2 teaspoons baking soda with enough water to make a paste. Apply the paste to the sting and leave it on for 15 to 20 minutes. Then rinse with cool water.

**Repel with tea tree oil.** This oil keeps bugs from bugging you. Use it straight from the bottle or, if you have sensitive skin, dilute 6 drops tea tree oil in 1 teaspoon vegetable oil. You can also use this natural antiseptic after the fact to help calm a sting and reduce pain, says Loughran.

## QUELLING THE ITCH OF POISON IVY AND POISON OAK

Contact with these pernicious plants can spoil any outdoor activity. Take this advice for soothing the resulting outbreak.

**Use booze as a balm.** Rubbing alcohol dissolves poison ivy's resin better than soap and water—though that combo works, too. In a pinch, any type of alcohol—even beer—will suffice, says Irons. For best results, administer treatment within 15 minutes of exposure, before the resin gets a chance to inflame the skin. But even applying rubbing alcohol within two hours can minimize the rash.

**Do your laundry.** Carefully remove your clothes and immediately wash them in hot water. Remember that the resin spreads easily, so wear gloves when handling the affected garments, suggests Loughran.

**Soak in oats.** Oatmeal helps soothe the itchy rash, says Dr. Kunin. Consider Aveeno's Oatmeal Bath Treatment (oilated), which contains about twice as much skin-soothing oil as most other brands.

## SOOTHING SUNBURN

You probably feel foolish enough that you got burned, so we won't make you feel any worse by preaching the value of sunscreen. (For those of you who still need to see the light, check out "The Truth About Sunscreens," below.) Meanwhile, try these suggestions for quenching that fire.

**Rub on aloe vera.** A member of the lily family, this cactuslike plant contains a gel that has long been prized as a sunburn remedy. Skin absorbs aloe four times faster than it does water, helping pores open up to hydration and nutrition, says Loughran. Keep a live aloe plant at home for such sun emergencies. Break off a juicy leaf and open it up whenever you've absorbed too many rays.

**Bathe in vinegar.** Pour a 32-ounce bottle of apple cider vinegar into a tub of warm water. Soak for at least 15 minutes. Vinegar takes the sizzle out of the burn and makes skin feel soft, says Irons. Substitute raspberry vinegar for an even more pleasant fragrance.

## THE TRUTH ABOUT SUNSCREENS

*You know the rule: Slather on the sunscreen before you go outside.*

The most effective way to prevent skin cancer is to avoid exposure to the sun as much as possible, especially between 10 a.m. and 2 p.m., when the ultraviolet (UV) rays are strongest. Whenever you go out, wear a sunscreen with sun protection factor (SPF) of 15 or higher, recommends *Dana Sachs, M.D.,* clinical assistant physician in dermatology at Memorial Sloan-Kettering Cancer Center in New York City.

### SUNSCREEN 101

There's a lot you may not know about sunscreens:

**Raise your awareness.** Sunlight that reaches the earth includes two types of UV radiation, known as UVA and UVB rays. Most sunscreens block only UVB rays, which are more likely to cause sunburn. UVA rays penetrate deeper into the skin than UVBs, though, causing more of the wrinkles and cellular changes that lead to skin cancer, says *Debra Jaliman, M.D.,* dermatologist and clinical instructor at Mount Sinai School of Medicine in New York City. UVAs can even penetrate the windows of a car or building, so these rays can hit you all day. The only products that protect against UVAs are sunblocks, which contain zinc oxide and titanium dioxide. Some sunscreens include the chemical avobenzone to absorb UVA rays, but studies suggest that it quickly degrades in the sun and, thus, offers limited protection.

**Do the math.** SPF indicates the level of defense a product provides against sunburn. SPF 10 or below is considered low, 10 to 20 is medium, and 20 to 40 is high protection. Cosmetics with sun protection are great if you're inside most of the day and don't want to wear sunscreen. But SPF foundation wears off quickly in the sun. If you'll be outside for longer than two hours, wear a true sunscreen underneath your foundation. But when you put

**Look to lavender.** Lavender oil, available at health-food stores, can be applied directly onto a sunburned area for relief. Dr. Jacknin suggests adding 40 drops to a tubful of cold water and immersing yourself in it for 15 minutes. The oil soothes the pain and helps speed healing.

## WISKING AWAY WARTS

If you have diabetes or problems with the nerves or blood circulation in your feet, always consult your doctor before attempting any home remedies. Otherwise, these pointers might help get rid of these nasty bumps.

**Rely on Retin-A.** The same prescription vitamin-A cream that fights wrinkles can also make warts vanish. "It works especially well with flat warts," says Dr. Jacknin. Retin-A (tretinoin) peels off the surface layers of skin, hastening cell turnover. More importantly, it disrupts growth of new wart cells and encourages healthy cells to grow instead.

SPF 15 sunscreen under SPF 10 foundation, 15 plus 10 doesn't add up to 25. You'll get coverage equal to the higher product, in this case SPF 15.

**SPF only measures UVB protection.** As impressive as SPF 50 sounds, it still blocks only UVB rays. To get full UVA/UVB coverage, look for a product that promises broad spectrum protection. Check the label for the ingredients zinc oxide and titanium dioxide.

### APPLY IT RIGHT

Research shows that most people fail to successfully cover their bodies when using sunscreen. Consider these tips from Dr. Sachs for the lowdown on proper application:

**Think ahead.** Apply sunscreen to all exposed skin 20 minutes before going outside. That's how long it takes to start working. Reapply every two to three hours.

**Hit the bottle.** Most people put sunscreen in their palms and then rub their hands together before covering their body with the lotion. This practice leaves you with more sunscreen on your palms than anywhere else. Instead, apply the lotion straight from the bottle and use your fingertips to smooth it into your skin.

**Use at least 1 ounce.** The amount of sunscreen needed to adequately cover an average person fills a shot glass. Use more if necessary.

**Be thorough.** Don't forget to put sunscreen on the tops of your ears and feet, your temple, and the back of your neck.

**Throw out the old.** Toss bottles older than two years, since sunscreen does expire.

### WEAR IT ALL WINTER

UV rays are not temperature-sensitive and so are just as strong in the winter as in the summer. Add snow to the ground and the danger increases: The sun's reflection off snow adds up to 40 percent more UV exposure. So a downhill skier is subjected to considerably more UVs than an urban pedestrian. On a clear day at noon, the skier risks sunburn after only six minutes on the slopes.

# Mix vitamin-A oil with lemon juice to treat warts on your feet.

—Jeanette Jacknin, M.D.

**Make lemon-aid.** Break open a soft vitamin-A capsule with a pin. Mix the contents with a few drops of lemon juice. Apply the mixture directly onto the wart, then cover it with a bandage, advises Dr. Jacknin. This treatment is especially beneficial for warts on the soles of the feet, since lemon juice—a natural alpha hydroxy acid—helps exfoliate tough skin and get the vitamin A down into the wart.

**Add garlic.** Mix the contents of a vitamin-E capsule with a crushed, raw garlic clove. Apply to the wart and cover with a bandage. Garlic's antiviral properties will burn the wart, causing it to blister and fall off within a week. Rub vitamin E into the area as needed to improve circulation and promote tissue repair. Everyone responds differently to natural self-care, so if this garlic mix doesn't work for you, give another treatment a try. Cedar leaf oil, tea tree oil, and essential oil of oregano also have antiviral properties. If you don't benefit from one of these oils after applying it daily for about two weeks, you can move directly on to another remedy, says Dr. Jacknin.

## ECZEMA: DON'T BE RASH

Is your skin irritated by perfumes, detergents, or dyes? If the answer is yes, you may have atopic dermatitis, better known as eczema. This is an inherited

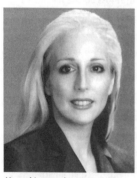

*Your skin may become more susceptible to irritation as you age, warns Lisa Donofrio, M.D.*

susceptibility of the skin to react strongly to certain natural or man-made chemicals, says *Robyn Gmyrek, M.D.*, dermatologist and assistant clinical professor at Columbia-Presbyterian Hospital in New York City.

The signs of eczema are unmistakable: red, dry, scaly skin that sometimes erupts with fluid-filled blisters. Patches pop up on the face, insides of elbows, and backs of knees—anywhere you've come in contact with an irritant. As they age, women are prone to such skin reactions, perhaps due to a weakened immune system, says *Lisa Donofrio, M.D.*, assistant clinical professor of dermatology at Yale University

School of Medicine in New Haven, Connecticut. One survey found that an astounding 75 percent of the women polled claimed to have sensitive skin.

Fortunately, the U.S. Food and Drug Administration recently approved Protopic (tacrolimus), the first topical nonsteroid treatment available for eczema. Dr. Gmyrek explains that traditional steroid creams are infamous for their numerous side effects, including thinning skin, stretch marks, and prominent blood vessels. Eczema sufferers often develop a resistance to steroid creams, requiring stronger medications over time—which then leads to even more side effects.

The most commonly reported adverse reaction to Protopic is a potential for initial irritation of the skin, says Dr. Gmyrek. You can even use Protopic around your eyes, something prohibited with steroids, since they increase the risk of cataracts and glaucoma. If you do notice any reaction and it lasts for more than three days, discontinue use of Protopic and consult your physician.

"This breakthrough has made a world of difference for eczema sufferers," says Dr. Gmyrek. Ask your doctor if Protopic is right for you.

If you have mild eczema, you may be able to control it on your own. Follow Dr. Gmyrek's advice for deterring flare-ups.

**Avoid fragrances.** Buy lotions and cosmetics labeled as hypoallergenic or specifically for sensitive skin. They usually contain few irritating chemicals, such as perfumes and preservatives. Fragrances tend to be more offensive than any other ingredient—and they're somewhat difficult to dodge since more than five thousand of them are put into skin-care products. Also shun soaps with antibacterial ingredients, as well as those touted as unscented that may contain chemicals that mask the soap's natural fragrance. Stick with fragrance-free products instead.

*To control eczema, keep your skin moisturized and avoid irritating chemicals.*—Robyn Gmyrek, M.D.

**Moisturize often.** Taking care of dry skin can prevent most rashes. Use petroleum-based ointments, which penetrate better than creams and offer a more protective barrier against the elements.

**Don't claw at it.** Dr. Gmyrek calls eczema "the itch that rashes." So the more you scratch, the itchier it gets. Even simply rubbing with a washcloth in the shower worsens the condition.

**Buy generic hydrocortisone.** Remember that the fewer preservatives, the better. Some hydrocortisone products contain fragrances that can irritate your skin.

**Remember that natural isn't always best.** Many ointments and oils that contain herbs—such as vanilla, clove, cinnamon, and tea tree—can cause strong reactions in sensitive people. Test a small amount on your inner forearm over a couple of days to check for an adverse response before applying it to the affected site. You're more likely to notice irritation if you have fair or dry skin.

**Delouse your house.** Pollens, molds, dyes, perfumes, and pet dander can make skin irritated and itchy. To reduce their presence in your home, wash bedding and clothing in hot water with a hypoallergenic detergent. Use a damp duster to clean in corners and under beds; vacuum carpets thoroughly and often. Always wash your hands after touching an animal.

### RING AROUND THE MOUTH

A rashlike dryness around your lips could be an allergic reaction to the dyes, fragrances, flavoring, or preservatives used in lipsticks and toothpastes. Dr. Gmyrek recommends that women be wary of the following triggers.

- Toothpastes that are tartar-control, cinnamon-flavored, or tinted blue, red, or green because they tend to contain more potentially irritating dyes, flavorings, and preservatives. Also look out for sodium lauryl sulfate, a preservative that is a common cause of this problem.
- Lipsticks with yellow dye #11 and red dyes #17, #19, #31, and #36 (#17 is no longer available in the United States because of its tendency to cause irritation). Problematic dyes are more often found in long-wearing lipsticks, so always check the ingredients to be on the safe side.
- Acidic foods, such as orange peels, coffee, and menthol
- Mangoes, which contain an oil similar to the resin found in poison ivy and oak

## DRY SKIN: HOW TO RESTORE MOISTURE

Along with a drop in temperature, winter often brings dry, scaly, shedding skin that no amount of hand cream seems to cure. Known by the medical term xerosis, this condition is more common as women age, since cells lose their ability to retain water with age, says **Robyn Gmyrek, M.D.,** dermatologist and assistant clinical professor at Columbia-Presbyterian Hospital in New York City.

The tendency toward dryness increases in the winter because artificial heat sucks moisture out of the air and can make the indoor climate as arid as a desert. Add to that the hot showers and baths you take to warm up, which strip away natural oils, and your skin is left even more thirsty.

Here are our top tips for keeping your skin from drying out.

**Chugalug, chugalug.** Drink at least 8 to 10 (8-ounce) glasses of water every day to hydrate your skin.

**Hydrate while you sleep.** Run a humidifier or place a shallow pan of water near a radiator in your bedroom. The evaporated water adds moisture to the air, which then helps to rehydrate your skin. If you can, humidify your environment during the day, too.

**Don't overwash.** Aggressive scrubbing or the use of harsh cleansers can leave your skin parched.

**Cover up.** When exposed to the cold, skin loses its moisture and can become flaky. Wear gloves, a hat, and scarf to protect as much skin as possible.

**Avoid abrasive fabrics.** Rough textiles can further irritate dry skin.

**Brush it off.** Dry-brushing your skin sloughs off dead cells and encourages oil production. Look for a soft paddle brush with natural plant fibers, such as sisal, at beauty boutiques and health-food stores with beauty departments, suggests **Ariane Saint-Martin,** director of massage therapies at Ona Spa in Los Angeles. Avoid plastic, nylon, or boar bristle brushes, which are too stiff. Use long upward strokes on your arms and legs. Pay special attention to rough areas, such as elbows and knees. Then shower away loosened dry skin. Don't store the brush in the shower, as constant moisture breeds bacteria.

**Buff your body.** Try a gritty scrub, such as Clinique's Sparkle Skin Body Exfoliator, suggests **Amy E. Newburger, M.D.,** assistant attending physician in dermatology at St. Luke's-Roosevelt Hospital Center in New York City and author of *Looking Good at Any Age.* Or treat yourself to an invigorating full-body rubdown with a coarse salt mixture or loofah, which softens rough, dry skin and smoothes bumps, while allowing your moisturizer to penetrate better.

**Shower first.** Since the whole point of moisturizer is to lock in moisture, applying it to dry skin doesn't do much good. For best hydration, slather on lotion within three minutes of bathing, suggests Dr. Gmyrek.

*The best treatment for dry skin might be found in your kitchen. Smear on a little Crisco for overnight moisturizing.*—Dee Anna Glaser, M.D.

**Dip into Crisco.** It may sound odd, but vegetable shortening is one of the best moisturizers for dry skin, says **Dee Anna Glaser, M.D.,** associate professor of dermatology at St. Louis University School of Medicine. It's especially beneficial to sensitive skin, since it doesn't contain irritating fragrances or preservatives. Bathe at night and then apply a light layer of shortening all over. Then put on some old pajamas you don't mind getting greasy. (You may want to forgo the satin sheets that evening.)

**Switch to a mild cleanser.** If your face feels taut 15 minutes after you wash it, your soap could be preventing your skin from naturally remoisturizing itself. Switch to a more gentle liquid cleanser, such as Cetaphil, says Dr. Gmyrek.

## HIVES: BUMP THEM OFF

Many things can cause an outbreak of hives, which manifest as red or pink bumps about the size of an eraser head or blotchy streaks the width of a dinner plate. They can appear after eating strawberries, basking in the sun, or popping an aspirin—to name but a few triggers.

If you experience one episode of hives that lasts weeks, a virus might be to blame, says **D'Anne Kleinsmith, M.D.,** cosmetic dermatologist at William Beaumont Hospital in Royal Oak, Michigan. But if you get them repeatedly, an allergic reaction is probably the cause. You'll know within hours of encountering something if it's a trigger for hives. Luckily, hives usually go away within a few hours, says Dr. Kleinsmith.

Chronic cases—involving hives that endure or recur over a period longer than six weeks—seem to indicate an overactive immune system. Try to identify those things that can set off an episode, such as these common triggers.

- Foods, particularly nuts, chocolate, fish, tomatoes, eggs, fresh berries, and milk
- Preservatives, like yellow dye #5, found in some toothpastes and chewing gum

## BANISHING A BOIL

*A skin abscess is caused by a bacterial infection, usually in a hair follicle. With proper care, most boils will clear up in a couple of weeks.*

A boil starts out red and tender, then hardens as the infection grows. Cystic acne blemishes are a type of boil, but even a splinter or ingrown hair can lead to such an unpleasant abscess, says *Amy E. Newburger, M.D.,* assistant attending physician in dermatology at St. Luke's-Roosevelt Hospital Center in New York City and author of *Looking Good at Any Age.*

As your body fights the infection, white blood cells gather and form pus, which eventually rises to the surface to form a whitehead. Most boils drain on their own in time. To speed the process, apply a warm compress to the inflamed spot for about 30 minutes every two to three hours. Once the boil drains, wash with antibacterial soap to prevent recontamination of the area, says Dr. Newburger.

Never squeeze or lance a boil yourself, or you risk spreading the infection. See a doctor if the boil hasn't improved in two to three weeks. Your doctor may drain it or prescribe antibiotics.

- Medications, such as aspirin and ibuprofen (Advil or Motrin), antibiotics, sedatives, antacids, and even vitamins. Indeed, any drug or supplement is a potential culprit.

For relief from hives, your doctor may prescribe antihistamines. Taken regularly, they can prevent future reactions from occuring, says Dr. Kleinsmith.

## FOLLICULITIS

You may never have heard of it, but chances are you've probably had folliculitis. That's the medical term for those red, pus-filled bumps you get on your rear after sitting for hours in a wet swimsuit. Women who wear panty hose also tend to get them on the backs of their thighs.

Folliculitis occurs when hair follicles become inflamed by trapped bacteria, explains Dr. Kleinsmith. If the infection grows deeper, these bumps become boils. (For more information, see "Banishing a Boil," above.)

Dr. Kleinsmith has this advice for preventing and treating folliculitis.

**Wear cotton.** Loose-fitting clothing made of natural fibers will circulate air better than garments featuring synthetics, which trap moisture. This choice is particularly important in exercise togs.

**Wash after a workout.** Use your hands or a washcloth to gently cleanse with an antibacterial soap. Never scrub, which can cause more openings in the skin to let in bacteria.

**Try 10-percent benzoyl peroxide.** Apply the product directly to affected areas. Benzoyl peroxide is available at drugstores under many brand names in liquids, lotions, creams, gels, and soaps. Your pharmacist may be able to recommend a specific product.

**SHAVING BUMPS** The red spots you sometimes see along your bikini line or on your legs after shaving are a type of folliculitis. To avoid getting them, throw out a razor after three or four uses, says Dr. Kleinsmith. A dull blade increases friction on your skin, increasing the chance of cuts and making it easier for bacteria to get in.

To keep your skin healthy after shaving, follow these recommendations from Dr. Kleinsmith.

**Warm up.** To thoroughly moisten hairs and make them easier to cut, shower for at least three minutes before shaving.

**Lather lavishly.** Use shaving cream to soften hair and decrease skin friction.

**Go with the flow.** To avoid irritation, shave in the same direction that the hairs grow.

**Don't repeat.** Try to run your razor over each area just one time.

**Don't shave before you swim.** To keep from irritating any tiny nicks, avoid salt or chlorinated water for a couple of hours after shaving.

## PSORIASIS: NEW AND BETTER TREATMENTS

Writer John Updike once referred to psoriasis as a curse. The approximate six million Americans who suffer from this skin condition would undoubtedly agree with his assessment.

Psoriasis results when cell reproduction goes haywire. Whereas cells regularly take 28 to 30 days to mature, with psoriasis the cells rise to the skin's surface every three to four days. These dead cells form distinct patches of red, raised skin that are covered with silvery-white flakes. And these lesions *itch*.

There is no known cure for psoriasis. Standard therapies do little more than reduce swelling, redness, and itching. Current research offers hope of better treatments featuring genetically engineered drugs, known as biologics.

It's generally accepted that faulty cues in the immune system are the underlying cause of psoriasis. And while current therapies interrupt the immune responses involved, biologic medications target a specific part of those responses. These drugs promise more benefits and fewer side effects, says *Alice Gottlieb, M.D., Ph.D.*, professor of medicine and director of the Clinical Research Center at the Robert Wood Johnson Medical School in New Brunswick, New Jersey.

One such medication is Amevive (alefacept), approved by the Food and Drug Administration (FDA) in January 2003. Even this new drug is far from the ultimate answer: A 2001 study published in the *New England Journal of Medicine* showed that 53 percent of patients with moderate to severe psoriasis saw significant improvement after receiving injections of Amevive, but only 23 percent were free or almost free of psoriasis after 12 weeks of treatment.

*Moisturize to keep psoriasis in check. The greasier your moisturizer, the less flaky your skin will be.*

—*Alice Gottlieb, M.D., Ph.D.*

Other approaches abound. Some research suggests that bacteria may cause psoriasis. Antibiotics may clear up psoriasis completely if this theory bears out. It certainly gained some acceptability from a study conducted at the University of Tennessee in Memphis. Findings showed that more than half of the participants who took the antibiotic clindamycin for 10 to 14 days showed substantial improvement within a month. Of course, more research is needed, but this course of treatment is worth discussing with your dermatologist.

In fact, that's the best advice there is: Talk to your doctor. "Find out what might be best for you," says Dr. Gottlieb. If your psoriasis is moderate to severe, your physician may suggest some of these standard topical therapies.

- Steroids: These synthetic drugs resemble naturally occurring hormones, such as cortisone. Steroids come in various forms, including ointments, creams, lotions, solutions, sprays, foam, and tape. They treat inflammation effectively, but the risk of side effects is substantial, says Dr. Gottlieb. Over- or misuse of steroids can lead to thinning of the skin, easy bruising, and stretch marks.

- Coal tar: Topical coal-tar preparations have been used for centuries to treat the scaling, inflammation, and itching of psoriasis. There are over-the-counter ointments, gels, and bath solutions available with tar concentrations ranging from 0.5 to 5.0 percent, as well as tar shampoos for psoriasis on the scalp. But Dr. Gottlieb warns that tar products have a strong odor, stain clothing and linens, and can irritate the skin.
- Calcipotriene: Sold in prescription form as Dovonex, this synthetic form of vitamin $D_3$ is used to ease mild to moderate psoriasis. Available in a cream, ointment, or scalp solution, this treatment doesn't work quickly. It is effective and safe for long-term control, though, with few side effects, says Dr. Gottlieb.
- Vitamin A: Tazorac (tazarotene) is a prescription topical retinoid for mild to moderate psoriasis. This once-a-day medication can also treat psoriasis affecting the scalp and nails. Many dermatologists prescribe it along with a topical steroid for the best results, says Dr. Gottlieb.

You don't always need a prescription drug to treat a mild case of psoriasis. Check out these do-it-yourself remedies.

**Slather it on.** Moisturizing your skin prevents cracking. "It's one of the best things you can do for mild psoriasis," says Dr. Gottlieb. "The greasier your moisturizer, the less dry and flaky your skin will be." Apply Bag Balm ointment as often as needed or raid your kitchen for some Crisco.

**Add salt.** People trek across the world to swim in the Dead Sea because its healing minerals help such skin diseases as psoriasis. To reap similar scale-removal and itch-relief benefits at home, add ½ to 1 cup Epsom salts to a tub of warm water, says Dr. Gottlieb. After you bathe, be sure to generously apply lotion to lock in moisture.

**Face up to cream.** Salicylic acid, also known as beta hydroxy acids (BHAs), is found in many wrinkle-fighting facial moisturizers, especially those made by Olay. In strengths of 1.8 to 3 percent, salicylic acid is FDA-approved as an over-the-counter treatment for psoriasis. It softens and removes scales, allowing topical medications to better penetrate the skin, says Dr. Gottlieb.

**Sun without screen.** Psoriasis treatment is the single exception to the no-sunbathing rule. The ultraviolet (UV) light from the sun prevents inflamed, scaling skin cells from multiplying. In fact, most people with psoriasis notice improvement with daily doses of sunshine. To protect fair skin, expose affected areas only 5 to 15 minutes a day for the first three or four days. Then you can stay out in the sun two to five minutes longer each day thereafter. Sunbathe until your outbreak disappears—and no longer—advises Dr. Gottlieb.

**See the light.** A device called an excimer laser delivers high-intensity UV light to patches of psoriasis. A study found that half the participants who underwent this treatment noticed a 90-percent improvement with fewer than 10 treatments; the remaining test subjects also benefited, although less significantly. The laser specifically targets the affected areas so you can avoid exposing your entire body to potentially harmful UV rays. The procedure is expensive, but it can be helpful for people who suffer with moderate psoriasis, says Dr. Gottlieb.

## ROSACEA: REDUCING THE REDNESS

Rosacea is an inherited skin disorder that affects an estimated 13 million Americans—nearly three times as many woman as men. The condition is often mistaken for adult acne because it usually strikes after age 30, but its red bumps are caused by enlarged blood vessels.

Many factors can bring on the telltale flush of rosacea by dilating blood vessels. Eating spicy foods, drinking alcohol, exercising strenuously, and exposing your skin to extreme temperatures are just a few of the known triggers. You may not even notice the initial symptoms, since they're subtle: distended pores, increased oil production, swelling from bacterial inflammation, and enlarged blood vessels. The blushing that results on the face eventually becomes more noticeable, especially on the nose, chin, cheeks, and forehead. In advanced cases, inflamed lesions can develop.

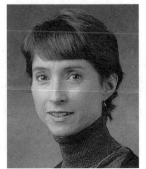

The hows and whys of rosacea are not fully understood, and there is no cure. But there are steps you can take to prevent or control flare-ups, says *Diane Thiboutot, M.D.*, staff physician at Pennsylvania State University College of Medicine in Hershey. First and foremost, see your doctor for a proper diagnosis. Rosacea is a progressive disorder, so you want to halt its advance. In addition to oral antibiotics, your physician may suggest a topical antibiotic, such as metronidazole, to diminish bumps and lesions, as well as hydrocortisone cream to reduce the redness.

*Keep a journal to help figure out what sets off your breakouts of rosacea, then avoid those triggers, says Diane Thiboutot, M.D.*

Take this advice from Dr. Thiboutot to get a handle on rosacea.

**Avoid your triggers.** Keep a journal of your flare-ups, making note of your mood, what you ate and drank, where you went, and what you did on that particular day. Look for clues as to what irritates your skin so that you can then practice avoidance. Some of the usual suspects are spicy foods, alcohol, sun exposure, hot and cold temperatures, stress, exercise, and products containing alcohol or fragrances.

**Be patient.** Triggers are highly personal: What elicits a response in the person sitting next to you in your dermatologist's waiting room may not affect you at all. Figuring out the various things that provoke your rosacea—and then making the necessary life changes—can take some time.

**Never scrub.** Don't clean with a loofah or rub your face with a washcloth. It's preferable to just use your hands.

**Conceal it.** A green- or yellow-tinted concealer, available at most makeup counters, camouflages redness well. Apply it under your foundation. You may also want to switch to a heavier foundation—but avoid powders, which can accentuate dry, flaky skin.


## SKIN CANCER: A SELF-EXAM CAN SAVE YOUR LIFE

If wrinkles are your greatest concern from sun exposure, perhaps you haven't heard that skin cancer is now the most widespread form of the disease in the United States. Nearly half of all Americans who live to age 65 will experience skin cancer at least once in their lives. And each year, about one million more will be diagnosed with it.

More alarming is that melanoma—the deadliest kind of skin cancer—has been rapidly on the rise for more than two decades, with about 51 thousand new cases occurring every year. If diagnosed and removed early, melanoma can be treated, says *Dana Sachs, M.D.,* clinical assistant physician in dermatology at Memorial Sloan-Kettering Cancer Center in New York City. But once it spreads, or metastasizes, to other parts of the body, melanoma can be lethal.

That's why it's so important to examine your body every month for suspicious spots and to protect your skin with sunscreen. (See "The Truth About Sunscreens," page 450). You are at high risk for skin cancer if you have any of the following.

- A family history of the disease
- Many moles

- Fair and freckled skin, blue or green eyes, and blonde or red hair
- A history of excessive sun exposure

If *any* of these risk factors apply to you, have your skin checked by your health-care provider each year or as often as your dermatologist recommends, says Dr. Sachs.

You might want to include a head-to-toe skin check when you perform your monthly breast self-exam. "Look for the black sheep on your skin," suggests Dr. Sachs. Check for any freckles that are new or have an unusual appearance, as well as moles that seem to have changed in shape, size, or color. If you have a family history of malignant melanoma, have

## ONE WOMAN'S STORY:MELANOMA

*Genetics and environment are two of the factors that determine a woman's risk for melanoma, the most common form of cancer.*

Susan Sullivan of Hobe Sound, Florida, was age 35 when she first noticed a pink patch of irritated skin on her inner knee. No bigger than a finger-nail, the pimplelike growth itched and bled. Sullivan questioned both her general practitioner and gynecologist about it, but neither considered it to be a cause for concern. The blemish wasn't a mole—the typical sign of skin cancer—but it bothered her nevertheless.

Six months later, Sullivan had a plastic sur-geon remove the annoyance. Then she got bad news: The routine biopsy tested positive for melanoma. Sullivan had the most deadly form of skin cancer.

A sequence of tragic events unfolded from that point on: One of Sullivans' sisters died from melanoma; a brother and another sister were subsequently also diagnosed with the disease. Sullivan steadfastly battled six recurrences over the next three decades, including one melanoma that metastasized, or spread, to other parts of her body.

Sullivan and her family learned the hard way that they had a considerable genetic risk for this form of cancer. A strawberry-blond with fair skin that freckled, Sullivan didn't really use sunscreen during her childhood. Even as an adult, she hadn't given much thought to the types she used.

Sullivan's experiences with melanoma changed her attitude toward skin protection. After years of researching sunscreens, she grew dissatis-fied with the products available. So she started her own company, www.birchtrees.com. It produces and sells nontoxic sunscreens that Sullivan believes do a better job of protecting against UVA and UVB rays than most commercial products.

Now in her 60s, Sullivan is free of cancer. She attributes this success to constant vigilance and the fact that she kept herself informed, asked pertinent questions, and sought out the right doctors. Otherwise, she might not be here today. Sullivan's advice to all women? If your doctor doesn't follow up on a skin problem that concerns you, get another opinion.

your doctor look at any new mole that appears after age 20. Also be on the lookout for these signs of possible trouble.

- A sore that doesn't heal for three weeks or more, particularly if it bleeds, oozes, or crusts
- A red, painful, itchy area
- A smooth growth with a raised border
- A white or yellow mark, similar to scar tissue
- A pearly nodule that resembles a mole (It can be red, pink, white, black, brown, or clear.)
- A rough, scaly patch that's red or brown

Some signs of skin cancer mimic skin complaints mentioned earlier in this chapter. Only a physician can determine the true nature of your condition.

*Check your body regularly for suspicious freckles and moles. Early detection is the key to successful treatment of melanoma.*—Dana Sachs, M.D.

In addition to using sunscreen, Dr. Sachs has these sun-smart suggestions.

**Invest in solar clothing.** If you're at high risk for skin cancer or spend a lot of time in the great outdoors, these special outfits are worth the money spent. Companies that offer garments on par with sun protection factor (SPF) 30 or greater include Solarveil (www.solarveil.com, 800-400-3377), Solumbra by Sun Precautions (www.sunprecautions.com, 800-882-7860), and SunGrubbies (www.sungrubbies.com, 888-970-1600).

**Love basic black.** Dark-colored clothing absorbs more ultraviolet rays than light garments and prevent rays from reaching your skin. If you'd rather not don black at the beach, remember that wearing a T-shirt of any color is better than not putting anything at all over your bathing suit.

**Go undercover.** At the beach, rent a big umbrella for shade or put on a wide-brimmed hat. Leave the straw hat at home, though, because the loose weave lets in too much light. Likewise, don't pack the baseball cap, since it won't protect your ears or the back of your neck—two common sites for skin cancer.

# 24 Urinary Tract

## Soothing Relief for Urgent Situations

*Have you ever heard that women have more urinary-tract problems than men because we're built funny down there? While such a statement may set your teeth on edge, in a strange way, it's true.*

There's nothing funny about a woman's anatomy. But the tube that empties urine from the bladder, called the urethra, is shorter in women than in men, so it's easier for bacteria to enter our urinary tracts and cause infections. Thus, women are twice as likely to have urinary-tract infections (UTIs) than men; in fact, one in five women will likely get a UTI in her lifetime. And because childbearing weakens pelvic-floor muscles, women are more likely to develop incontinence, that unintentional—and embarrassing—leakage of urine.

As if that weren't enough, women are also more prone to interstitial cystitis, a painful bladder condition that has symptoms similar to those of a UTI and results in frequent urination. The fact is that when it comes to urinary conditions, only kidney stones affect men more often than women.

On the plus side, women tend to be more pro-active about their health, and there is much we can do to treat, improve, or prevent urinary conditions, says *Carmen Ripley, N.D.*, a naturopath at A Woman's Time in Portland, Oregon, who specializes in women's urological health. "There's something wonderfully powerful and healing about taking care of one's health. And urinary-tract problems respond well to self-initiated care."

Before you read on, it might help to understand the mechanics: The urinary tract consists of the kidneys, ureters, bladder, and urethra. The kidneys are two bean-shaped organs located below your ribs at the middle of your back.

They remove extra water and waste from your blood and convert them to urine. From your kidneys, narrow tubes called ureters carry urine to your bladder, a triangle-shaped reservoir in your lower abdomen. The bladder's elastic walls stretch and expand like a balloon to store urine, then flatten when urine empties through the urethra.

Got the picture? Good. Now you'll be able to visualize more clearly how the things that help you go can sometimes go wrong.

## BLADDER INFECTIONS: BANISH BACTERIA

Although your urinary tract usually does a great job of filtering impurities from your bloodstream, it occasionally serves as an entry point for impurities. And bacteria find the warm, moist environment most hospitable. You know you have unwanted company if urinating becomes painful.

When bacteria multiply in your bladder, you feel burning and pressure, as well as the frequent need to urinate, says *Larrian Gillespie, M.D.*, a urogyne-cologist in Beverly Hills and author of *You Don't Have to Live With Cystitis*.

"We are built like French bidets: We thoroughly cleanse ourselves as we urinate," she says. "In a woman's body, the urethra is placed so that urine streams down over the labia, vagina, and perineum (the skin bridge between the vagina and rectum), then exits over the anal sphincter. Because urine is sterile, any bacteria adhering to surrounding tissues is washed away."

### SHOULD I SEE A DOCTOR?

*The signs of a urinary problem are usually hard to miss for most women.*

Most kidney stones are small enough to pass out of the body without the help of a doctor, says *Larrian Gillespie, M.D.,* a urogynecologist in Beverly Hills. However, you should call your doctor to see her the same day if any of the following apply to you:

- Your urine is bloody, cloudy, or foul smelling.
- You have a frequent urge to urinate and a burning sensation.
- You experience nausea or vomiting.
- You have chills or a fever over 100 degrees.

- You have severe pain in your lower back or side, which may move to the lower abdomen and last for minutes or hours.

These symptoms could be warning signs of a severe kidney infection or indicate a problem related to your ovaries, uterus, bladder, or appendix. If the diagnosis is a urinary-tract infection, an antibiotic can often clear it up and put an end to the discomfort. If not treated promptly, a severe infection can develop into a more serious problem with your kidneys.

If the bladder does not empty efficiently, however, bacteria remains. And that sets the stage for an infection called cystitis. A variety of factors can cause this inefficiency, ranging from a poorly fitted diaphragm to an overly perfumed bubble bath. One thing is certain: When the pain and burning starts, you want it to stop—*immediately.*

A urine culture, performed in your doctor's office, indicates which bacteria are to blame and enables your physician to prescribe an antibiotic specifically targeted to that strain. Don't expect your doctor to guess the cause and prescribe an antibiotic over the phone—this shortcut may only serve to prolong your infection, warns Dr. Gillespie.

The standard treatment for a urinary-tract infection (UTI) is antibiotics for two days to two weeks, depending on the severity of your symptoms, whether you have other medical or urinary-tract problems, or if you're pregnant. But Dr. Gillespie recommends taking a one-time dose of three pills of cephalosporin (such as Ceclor or Keflex) or sulfonamide trimethoprim (such as Bactrim or Septra) to fight an infection. "Why expose your entire body to 10 days of antibiotic therapy when a single large dose will knock the infection out rapidly and effectively?" she says. "As long as your bladder is capable of normal function and empties properly, you should feel better in a few hours."

## HOME REMEDIES FOR A COMMON PROBLEM

If you've had past infections, you'll know whether the pain of a new one is more or less intense than those you've experienced before. Antibiotics are available if needed, but improper use can lead to antibiotic-resistant bacteria in your bladder, warns *Carmen Ripley, N.D.,* a naturopath at A Woman's Time in Portland, Oregon. She says a naturopathic doctor can successfully treat most UTIs using nonpharmacological treatments, such as botanical medicine and nutritional recommendations.

*To knock out a urinary infection, load up on vitamin C at the first sign of trouble.*—Deborah L. Myers, M.D.

So before you opt for a prescription, you might want try these remedies.

**Drink up.** Urinating more often may seem like the last thing you want to do. But women with UTIs who drink an extra gallon of water a day can clear the infection in about two days, *without* the aid of antibiotics, says Dr. Ripley. If your symptoms don't improve within 24 hours, then contact your physician.

**Add vitamin C.** Taking in additional vitamin C increases the acidity of your urine, which in turn inhibits the growth of bacteria, says **Deborah L. Myers, M.D.**, an obstetrician and gynecologist at Women & Infants' Hospital of Rhode Island in Providence. At the first hint of infection, start taking 500 milligrams vitamin C twice a day, she says. If you're not better after three days, see your doctor.

## TAKING PREVENTIVE MEASURES

Prevention is usually the best medicine. To steer clear of bladder infections, follow this expert advice.

**Clean right.** Wipe yourself from front to back after all eliminations, says Dr. Ripley. While this may feel awkwardly opposite from the way you were taught to clean yourself, she says it's the best way to keep bacteria from entering the urinary tract.

> *It's not just an old wives' tale: Cranberry juice really can help prevent a bladder infection.*
>
> —*Larrian Gillespie, M.D.*

**Ditch douching.** "The vagina doesn't like smelling like flowers or soap," says Dr. Ripley. There's no need to clean the vagina internally, she says, much less introduce perfumes that can lead to irritation and infection. Plus, douching can dry out vaginal tissues, giving bacteria a better surface on which to adhere. You can wash the pubic hair with soap if you take care to rinse thoroughly, Dr. Ripley says, "but avoid using soap intravaginally."

**Drink cranberry.** Cranberry juice can work as a preventive, says Dr. Gillespie. She recommends you drink 8 ounces sugar-free juice every day. The hippuronic acid in the juice is an antiseptic that prevents *E. coli* bacteria from adhering to the lining of your bladder. Hate the red stuff? Then substitute ½ cup blueberries or 8 ounces unsweetened blueberry juice. Sugar-free juices are available at many grocery stores and health-food stores.

## INTERSTITIAL CYSTITIS: INFLAMMATION, NOT INFECTION

What you think is a bladder infection may actually be a condition called interstitial cystitis. This is not an infection at all, but rather it is an inflammation of the bladder lining that mimics the symptoms of a bladder infection, says *Deborah L. Myers, M.D.,* an obstetrician and gynecologist at Women & Infants' Hospital of Rhode Island in Providence.

Researchers are still investigating the causes of this condition, which typically involves recurrent bouts of inflammation, says *Larrian Gillespie, M.D.,* a urogynecologist in Beverly Hills and author of *You Don't Have to Live With Cystitis.* Factors linked to the problem include previous bladder infections, the effect of female reproductive hormones on the bladder lining, and lower back problems that strain the nerves in the bladder area.

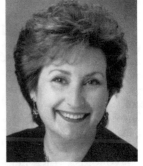

*Watch what you eat and drink if you have interstitial cystitis, warns Larrian Gillespie, M.D. Avoid anything acidic, including cranberry juice, citrus fruits, chocolate, coffee, and wine.*

Bacteria, however, is not a culprit, so antibiotics won't provide relief. Try these solutions instead.

**Drink more water.** Women who have interstitial cystitis should drink six to eight 8-ounce glasses of water a day to help relieve symptoms, says Dr. Myers. This flow of $H_2O$ will keep your urine from becoming too acidic, preventing irritation of your bladder.

**Avoid acidic liquids.** Cranberry juice and citrus fruits may help combat bacterial cystitis, but they only ramp up the misery if you have interstitial cystitis, says Dr. Gillespie. Avoid such foods and drinks as chocolate, coffee, and wine, which also increase the acidity of your urine, irritating the already damaged protective layer of your bladder.

**Try glucosamine and chondroitin.** These supplements—known for easing the inflammation in joints associated with arthritis—can also reduce inflammation in the bladder. Dr. Myers recommends a daily supplement containing 1,500 milligrams glucosamine and 1,000 milligrams chondroitin sulfate to curtail a bout of interstitial cystitis and minimize flare-ups.

**Build GAGs.** The lining of a healthy bladder is covered with a mucouslike protective layer that is mostly made up of a substance called glycosaminoglycan (GAG). When this protective layer is damaged, the underlying cells of your bladder tissue interact painfully with your urine, says Dr. Ripley. To help your body improve its GAG layer, Dr. Ripley suggests you take 400 milligrams L-arginine three times a day. She also suggests eating foods rich in omega-3 fatty acids, which are an important component for decreasing inflammation. To get enough omega-3s in your diet, Dr. Ripley recommends 1 tablespoon flaxseed daily or three to four servings a week of cold-water fish, such as salmon, sardines, and tuna.

*Glucosamine and chondroitin, known for easing arthritis pain, may also curb interstitial cystitis.—Larrian Gillespie, M.D.*

**Sip licorice.** Licorice contains anti-inflammatory glycyrrhizin, as well as flavonoids, which help heal inflamed and damaged cells. So Dr. Ripley recommends drinking a cup of licorice tea three times a day to ease the burning and help calm the spasms that sometimes accompany interstitial cystitis. Use licorice tea bags or steep ½ ounce fresh licorice root (available at health-food stores) in 1 pint boiling water for 15 minutes.

## INCONTINENCE: THERE'S NOTHING TO BE ASHAMED OF

About half of all elderly Americans are incontinent, but you don't have to be old to have the problem of not being able to control the flow of urine. It affects millions of women of all ages. For some, the leaking starts after childbirth. Others develop the condition in the years leading up to menopause and beyond. Being overweight can also sometimes bring on incontinence.

There's no reason to be embarrassed about flagging bladder control, says *Larrian Gillespie, M.D.,* a urogynecologist in Beverly Hills. "It's a medical condition and it's not your fault."

There are two types of urinary incontinence.

- Stress incontinence: This most common form of incontinence occurs if pelvic-floor muscles become stretched and weakened by childbirth, menopause, or obesity. When these sling-shaped muscles no longer hold the bladder and urethra in place properly you can experience difficulty controlling your urine flow. Any physical stress or pressure on the bladder, such as a cough or sneeze, can cause leakage.

- Urge incontinence: With this type, sudden, strong, and uncontrollable contractions cause the bladder to empty on its own accord. Older women have this type of incontinence more often than younger women. The cause may be the diminished supply of estrogen, which helps keep the muscles surrounding the bladder limber. Still, this condition is not an inevitable fate of aging. Urge incontinence may also be caused by a urinary-tract infection. More often, though, the problem results from strokes, neurological disorders, or damage to nerves in the upper back, says Dr. Gillespie. When brought on by a stroke or brain damage, urge incontinence can be controlled with medication, she says. If an infection or back injury is to blame, the condition will go away once that problem is resolved. Existing remedies can correct the problem in 8 out of 10 cases, but fewer than half of women with the condition discuss urge incontinence with their physicians.

## ONE WOMAN'S STORY: INCONTINENCE

*Incontinence isn't something most women feel comfortable talking about, even with their doctors.*

At age 35, soon after the birth of her second child, Amy Jones (not her real name) started "having little leaks" when she laughed or coughed. Although annoyed at first, she expected this stress incontinence to go away as her body returned to normal. But the problem continued.

Tired of changing soggy panties once or twice a day, Jones began wearing sanitary pads for light days around the clock. Then one day, her 4-year-old daughter dramatically sniffed and proclaimed, "Mommy, you smell like the baby when he needs his diaper changed!"

Flustered and embarrassed, Jones tried to explain away the scent, but she determined then that she would take this problem up with her gynecologist—pronto.

Her doctor recommended exercises to strengthen her pelvic-floor muscles and advised Jones to lose weight. Carrying 250 pounds on her 5'3" frame stressed Jones' pelvic-floor muscles every time she walked.

"My doctor told me that, in a nutshell, gravity is to blame," says Jones. "As these muscles get pulled down over time by babies, excess weight, and the sheer force of living, the bladder and urethra get slack." In addition to Kegel exercises, her doctor suggested vaginetics. (For more information on both exercises, see "Exercise internally," page 472.) After a month of exercising regularly, Jones lost 15 pounds and her incontinence problems disappeared. Today, her weight is down a total of 35 pounds, and she does her pelvic-floor exercises daily. "I hated the way incontinence made me feel about myself—that I was gross and out-of-control," says Jones. "Solving the problem was simple, really. But until I learned what was causing the problem, I didn't have a clue how to solve it."

Use these recommendations, treatments, exercises, and devices to help stop the uncontrolled flow of urine.

**Urinate often.** Many women sometimes hold their urine too long, says *Deborah L. Myers, M.D.,* an obstetrician and gynecologist at Women & Infants' Hospital of Rhode Island in Providence. This practice puts a great strain on your bladder, causing urine to dribble out. She suggests voiding regularly, about every three hours, whether you feel the urge or not.

**Nix stimulants.** Reduce your consumption of caffeine, artificial sweeteners, and acidic juices, which can stimulate the need to urinate, says Dr. Myers.

*Forgo the java and artificial sweeteners. Coffee and other stimulants can make incontinence worse.—Deborah L. Myers, M.D.*

**Avoid overdrinking.** Women with incontinence are the exception to the rule of drinking eight 8-ounce glasses of fluid every day. Dr. Myers advises them to drink no more than four 8-ounce glasses of fluid—preferably water—a day.

**Explore estrogen replacement.** When estrogen production wanes after menopause, the bladder and urethra muscles and nearby vaginal tissue become drier and may weaken. Estrogen replacement bolsters the nerve receptors to this area and provides more natural lubrication and muscle support, says *Carmen Ripley, N.D.,* a naturopath in Portland, Oregon, who specializes in women's health. Because there are risks associated with estrogen and hormone replacement, talk with your doctor to weigh the pros and cons of using either oral or vaginal hormonal support. Dr. Ripley suggests talking with your doctor about a bioidentical hormone. (For more on selecting the best estrogen for you, see page 256.)

**Exercise internally.** Think of the bladder as a balloon and the urethra as the knot that keeps the balloon's contents from leaking out. "If the knot has become slack, you can tighten it with exercises," says Dr. Ripley. To strengthen your urinary-tract muscles, practice tightening and relaxing the muscles that stop the flow of urine while you're voiding. These moves are known as Kegel exercises, and you can perform them anywhere, anytime, and no one will know. Dr. Ripley recommends doing five sets of 10 repetitions every day.

For 20 of the repetitions, hold the squeeze for three seconds; for the remaining 30 repetitions, hold for one second and relax for one second. You should notice improvement after about a month. But as with any workout, the benefits last only as long as you continue the exercises. Not sure if you're doing them right? Stop your urine midflow and hold it for a second before you let the flow continue. That action requires using the targeted muscles. Once you get the hang of it you can simply imagine that you're stopping the stream to perform the exercise.

Dr. Gillespie suggests you also try a technique called vaginetics: Lie faceup on the floor, with your knees bent, arms straight at your sides, and palms down flat. Lift your buttocks and pelvis off the floor to a tilt position, counterbalancing with your hands. In this position, which simultaneously tightens your stomach and back muscles, pull up and in with your vagina; hold, while you slowly count to three. Repeat as often as you can, but note that this action automatically contracts the pelvic-floor muscles so effectively that Dr. Gillespie admits she can do only five repetitions at a time.

**Try cones.** Vaginal weight training may sound odd, but it can strengthen urinary-tract muscles, says Dr. Ripley. She recommends you insert a vaginal cone, a tamponlike weight of 10 to 70 grams, and carry it inside you for only 15 minutes a day. (Hold 20 paper clips in your hand to get a sense of what 10 grams feels like.) These cones—as well as Kegel exercises—are a major help with stress incontinence. They may also help with urge incontinence, even though its underlying cause tends to be more neurological than muscular, says Dr. Ripley

**Turn yourself upside down.** Any exercise that strengthens the abdominal and lower back muscles also strengthens the urinary tract, says Dr. Ripley. She recommends practicing yoga, particularly inverted poses that use reverse gravity to "get things 'up' into the body, temporarily," and standing poses that work the center of the body.

Viparita Karani is an inverted pose that uses a bolster pillow or pile of folded blankets to support the body: Place the bolster against the wall and sit sideways on it, with one hip against the wall. Keep your hands on the floor for support as you lower your head and shoulders to rest on the floor and swing your legs up onto the wall. Then push your buttocks up against the wall as well. The small of your back should be supported by the bolster as you stretch your legs up, resting your heels against the wall. Let your body relax into the bolster and release all tension from your shoulders and neck.

Bring your arms out to your sides, with palms facing up, or encircle your head with your arms. Close your eyes, breath softly, and relax for 5 to 10 minutes. To come out of the pose, raise your hips just enough to pull the bolster out from under you. Rest your spine on the floor for a few seconds, then pull your knees into your chest and roll onto one side. Use your arms to push up to a sitting position.

**Encourage regularity.** Constipation can put undue pressure on the bladder, so you should empty your bowels regularly, without straining, says Dr. Ripley. She suggests gradually increasing the amount of fiber you eat to 15 to 25 grams a day. You can bulk up your diet by eating high-fiber vegetables, such as broccoli, or by taking a daily fiber supplement.

## *Tighten pelvic floor muscles with 50 repetitions a day of Kegel exercises.*
### *—Carmen Ripley, N.D.*

**Ask about a pessary.** If the remedies suggested so far don't ease your incontinence problem, Dr. Ripley suggests you ask your physician about a pessary. Inserted like a tampon, this plastic device puts pressure on the urethra, keeping urine from leaking out. You need to see a doctor to get the right fit for the pessary. Then you wear it all the time, removing it only during menstruation, before sexual intercourse, and for a weekly washing.

**Try a medication.** Antispasmodic drugs, such as Detrol (tolterodine) or Ditropan (oxybutynin), can help urge incontinence by reducing the frequency and intensity of bladder contractions, says Dr. Gillespie.

**Consider surgery.** In a few cases, stress incontinence can have an anatomical cause. A physical exam can reveal if the supportive tissue that closes the neck of the bladder has become slack. In such a case, surgery may be required to resupport the urethra. "It's like a face-lift for the bladder, in which saggy muscles that no longer support the bladder are surgically tightened," says Dr. Gillespie. "Once you find out what's causing the problem, discuss your treatment options with your doctor."

**Protect yourself.** If you're prone to leaking, try absorbent pads, advises Dr. Myers. Change pads often to avoid irritating your skin. You can also use a skin salve to protect delicate genital tissue. Try petroleum jelly or such zinc oxide products as Balmex or Desitin.

# KIDNEY STONES: ROCKS YOU DON'T WANT

A kidney stone is a mass that builds up on the inner surface of the kidney when combinations of chemicals crystallize abnormally, says *Jill S. Lindberg, M.D.*, director of Ochsner Medical Institution's Metabolic Bone and Stone Clinic in New Orleans. The most common chemical combinations are calcium with either oxalate or phosphate. Less common are stones composed of uric acid or magnesium phosphate. You ingest these chemicals in a normal diet. They make up such vital body parts as bones and muscles. Unfortunately, in some people, these chemicals behave weirdly and form stones. And you won't know you're among the unlucky few until your first attack.

Kidney stones are one of the most common urinary-tract disorders, affecting about 10 percent of adults at some point in their lives, typically between ages 20 and 40. And once you've had one, more will likely follow.

Extreme pain is usually the first symptom of a kidney stone. As the stone moves into the urinary tract, it can cause irritation or a blockage. You feel a sharp, cramping pain in your back and side, near the affected kidney or in your lower abdomen. You may also feel nauseous or vomit, and the pain may spread to your groin. As the stone moves down the ureter and closer to the bladder, you may feel a burning sensation when you void or see blood in your urine.

With sufficient fluid intake, most kidney stones can be passed naturally with the urine, says Dr. Lindberg. But you may require one of the following medical treatments if the stone is too big to pass, particularly if it is causing an ongoing urinary-tract infection, pain, or constant bleeding.

- Extracorporeal shockwave lithotripsy (ESWL): This noninvasive outpatient procedure is the one most frequently used to treat kidney stones that are too large to pass on their own. ESWL sends high-energy shock waves through your body, smashing a kidney stone into sandlike particles that easily pass through the urinary tract. Although there is only minimal discomfort, patients are placed under anesthesia to make sure they don't move during the procedure. Over the course of about an hour, 1,000 to 2,000 shockwaves hit the stone, then hit its fragments as the stone breaks up.

- Surgery: Cutting into the kidney to remove a stone is an option of last resort today, performed in less than 5 percent of cases, says *Larrian Gillespie, M.D.*, a urogynecologist in Beverly Hills. It is done only when a stone is too large to be broken up with ESWL (larger than 2 centimeters) and threatens kidney function. Even then, less invasive surgical techniques are often favored. These include:

— Ureteroscopy, performed under general anesthesia, usually involves the insertion of an instrument through the urethra and bladder, and directly into the ureter to locate the stone and pull it out. Another ureteroscopy method eases a laser tool along the same route, and the laser vaporizes the stone inside the ureter.

— With percutaneous nephrolithotomy, a small incision is made through the patient's back and into the affected kidney. Special tools are inserted to locate and grab the stone. The advantage to this surgery is that the tissue of the kidney is relatively undisturbed, says Dr. Gillespie.

## STOPPING STONES BEFORE THEY START

If you've ever had a kidney stone, you won't need to be convinced to do everything you can to prevent another from forming. First, your doctor needs to determine what caused that first stone, says Dr. Lindberg. To figure that out, your doctor will perform a series of urine and blood tests, review your medical history and eating habits, and study a laboratory analysis of the stone, if possible.

Genetics play a major role in the formation of kidney stones. "Everyone makes crystals in their urine, but not everyone's crystals turn into stones," says Dr. Lindberg. Most people produce chemicals that prevent crystals from becoming stones, but about 10 percent of the population don't. So if anyone in your immediate family had kidney stones, you're more likely to have them. And as we said before, once you've had one, you're susceptible to more. To help prevent recurrences, your doctor may suggest one of the following medications, which prevent formation of calcium and uric-acid crystals.

• Allopurinol: Sold under the brand name Aloprim or Zyloprim, this gout medication is used to control uric-acid levels in the blood and urine. It is also prescribed to combat uric-acid stones, which account for 1 to 2 percent of cases. Doctors give allopurinol to patients who continue to have high uric-acid levels in their blood despite dietary changes, says Dr. Lindberg.

• Polycitra-K (potassium citrate): Your doctor may prescribe this drug to make your urine less acidic, if your urine has low citrate levels, high uric levels, or high calcium levels. Changing the acidity of urine helps prevent crystal compounds from clustering into stones, says Dr. Lindberg. Potassium citrate naturally occurs in citrus fruits, she says, "but it would be impossible to eat the amount needed to prevent kidney stones," hence the prescription formulation.

- Thiazide: This diuretic—sold under brand names such as Aquatensen and Esidrix—can prevent the recurrence of calcium kidney stones in people genetically predisposed to them, says Dr. Gillespie. It works by decreasing the excretion of calcium in the urine.

Lifestyle changes can also go a long way toward keeping you free from the agony of kidney stones. To avoid getting future stones, try out these nonpharmacological remedies.

**Drink up.** Drinking more liquids is a simple way to prevent kidney stones, says Dr. Lindberg. She recommends drinking at least two quarts fluid—water is best—each day. She suggests you should avoid iced tea because it can encourage urinary oxalate excretion, leading to stone formation.

*Limit how much chocolate and black tea you consume to help avoid those painful kidney stones.—Jill S. Lindberg, M.D.*

**Eat wisely.** A commonsense diet may be the ticket to keep kidney stones at bay, says Dr. Lindberg. A diet high in meat may encourage stone formation, she says, noting that when Third World countries adopt a Western-style diet built around meat, kidney stones become a never-seen-before medical problem. She recommends eating no more than 6 ounces of red meat, fish, or poultry a day if you're prone to forming kidney stones. Also avoid such high oxalate-containing foods and beverages as chocolate and black tea.

Contrary to popular belief, there's no need to avoid calcium if you tend to get kidney stones, assures Dr. Lindberg. Low-calcium diets lead to an increase in urinary oxalate, promoting stone formation. "In addition, stone-formers are prone to bone loss, and calcium restriction may exacerbate this," she says.

# 25 Weight Control
## Winning the Battle
## of the Bulge

*If you want to get a grip on your magnified midriff, the formula for success is as elementary as grade school arithmetic: Eat less and move more.*

In ancient times, fat was a rare and valuable asset. Having a few extra pounds to draw upon during periods of famine could be the difference between life and death. But times have changed, and more than half of all Americans are now overweight.

No people on earth have ever been as well-fed as Americans are today. Across the United States are thousands of neighborhood grocery stores, overflowing with plenty. Restaurants routinely serve up to five times what you should eat as a serving size. And all those super-sized fries add up: The average American woman eats more than a ton of food a year. But at least 75 percent of women don't get enough exercise to compensate for the culinary overload. The risk we face is no longer one of starving, but of eating ourselves to death.

The good news is that getting your weight under control requires just one simple strategy: Eat less and move more. "This may be boring advice, but it's what works," says **Lisa R. Young, Ph.D., R.D.,** a nutrition consultant and adjunct assistant professor in the department of nutrition and food studies at New York University.

Few women go through life without ever worrying about their weight. But how much should you weigh? What does it really mean if you weigh in at a higher number? And the big question: What does it take to get excess weight off and keep it off? Our experts have the answers that will help you make peace with your weight.

# BODY MASS INDEX: ARE YOU OVERWEIGHT?

If you're overweight, chances are you already know it by the bulges around your waist and in your thighs. But there are more scientific clues.

The body mass index (BMI) evaluates your weight in relation to your height. Here's how to find your BMI in the chart below: Find your height on the top line, then run your finger down that column to the row that aligns with your weight in pounds. If your BMI is:

- less than 18.5, you are considered underweight;
- between 19 and 24.9, you are in good shape;
- between 25 and 29.9, you are overweight;
- between 30 and 39, you are obese;
- 40 or higher, you are considered extremely obese.

Keep in mind that muscle weighs more than fat. If you are very muscular, a high BMI isn't necessarily unhealthy.

| Height | 5'0" | 5'1" | 5'2" | 5'3" | 5'4" | 5'5" | 5'6" | 5'7" | 5'8" | 5'9" | 5'10" | 5'11" | 6'0" |
|---|---|---|---|---|---|---|---|---|---|---|---|---|---|
| Weight (lbs) | | | | | BODY MASS INDEX | | | | | | | | |
| 120 | 23 | 23 | 22 | 21 | 21 | 20 | 19 | 19 | 18 | 18 | 17 | 17 | 16 |
| 125 | 24 | 24 | 23 | 22 | 21 | 21 | 20 | 20 | 19 | 18 | 18 | 17 | 17 |
| 130 | 25 | 25 | 24 | 23 | 22 | 22 | 21 | 20 | 20 | 19 | 19 | 18 | 18 |
| 135 | 26 | 26 | 25 | 24 | 23 | 22 | 22 | 21 | 21 | 20 | 19 | 19 | 18 |
| 140 | 27 | 26 | 26 | 25 | 24 | 23 | 23 | 22 | 21 | 21 | 20 | 20 | 19 |
| 145 | 28 | 27 | 27 | 26 | 25 | 24 | 23 | 23 | 22 | 21 | 21 | 20 | 20 |
| 150 | 29 | 28 | 27 | 27 | 26 | 25 | 24 | 23 | 23 | 22 | 22 | 21 | 20 |
| 155 | 30 | 29 | 28 | 27 | 27 | 26 | 25 | 24 | 24 | 23 | 22 | 22 | 21 |
| 160 | 31 | 30 | 29 | 28 | 27 | 27 | 26 | 25 | 24 | 24 | 23 | 22 | 22 |
| 165 | 32 | 31 | 30 | 29 | 28 | 27 | 27 | 26 | 25 | 24 | 24 | 23 | 22 |
| 170 | 33 | 32 | 31 | 30 | 29 | 28 | 27 | 27 | 26 | 25 | 24 | 24 | 23 |
| 175 | 34 | 33 | 32 | 31 | 30 | 29 | 28 | 27 | 27 | 26 | 25 | 24 | 24 |
| 180 | 35 | 34 | 33 | 32 | 31 | 30 | 29 | 28 | 27 | 27 | 26 | 25 | 24 |
| 185 | 36 | 35 | 34 | 33 | 32 | 31 | 30 | 29 | 28 | 27 | 27 | 26 | 25 |
| 190 | 37 | 36 | 35 | 34 | 33 | 32 | 31 | 30 | 29 | 28 | 27 | 26 | 26 |
| 195 | 38 | 37 | 36 | 35 | 33 | 32 | 31 | 31 | 30 | 29 | 28 | 27 | 26 |
| 200 | 39 | 38 | 37 | 35 | 34 | 33 | 32 | 31 | 30 | 30 | 29 | 28 | 27 |
| 205 | 40 | 39 | 37 | 36 | 35 | 34 | 33 | 32 | 31 | 30 | 29 | 29 | 28 |
| 210 | 41 | 40 | 38 | 37 | 36 | 35 | 34 | 33 | 32 | 31 | 30 | 29 | 28 |

These numbers are rounded off due to space limitations. For a more detailed BMI chart, log on to www.nhlbi.nih.gov/guidelines/obesity/bmi_tbl.htm.

More and more, doctors are finding that it's not simply extra weight that causes problems but where that weight settles. The more fat you carry around your abdomen, the more likely you are to develop obesity-related health problems, such as diabetes, heart disease, and high blood pressure. A woman's waist should measure 35 inches or less. (A man's waist should be 40 inches or less.) Exceed these measurements, and your health risks also increase.

## FAT FACTORS: WHY ARE YOU OVERWEIGHT?

It's not hard to figure out the reason that most people become overweight: They consume more calories than they burn. The fat cells that store these extra calories expand as you pack on the pounds, as do the areas of your body in which these cells reside, usually the hips, thighs, and waist.

This storage process can be affected by genetics, environment, emotions, some medical problems (such as an underactive thyroid), and some medications (such as birth control pills and antidepressants). Age also plays a role because your metabolism gradually slows after about age 25, although you have a good shot at combating this cause with the right amount of exercise and a healthy diet. But there's little doubt that overeating is the number-one reason for those ever-tightening jeans.

*You're more likely to inherit bad habits from your parents than bad genes. Overeating is the number-one reason for obesity.*—Terry Maratos-Flier, M.D.

### NATURE OR NURTURE?

Don't be too quick to point a finger at Mom or Dad as you gaze at your girth in the mirror. Obesity does tend to run in families, but that may be because children adopt the diet and exercise habits of their parents—for better or for worse. "People with a body mass index (BMI) at the lower end of the obese category probably gain weight because of a combination of overeating, lack of exercise, and lack of awareness about their diet," says *Terry Maratos-Flier, M.D.*, associate professor of medicine at Harvard Medical School and an investigator at the Joslin Diabetes Center in Boston.

It's true that people who are extremely obese, with a very high BMI, may have a genetic problem, says Dr. Maratos-Flier. Research indicates that genes seem to affect your body's ability to produce and use certain hormones. An obese individual may have a genetic imbalance in the hormones that suppress appetite (and, thus, help control your weight) or that stimulate the urge to eat when your body doesn't have enough fat.

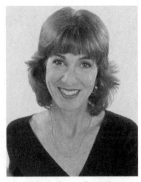

You can use diet and exercise to fight your obesity genes, says Susan Burke, M.S., R.D., C.D.E.

But don't despair: Obesity-prone genes don't condemn you to a life sentence of excess pounds. "Although your genes will determine your metabolism to a large extent, you can fight the odds by eating well, exercising, and building muscle," says *Susan L. Burke, M.S., R.D, C.D.E.,* director of nutrition services at eDiets.com.

## WEIGHTY RISKS: WHY YOU NEED TO TAKE ACTION

The health consequences of being overweight or obese can be dire. According to the National Institutes of Health, overweight and obese women are at high risk of dying from ovarian, cervical, uterine, and breast cancers. They also have high rates of infertility, menstrual difficulties, breathing problems, and gallbladder disease. In addition, excess weight increases strain on the joints, contributing to osteoarthritis.

Then there are the emotional struggles that heavy women face. In today's world, to be attractive is to be thin. Overweight people are often perceived as gluttonous or lazy, and may encounter discrimination in social situations and the workplace. All this can lead to feelings of depression, shame, and rejection.

Fortunately, even a small weight reduction can pay off in big ways. "Overweight women who lose only 5 to 10 percent of their body weight will see their health improve," says *Kim Crawford, M.S., R.D.,* program director for clinical dietetics and nutrition at the University of Pittsburgh. High blood pressure and cholesterol levels decline, and women with diabetes begin to have more manageable blood-sugar levels.

The best way to prevent or fight becoming overweight is to modify your lifestyle *gradually.* "You don't necessarily need to join a health club or

# Losing just 5 to 10 percent of your body weight can improve your overall health.—Kim Crawford, M.S., R.D.

change every food habit you ever had," says **Bonnie Brehm, Ph.D., R.D.,** assistant professor in the college of nursing at the University of Cincinnati. "You just need to make small adjustments in your daily routine."

Think of successful weight loss as a three-legged stool, with the legs representing attitude, dietary changes, and exercise. The stool won't stand without all three legs to support it.

## ATTITUDE: MAKE UP YOUR MIND TO SUCCEED

"Almost any professional approach—be it through a dietician or weight-loss organization—can provide you with a healthy weight-loss plan. But you must be prepared to follow it," says **Susan Burke, M.S., R.D, C.D.E.,** director of nutrition services at eDiets.com. Learn how to foster a healthy attitude that can pave the way to a slimmer way of life.

**Know yourself.** "You can't fix something if you don't know what's wrong with it," says **Franca Alphin, M.P.H., R.D., L.D.N.,** chief dietitian for the Duke University Sports Performance Program in Durham, North Carolina.

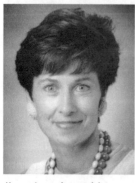

*Keep a journal to track how much you eat and exercise, suggests Franca Alphin, M.P.H., R.D., L.D.N. You probably don't realize how it really adds up.*

So you need to take a hard look at your habits for the causes of your weight gain or inability to lose weight. Alphin suggests you start by keeping a written account of *everything* you eat and drink. At the same time, record what you do for exercise. After a few days—including at least one weekend day—you should have enough information to study. Look for the trouble spots: How many times did you eat more than you should because you just *had* to clean your plate? How much did you exercise? If you're like most people, your patterns will be fairly evident, and you can work out what you need to change.

**Set realistic goals.** "If you're in your 40s or 50s, it just isn't realistic to strive for your high school weight," says *Kim Crawford, M.S., R.D.,* program director for clinical dietetics and nutrition at the University of Pittsburgh. Instead, set your sights on losing just 5 to 10 percent of your weight at a time. "If you weigh 200 pounds, that's 10 to 20 pounds, which is doable and a good start," says Crawford. Success achieved through small goals will help you feel motivated and competent to tackle larger ones.

**Start slowly.** Resolve to take one small step at a time. If you're used to eating out five times a week, you're likely to fail if you swear off restaurants all of a sudden. "You can still eat out but try to do it less often," advises Burke. And make a few changes when you do: Choose restaurants that offer a menu with some sensible options. (Fast-food joints usually don't qualify.) Avoid that smorgasbord of temptation, the all-you-can-eat buffet. Instead of filling up on fattening nachos or buttered bread, start your meal with a salad with dressing on the side. Then share your entrée or ask the waiter to doggie-bag half your meal. Little changes can reap big benefits, says Burke.

**Shop for success.** An organized plan for the grocery store is one key to succeeding. Carefully map out meals for the week, then buy only the foods on your list. Burke suggests you challenge yourself with fun food games (besides avoiding the bakery section): See how many different colored fruits and vegetables you can buy this trip. Discover which bread or cereal packs the most fiber per serving. Find a new low-fat product to try. Choose foods that will satisfy as well as give you the nutrients you need. Enjoying such good-for-you foods as fresh raspberries or low-fat ice-cream sandwiches entice you to stick with your plan much better than foods that make you feel deprived.

**Believe in yourself.** Remember that you've chosen to lose weight and that you have the power and responsibility to succeed in your efforts, says Burke. Make the decision to eat grilled veggies instead of a hamburger because it's a wise choice that helps you feel good about yourself, not because you feel you must deprive yourself. On the other hand, you shouldn't beat yourself up if you slip up and have a cookie or some ice cream, adds *Lisa R. Young, Ph.D., R.D.,* a nutrition consultant and adjunct assistant professor in the department of nutrition and food studies at New York University. Just know that you have the strength to get back on track. So instead of grumbling as you go out the door for your daily walk, try smiling. Celebrate your health, as well as your ability to set goals and meet them.

## HEAVY FEELINGS: THE EMOTIONAL CAUSES OF OVERWEIGHT

*The tendency to overeat is often fueled by emotions. You must recognize and deal with negative feelings in order to overcome a weight problem.*

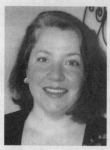

*Try exercise and body therapy, such as yoga or tai chi, to eliminate the stress in your life that prompts you to overeat, says Ana Squellati, N.D.*

Making people confront the emotions that spur them on to overeat is one of the first steps in effectively treating a weight problem, says *Ana Squellati, N.D.,* of diMedici Natural Family Medicine in Gresham, Oregon. Emotions can cause us to eat to excess for a variety of reasons, which may include the following:

**Numb negative emotions.** "Some people eat to relieve anger or frustration, or to distract themselves from thoughts they do not wish to pursue," says *Judith Wurtman, Ph.D.,* research scientist at the Massachusetts Institute of Technology and founder and director of Harvard University's TRIAD Weight Management Center. An emotional eater uses food to deal with depression, loneliness, or emotional exhaustion, she says. They often eat in direct response to the feelings they are trying to quell.

**Boost low self-esteem.** "Overweight and obese women often lack the self-esteem and self-confidence needed to attempt and continue weight-loss efforts," says *Bonnie Brehm, Ph.D., R.D.,* assistant professor in the College of Nursing at the University of Cincinnati. "Their past failures with weight loss and in other facets of their lives lead to negative self-talk, which reinforces their negative self-image and leads women to give up on being healthy," she says. "They use food as comfort."

**Relieve stress.** "When I work with a client, we really look at the person's relationship with food and what it means to them," says Dr. Squellati. "We find that stress is often a big component of overeating."

**Ease boredom.** "Eating is a quick, relatively cheap form of recreation," notes Dr. Wurtman.

Try these tactics to combat your emotional overeating:

**Tackle the stress.** Find a calorie-free means of winding down. "Partake in some sort of body therapy, such as yoga, tai chi, or meditation," suggests Dr. Squellati. "Do all three or pick the one you resonate with." Add two or three of these sessions to your weekly fitness routine to help you relax and address stress.

**Nourish your spirit.** Don't neglect yourself in the daily grind of caring for everyone else. "Create some space in your day that's just for you," says Dr. Squellati. You may be challenged to fit time into your busy schedule, but you'll benefit from the effort. Shut your office door for 15 minutes and just relax, or soak in a hot bath after the kids are in bed.

**Consider counseling.** You may need to consult a therapist to help you identify, avoid, or eliminate the emotional issues that are causing you to overeat, advises Dr. Wurtman.

## DIETARY CHANGES: FIND NEW FAVORITES

Trim your diet and your waistline will soon follow. Learn to make better food choices and forge new eating habits.

**Choose nutrient-dense foods.** If you're eating less, you also have to eat smart to get the appropriate nutrition. "When you're trying to lose weight, the best thing you can do is select foods that pack the most nutrients," says *Lesley White, Ph.D.,* assistant professor in the department of Exercise and Sports Sciences at the University of Florida in Gainesville. "A 500-calorie cinnamon bun provides minimal nutrients. For 100 calories *less,* you can eat a piece of whole-grain bread, a banana, *and* a glass of skim milk—and get fiber, potassium, and calcium."

*Measure to make sure you eat an accurate portion. Recommended servings are often smaller than you think.—Terri Maratos-Flier, M.D.*

**Measure first.** Few people recognize correct portions by sight, says *Terry Maratos-Flier, M.D.,* associate professor of medicine at Harvard Medical School and an investigator at the Joslin Diabetes Center. "You'll find that most recommended portions are smaller than you think," she says. For example, a serving of meat equals the size of a deck of cards, bar of soap, or audio cassette tape. A serving of rice is the size of a small fist; a slice of bread is approximately the width and height of a CD case. A baked potato should be the size of a computer mouse, a serving of cheese is about equal to four dice, and a serving of fruit is roughly the size of a tennis ball.

Use measuring cups and a kitchen scale to measure out your servings. Soon you'll be able to judge proper portions when your scale isn't handy.

**Watch the carbs.** Americans eat at least 100 calories more a day from carbohydrates than they did in 1970 and have been getting proportionately fatter ever since. "It's my personal view that high-carbohydrate diets cause a rise in blood sugar," says Dr. Maratos-Flier. A meal high in simple carbohydrates, such as pasta or white bread, can send your blood sugar soaring—and when it crashes a few hours later, the landing isn't soft. "The low blood sugar then makes you hungry again," says Dr. Maratos-Flier. But only simple carbs are bad. Complex carbohydrates, such as those in whole-grain oats and legumes, provide fiber and nutrients. And because these foods are digested more slowly, they stay in your bloodstream longer and prevent that blood-sugar crash.

"Nutritional guidelines recommend that you get approximately 55 to 60 percent of your calories from carbohydrates," says *Lisa R. Young, Ph.D., R.D.,* a nutrition consultant and adjunct assistant professor New York University's department of nutrition and food studies. That translates to 300 grams carbohydrates for a 2,000-calorie diet or 225 grams for a 1,500-calorie diet. Many people think of carbohydrates in terms of bread and potatoes,

## SHOULD I SEE A DOCTOR?

*Being overweight hurts more than your pride. Those extra pounds can be a major threat to your health.*

Call for a doctor's appointment if any of the following are true for you:

**I'm obese.** "If your body mass index, or BMI, is over 30, you should definitely be seeing your doctor annually," says *Bonnie Brehm, Ph.D., R.D.,* assistant professor in the College of Nursing at the University of Cincinnati. "You have a substantial risk of developing high blood pressure and high blood sugar." These conditions have hidden signs and symptoms that can be detected only with a blood pressure check or a blood test.

**I'm overweight.** "The risk of significant health problems—such as high blood pressure, Type II diabetes, and high cholesterol—begins with a BMI of 26," says *Jana Klauer, M.D.,* research fellow at the New York Obesity Research Center at St. Luke's-Roosevelt Hospital Center at Columbia University. "When you exceed that number, you should consult your doctor." Aim to keep your BMI within a range of 18.5 to 24.9. (See page 479.)

**I've recently gained 10 pounds or more.** A sudden and unexplained weight gain can indicate a medical condition. "If you're at a normal weight and you gain 10 pounds all of a sudden, address it with your doctor," suggests Dr. Klauer.

"You could be developing hypothyroidism, or your weight gain could be caused by a medication you take, such as antidepressants or birth control pills."

**I regularly binge.** "When a woman realizes that she's binging regularly, she should see a doctor," says Dr. Klauer. "That's not normal behavior."

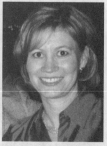

*If you are overweight, your doctor should check your blood pressure and blood sugar once a year, advises Bonnie Brehm, Ph.D., R.D.*

**I've done everything right, but....** What if you do everything right to lose weight in a healthful way and have no success? If you haven't lost a pound after six to eight weeks of healthy eating and moderate exercise, you may want to have a medical screening. You could have a medical problem, such as hypothyroidism, that can limit your ability to lose weight, says *Franca Alphin, M.P.H., R.D., L.D.N.,* chief dietitian for the Duke University Sports Performance Program in Durham, North Carolina.

but carbs are found in a range of food groups: grains, rice, cereals, fruits, vegetables, dairy, and beans. Aim for 6 to 11 servings of carbohydrates per day, which could include the following.

- One slice of bread
- 1 ounce ready-to-eat cereal
- Two to four fruits, or one medium fruit and 6 ounces juice
- Three to five vegetables, 1 cup raw or ½ cup cooked
- Two to four dairy products, such as 8 ounces milk or yogurt

**Forgo your fear of fats.** Contrary to what you might have heard, fat is not your enemy, even when it comes to weight loss. You *need* fat in your diet. "Fat contributes to satiety and fullness, enhances flavor, transports fat-soluble nutrients, and becomes part of cell membranes," says Dr. Young. She says that about 30 percent of your daily calories should come from fat, meaning you can have 67 grams with a 2,000-calorie diet or 53 grams with a 1,500-calorie diet. The following sampling of foods contain a *total* of about 65 grams of fat.

- Walnuts, 1 ounce: 18.5 grams
- Peanut butter, chunky-style, 2 tablespoons: 16 grams
- Sunflower seeds, 1 ounce: 14.1 grams
- Oil-and-vinegar salad dressing, made with olive, canola, soy, or safflower oil, 2 tablespoons: 13.5 grams
- Cheddar cheese, 1 ounce: 9.4 grams
- Salmon, canned, 3 ounces: 5.1 grams

**Know which fats are friendly.** All fats contain the same number of calories and affect weight in the same way. But the fats you eat can make all the difference to your heart's health, and obesity is a major risk factor for heart disease. Certain fats are fine in the right portions, such as the unsaturated fat in a 1-ounce serving of walnuts or pecans, or 1 tablespoon olive, canola, soy, or safflower oil. The omega-3 fatty acids in a 3- to 4-ounce serving of tuna or salmon are also good for your heart, says Dr. Maratos-Flier. Unsaturated fats and omega-3 fatty acids lower levels of LDL, the bad cholesterol, and raise levels of HDL, the good cholesterol.

Steer clear of saturated fat and trans fats. Eating foods high in saturated fat puts you at risk for atherosclerosis, better known as clogging of the arteries. That's why you need to limit how often you eat high-fat dairy products, red meat, and poultry skin, which are all high in saturated fats. Eating trans fats, found in margarine and commercial baked goods, puts you at an even greater risk for heart disease because they raise LDL and lower HDL. Healthy alternatives to butter and margarine include such plant-based products as Take Control and Benecol, available at most grocery stores, says *Jana Klauer, M.D.*, research fellow at the New York Obesity Research Center at St. Luke's-Roosevelt Hospital Center at Columbia University.

**Eat protein appropriately.** When you're trying to lose weight, you should eat the recommended daily allowance of protein—no more and no less, says *Barbara Rolls, Ph.D.*, professor of nutrition at Pennsylvania State University and co-author of *The Volumetrics Weight Control Plan*. Protein helps you feel full, and

| Protein Requirements | |
|---|---|
| Weight (pounds) | Recommended protein consumption per day (grams) |
| 110 | 40 |
| 130 | 47 |
| 150 | 54 |
| 180 | 65 |
| 210 | 76 |

its chemical composition requires your body to use energy to metabolize it. (Translation: You burn calories!) But that's not an excuse to eat unlimited amounts because you can get too much protein. Recommendations, determined by your body weight, are shown in the chart above.

*Protein helps you feel full and you burn calories metabolizing it, says Barbara Rolls, Ph.D.*

Check product labels for protein content or reference a book that lists nutritional values. (There are many such books available. A good choice is *The Complete Book of Food Counts* by Corinne T. Netzer.) Look at how much protein the following foods contain.

- Sirloin steak, 3 ounces: 26 grams
- Chicken breast, roasted, 3 ounces: 26 grams
- Tuna, white, canned, 3 ounces: 20.1 grams
- Low-fat yogurt, plain, 1 cup: 12 grams
- Kidney beans, boiled without salt, ½ cup: 7.6 grams
- One egg, hard-boiled: 6.3 grams

**Veg out.** "If you munch on broccoli, celery, and carrots, you'll fill up and be less likely to eat too many calories," says Dr. Maratos-Flier. Other healthy choices include cauliflower, zucchini, tomatoes, eggplant, spinach, and mushrooms. But don't overindulge in starchy vegetables. "Corn, potatoes, peas, butternut or acorn squash, and sweet potatoes each have 80 calories per serving, versus the 25 calories in a serving of a nonstarchy vegetable," says *Kim Crawford, M.S., R.D.*, program director for clinical dietetics and nutrition at the University of Pittsburgh. They are still nutritious, but you shouldn't eat them as freely as their less caloric cousins. Add more veggies to your diet by incorporating them into pasta dishes, pizzas, omelets, and soups. If you cook your veggies, go easy on the butter or oil.

**Pick lots of fruits.** Most fruits are high in fiber and nutrients, as well as relatively low in calories. To ensure variety, eat plenty of fresh apples, pears, grapes, and bananas. Try to eat at least one daily serving of citrus fruit, such as orange, tangerine, or grapefruit. In the summer, you can enjoy fresh blueberries, strawberries, cherries, and plums. Dr. Klauer recommends keeping your freezer stocked with frozen fruits—just make sure they don't contain sugar or preservatives. Then you can snack on fruits year-round. Try adding them to your favorite smoothie.

*Eat plenty of fiber. It fills you up, helps reduce bad cholesterol, and lowers your risk for colon cancer.*
*—Jana Klauer, M.D.*

**Roughage up.** High-fiber foods are digested and absorbed more slowly than other foods, so you feel full longer when you eat them. And fiber moves food through your intestines, which lowers your risk for colon cancer. "Fiber also helps reduce LDL, the bad form of cholesterol," says Dr. Klauer.

Try to eat at least 25 to 35 grams fiber a day. Fruits, vegetables, and whole grains are excellent sources of fiber. Check out the amount of fiber in these common foods.

- Corn bran, 2 tablespoons: 7.9 grams
- Raspberries, 1 cup: 6 grams
- Whole wheat spaghetti, 1 cup: 5.4 grams
- Succotash (corn and lima beans), ½ cup: 5.2 grams
- Pear, one medium: 4.3 grams
- Wheat germ, toasted, ½ cup: 3.7 grams
- Apple, one medium: 3 grams
- Squash, baked, ½ cup: 2.9 grams
- Spinach, boiled, ½ cup: 2 grams

"Buy bread with more than 3 grams fiber per slice and cereals with at least 5 grams per serving," says Dr. Klauer. She recommends Kashi's Good Friends and Go Lean as excellent high-fiber cereals. With a whopping 13 grams fiber per serving, All-Bran with Extra Fiber also packs a powerful punch.

*Water helps flush out fat, so drink up. Cut back on fruit juices and soft drinks, which are loaded with calories.*—Lisa R. Young, Ph.D., R.D.

**Wash it down.** "Drink at least 10 (8-ounce) glasses of water per day," advises Dr. Young. "Water may help flush fat out of your system and, more importantly, contributes to feelings of fullness." To help you meet your daily quota, keep a water bottle with you at all times.

**Be judicious with other liquids.** Believe it or not, that shot glass–sized serving of orange juice you get at most diners is exactly how much you should be drinking. "You can easily consume 10 percent of your daily calories just by drinking an 8-ounce glass of apple or orange juice," says Dr. Maratos-Flier. Other beverages also serve up a load of calories, while not filling you up: Eight ounces (less than a can) of cola contains 100 calories, and 6 ounces of wine is about 120 calories (red varieties serve up a few more calories than white). "If you forgo a single can of soda or bottle of sweetened iced tea or lemonade each day, you could lose up to 16 pounds in a year," adds *Franca Alphin, M.P.H., R.D., L.D.N.*, chief dietitian for the Duke University Sports Performance Program in Durham, North Carolina.

**Look out for imposters.** If you thought a bran muffin was a healthful, calorie-wise choice for breakfast on the go, think again. "Each muffin can have up to 500 calories and 25 grams fat, which is equivalent to a bacon cheeseburger," says Crawford. "If you're trying to diet, would you eat a bacon cheeseburger for breakfast?" Other calorie-dense foods that hide behind a healthful façade include turkey or chicken hot dogs, fruit and grain bars, granola, and frozen yogurt. "There are some lower calorie versions of all these foods, like a smoked turkey hot dog with 45 calories," says Crawford. "The point is, you must read labels. Don't let the names fool you. Know the calorie counts of the foods you're eating."

**Recognize your Achilles' heel.** We all find some foods hard to resist. "Whether your weakness is ice cream, cookies, chocolate, or bread, identify it," says Crawford. "Then get it out of your house, at least at the beginning of your weight-loss program." You may or may not be able to exercise willpower. So why test yourself? Remove temptation to make it easier for you to lose weight.

**Think small.** When you want an occasional indulgence, go for a small portion. "Instead of buying a giant bag of chips that you can gobble mindlessly, buy a little individual bag and eat only that amount," says Crawford. It may be more expensive to buy small, but if you lose weight and become healthier, you'll save more money in the long run.

**Start the day right.** "A large percentage of women skip breakfast, which is a mistake," says Crawford. Eating actually increases your metabolism. So when you don't have breakfast, you burn fewer calories. And if the skipped meal leaves you hungry, you're more likely to overeat as the day unfolds. This is particularly true in the late afternoon and evening when you lose concentration and focus, increasing the tendency to make poor food choices. "People think, 'Hey, I didn't eat breakfast so I can have an ice-cream sundae or chips and a beer after dinner,' " says Crawford. "But they probably never would have eaten that type of food or that many calories at breakfast."

*Skipping breakfast is a misguided strategy that often results in making inappropriate food choices later in the day.*—Kim Crawford, M.S., R.D.

**Have a strategy.** "Generally, the recommendation is for people to eat one-third of their calories at breakfast, one-third at lunch, and one-third at dinner," says Crawford. If you're a snacker or not very hungry at breakfast, you can save some of those calories for a midmorning snack. "For example, if you were planning to eat two pieces of wheat toast, a cup of yogurt, and a glass of orange juice for breakfast, you could save the yogurt for a snack," she says. Use the same approach with your lunch and dinner calories.

**Eat more than once a day.** "Calories eaten all at once are probably more readily converted to fat than the same number of calories distributed throughout the day," says Dr. Maratos-Flier. You're also better off eating multiple meals if you exercise. A British study found that eating light and often is a more effective eating pattern for physically active people than eating large meals. This doesn't mean you should force yourself to snack if you don't want to, adds Crawford. But, in general, you shouldn't go more than about four hours without eating.

**Snack smart.** A snack should be a bridge between meals, not a full meal in itself. "Aim for no more than 200 calories in a snack," recommends Crawford. "Eat things that satiate you, like fruits, vegetables, and low-fat yogurt." Here are some examples of snacks that fit that bill.

- Peanut butter, 1 tablespoon, spread on 5 whole wheat crackers: 185 calories
- Fresh blueberries (½ cup) with low-fat plain yogurt, 1 cup: 183 calories
- Low-fat (1-percent milk fat) cottage cheese, 1 cup: 163 calories
- Part-skim mozzarella cheese, 2 ounces: 158 calories
- Minestrone soup, 1 cup: 123 calories

**Beware of huge food.** Calorie catastrophes can lurk in unsuspected places. "The average bagel is equal to *five* servings of bread," says Dr. Young. "The average deli cookie can be up to 700 percent larger than the government's definition of a cookie." Yikes! Other dangerous items include muffins, chocolate bars, and sodas, which are sometimes much bigger than a recommended serving. If a serving seems very large, share it. Better yet, just pass it by.

**Head straight for dessert.** If you're looking forward to having a dish of ice cream or sliver of cheesecake for dessert, go ahead and eat it. But do so immediately after you take your last bite of dinner, advises Crawford. If you're still feeling full from dinner, you'll be better able to eat a serving within your weight-loss guidelines.

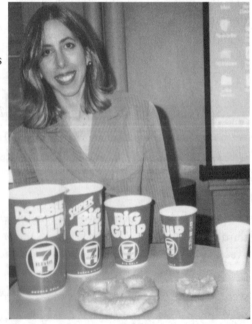

*Can you spot the recommended serving size? An overly large portion can be a calorie catastrophe, warns Lisa R. Young, Ph.D., R.D. Share a super-size meal with a friend, take half of it home for another meal, or just leave it on the table.*

**Eat by sunlight.** "You're more physically active during the day—and, thus, more likely to burn off calories—so eat proportionately less as the day goes on," recommends *Franca Alphin, M.P.H., R.D., L.D.N.*, chief dietitian for the Duke University Sports Performance Program in Durham, North Carolina. "Start with a good breakfast and lunch, then go light on dinner and dessert." If you want an after-dinner snack, keep it small and simple.

*Eat early in the day when you're active enough to burn off calories. Go light on dinner and late-night snacks.*—Franca Alphin, M.P.H., R.D., L.D.N.

**Keep your mind on it.** "Distinguish between mindful eating and the mind*less* eating you sometimes do to join in with a group or meet some kind of emotional need," says Crawford. Ask yourself these questions: Am I really hungry? Has it been three to four hours since I last ate? Am I eating simply because someone else is eating? Am I just bored? Let the answers to these questions determine whether you take a bite.

## DINING OUT

Going out for a meal is one of life's pleasures. It's a festive and social event, and somehow the food tastes all the better because you didn't have to prepare it. Unfortunately, dining out can also pack on the pounds. "If you go out to eat on a regular basis, chances are it's contributing significantly to your caloric intake and, thus, your weight," says Crawford.

One key is to recognize that you don't have to order rich foods to have a satisfying dining experience. Here are other ways to avoid cooking and cleaning up, have a nice time, and still eat healthfully.

**Split it.** Portions in most American restaurants are enormous, and they keep getting bigger. "Cut the meal in half before you put a bite of it in your mouth," suggests Dr. Klauer. Share the entrée with your dining companion, save half for the next day, or just throw the remainder away.

**Don't be fooled.** In some cases, the seemingly healthier restaurant option may actually not be such a wise choice. Let's say you opt for a baked potato instead of French fries. Good move? Maybe not. "A large baked potato at some restaurants could have as much as 300 calories—and that's *before* you add butter, cheese, or sour cream," says Crawford. "A small order of fries ranges from 210 to 235 calories." So you actually *save* 100 calories by choosing the smaller portion of fries, right? Yes, but then there's the extra 10 to 12 grams fat that the fries contain. Crawford says your best bet is probably to get the baked potato but eat only half of it. Bottom line: Be aware of the calories and fat in restaurant foods so that you can make healthful choices.

**Ban the bread.** It's easy to mindlessly munch on bread while your meal is being prepared. Crawford suggests, "If you tend to overindulge on pre-dinner bread, ask the waiter not to even bring it out."

**Read between the lines.** The menu description of an entrée provides clues about its fat and calorie content. "Watch out for items described as 'creamy,' 'grande,' or 'supreme,' " says Crawford. Scan for diet-friendly items, which are often marked with such symbols as smiley faces, hearts, or leaves. If the menu doesn't give such visual cues, look for "grilled," "steamed," or "broiled," but pass on any choice that is broiled in butter. "Petite" usually indicates a small portion.

**Eat an appetizer for dinner.** This advice doesn't mean you should chow down on buffalo wings, nachos, or fried calamari. But having an appetizer makes portion control easy. Instead of ordering an entrée-sized pasta dish, ask for an appetizer portion and a side salad. "If the restaurant has shrimp cocktail or clams on the half shell, order one of those as your dinner," suggests Crawford.

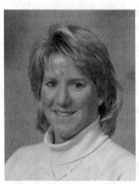

Alcoholic beverages are high in calories and can lower your reistance to temptation, warns Kim Crawford, M.S., R.D.

**Veto the vino.** Alcohol has a lot of empty calories and can lower your resolve to eat healthfully. "People usually make the worst food choices after drinking alcohol," says Crawford. If you want to stay in control, make your tea iced instead of Long Island.

**Have it your way.** Restaurants typically offer large servings of protein and simple carbohydrates, but only small portions of vegetables—the opposite of what you should eat. "So build your own meal," advises Dr. Young. Order a salad, share the main dish (or take half home), and order an extra side dish of grilled veggies. "You may have to pay a small sharing charge, but this choice is better for your health in the long run," she says. Most restaurants strive to fulfill your requests. If an eatery is not accommodating, find another that satisfies all your culinary desires.

**Don't eat the whole cow.** A trip to the steakhouse can add up to a 1,300-calorie slab of meat on your plate, and that's not counting the buttered veggies and baked potato with sour cream. "The bigger the steak, the fattier it is," says Dr. Young. Instead of succumbing to bigger-is-better brainwashing, order a 6- or 8-ounce steak, which is probably a leaner cut.

*Weight-bearing exercise keeps on giving: It revs your metabolism so that you'll continue to burn calories even after your workout is finished.*
—*Michele S. Olson, Ph.D.*

## EXERCISE: YOU GOTTA MOVE TO LOSE

If losing weight were easy, everybody would be doing it at will. One of the challenging elements of weight loss is real exercise—not strolling through the mall, mind you, but activity that makes you *sweat*.

The best exercise for weight loss is a combination of heart-healthy aerobic exercise and muscle-building weight training. Nobody is suggesting that you should bulk up like a female Arnold Schwarzenegger. But a little weight-bearing exercise does you a world of good beyond the calories you burn while exercising, explains **Michele S. Olson, Ph.D.**, professor of exercise science at Auburn University Montgomery in Montgomery, Alabama. "Your muscles are metabolically active tissues," she says. "They continue to burn calories once you've stopped lifting weights for the day." So the more muscle you develop, the higher your metabolism and the more energy—or calories—you'll burn as you sit at your desk or in front of the television.

"Consult your physician before you initiate an exercise program, especially if you are over age 55

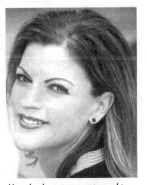

*Your body gets accustomed to the same old fitness routine, so now and then you have to pump it up with high-energy intervals, says Michele S. Olson, Ph.D.*

or have more than one risk factor for coronary artery disease (CAD)," says *Lesley White, Ph.D.,* assistant professor in the department of Exercise and Sports Science at the University of Florida at Gainesville. Your risk of CAD increases if you have gone through menopause, have a close relative with heart disease, smoke, are overweight, or have high blood pressure, high cholesterol, or diabetes.

With your doctor's approval, plan an exercise program suitable to your current fitness level, schedule, and available resources. Start out by walking or cycling in your neighborhood for 5 to 10 minutes a day. Add some time and distance to your route each week. "You don't have be able to run a 10-K race in a month to consider your exercise plan successful," says Dr. White. "In fact, aiming too far too fast can cause injury and burnout." Your program should fit your lifestyle so that you'll stick with it long-term. "You cannot successfully maintain weight loss without exercise," adds Dr. Olson.

## HEART-HEALTHY STRATEGIES

The American College of Sports Medicine recommends a moderate level of aerobic exercise for a minimum of 2½ to 5 hours a week to achieve weight loss. That's an average of 30 to 45 minutes, five days a week. "Continuous activities—such as walking, jogging, biking, or using an elliptical or stair machine—are the most robust in burning calories," says Dr. Olson.

Here are some suggestions on how to get your program started.

**Give it time.** There's no telling how many women sign up at gyms because of well-meaning New Year's resolutions. But for most of them, going to the gym is a thing of the past before the first daffodils bloom. These women got sore, tired, and fatigued, then lost interest when they didn't see any immediate results. "You need to stick with an exercise program for a period of time to see results," advises Dr. White. "Once you get through the initial soreness and adjust to the shift in your schedule, you'll start to feel the beneficial effects of the activity, which will motivate you to continue to exercise."

*No fitness plan will give you instant results, but persistence* will *pay off.*
—*Lesley White, Ph.D.*

# Brief intervals at a more vigorous pace can make your workout seem to go by faster.—*Michele S. Olson, Ph.D.*

**Count your steps.** "Wear a belt pedometer to see how many steps you take during the course of a typical day," suggests **Kim Crawford, M.S., R.D.,** program director for clinical dietetics and nutrition at the University of Pittsburgh. "Then try to increase your steps by 500 each week." Anything you can do to gradually increase your physical activity will help you burn more calories and bring you closer to your weight-loss goal. Once you start tracking your steps, you'll be eager to challenge yourself each day. While Crawford doesn't recommend a specific brand, she says you can expect to spend about $30 for a good-quality pedometer.

**Kick it up a notch.** If exercising is an alien concept to you, you may find it hard to believe that your body will eventually become accustomed to a routine workout. So every now and then you have to break loose. This interval approach encourages you to work out at a steady rate, then exercise more strenuously for a brief time before returning to your usual pace. "A growing body of research shows that the interval approach to aerobic exercise may actually be superior to continuous aerobic exercise," says Dr. Olson. "There's also something about the dynamic nature of intervals that keeps exercise interesting and makes the workout seem to go faster than if you just plod along." To insert intervals into a workout, Dr. Olson suggests you try the following routine for a total of 30 to 45 minutes.

- Walk on a level treadmill at your usual pace for three minutes. Then increase the treadmill's incline to 2 percent to simulate walking up a hill and continue for two minutes. Alternate the grade every three minutes. Gradually increase the grade and length of time you walk uphill as you get in better shape. Walking at a 5-percent grade for 10 minutes burns about as many calories as jogging a 10-minute mile, while strengthening muscles in your butt, thighs, and back.
- If you'd rather jog, perform the same workout at a jogging pace.
- If the treadmill isn't your favorite machine, try the interval approach while working out on a stair climber or stationary bike. Start at a middle level of difficulty, then push it up to a higher level for a minute every two to three minutes.

You can also work intervals into outdoors exercise: On flat terrain, walk at a steady pace for three minutes; then walk as fast as you can for 30 seconds to a minute. Or walk for three minutes and then do a set of walking lunges for a minute. (For tips on walking lunges, see page 503.) To pump up your workout, move on to hilly terrain, where you'll have to work harder to maintain a steady pace and not slow down going up hills.

### PUMP IRON

Dr. Olson recommends that women strength-train all major muscle groups three times a week. "Generally, free weights are better for women than machines," she says. "Nautilus machines are often designed based on the limb lengths of a typical male, so women face possible strain and injury." Free weights also allow you to increase the amount you lift in precise increments as low as 2.5 pounds, versus the 10-pound increments most machines offer.

*Use free weights rather than weight machines, which are designed for men's limb lengths.*—Michele S. Olson, Ph.D.

Look for fitness clubs that cater exclusively to women, where you're more likely to find female-friendly weight machines with small weight increments.

Try out some of the weight-bearing exercises described in "Tackling Problem Spots and Trouble Zones," below. Dr. Olson suggests that for each activity you work up to three sets of 10 to 15 repetitions. Your goal when you reach the last two or three repetitions of each set is that you reach failure, meaning you have to really exert yourself to finish those last repetitions. If you're not reaching failure, you probably need to lift heavier weights. Start with 5-pound weights and increase the poundage as necessary.

### TACKLING PROBLEM SPOTS AND TROUBLE ZONES

Most women would like to change select parts of their bodies. If only wishing made it so.

Your body converts surplus calories into fat, which always seems to find its way to your abdomen, hips, and thighs. If you lose weight, the *overall* fat storage drops, but you can't target removal from a specific storage area.

"If you want to lose abdominal fat, for instance, you must lose fat from your whole body," says *Lesley White, Ph.D.,* assistant professor in the department of Exercise and Sports Science at the University of Florida at Gainesville.

So the bad news is that you can't spot-reduce. But there's also good news: The exercises described below may help to improve the appearance of those problem parts. (Always check with your doctor before beginning any fitness program.)

**DOUBLE CHIN** The makings of a double chin can be in your genes or caused by being overweight—or both—says *Tanya Humphreys, M.D.,* director of cutaneous surgery, department of dermatology at Thomas Jefferson University in Philadelphia. Here's what you can do to make your chin single again.

**Wear sunscreen.** Sunlight can break down skin's collagen and elastin, which keep your face taut. To preserve the elasticity in your skin, wear sunscreen with sun protection factor (SPF) of at least 30 on your face and neck every day, says Dr. Olson.

**Contract it.** Try this daily exercise to tone your facial muscles: Looking straight ahead, pull your chin back and push the crown of your head up toward the ceiling at the same time, suggests *Marilyn Moffat, Ph.D., P.T.,* professor in the department of physical therapy at New York University. Then relax. Repeat 10 times, working up to 50 a day as you get stronger.

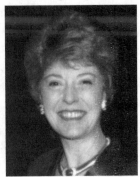

*Give your facial muscles a daily workout to keep your chin in shape, advises Marilyn Moffat, Ph.D., P.T.*

**FLABBY ARMS** "Arm fat is a big concern for some women as they grow older," says Dr. Humphreys. Sun exposure and weight gain may cause your skin to lose elasticity, giving your upper arms that saggy, flabby look. Our experts have this advice to help restore your right to bare arms.

**Slap on SPF.** To prevent further skin damage, Dr. Olson recommends applying sunscreen with a minimum SPF of 30 whenever you will be exposed to the sun. (For more information, see "The Truth About Sunscreens," page 450.)

**Get pumped.** "Strength-training exercises for your upper body can dramatically improve the appearance of your arms," says Dr. Olson. "Do three sets of 10 to 15 repetitions so you reach failure at the last couple of reps," says

Dr. Olson. The following exercises help tone your upper arms, where women tend to carry fat.

- Alternating curls: Use 5-pound weights to start and increase the weight as you get stronger. Stand with your feet shoulder-width apart and knees slightly bent. Holding a dumbbell in each hand, let your arms hang at your sides, with your palms facing forward. Bend the elbow of your right arm to slowly bring the weight up to your shoulder; then slowly lower the weight until your right arm is hanging straight by your side again. Repeat with the left arm. Continue alternating arms until you have curled each arm 15 times to complete a set. Your movements should be slow and controlled. Be sure to keep your back straight and your upper arms against your sides throughout.

- Bar curls: You can lift a dumbbell in each hand or use a single curling bar. If you usually lift 5-pound dumbbells, then select a 10-pound curling bar, which weighs twice that of one dumbbell. Stand with your knees shoulder-width apart and slightly bent. Hold the dumbbells or bar with an underhand grip, palms facing forward. Slowly bend both arms at the elbows, curling toward your shoulders. Keep your upper arms against your sides and back straight. Lower the dumbbells or bar slowly to the starting position.

- Dips: Place a sturdy kitchen chair with its back against a wall so that it won't tip backward. Sit on the chair and then grip the front edge of the seat. Slide your bottom forward off the chair, distributing your weight between your hands and feet. This is the starting position for each repetition: arms straight, knees bent, and thighs parallel to the floor. Keeping your back straight, slowly bend your elbows as you lower your bottom as far as possible toward the floor. Then slowly straighten your arms to raise your body back to the starting position.

**ABDOMINAL FAT** "This is an especially important problem area to fight because women who have abdominal obesity also have an increased risk of heart disease and related conditions," says Dr. Olson. She offers this advice to help you whittle your waistline.

**Burn it off.** Engage in some form of aerobic activity for a minimum of 45 minutes at least four times a week.

**Build it up.** Strength training trims abdominal fat in the long run because more muscle burns more calories continuously.

**Be strong.** Great abdominal muscles don't just look good; they also help you stand taller and appear leaner. Crunches strengthen these muscles and improve endurance, both of which benefit your back. To do crunches properly, lie on your back with knees bent and feet on the floor. Support your head with your hands but be careful not to pull on your neck. Lift your shoulder blades off the floor, raising your upper body toward your knees; breathe out. Then breathe in as you lower your shoulders to the floor. Perform three sets of 10 to 15 crunches to start and build up to more. These crunches are beneficial, but remember that they won't melt fat. "I did some studies that showed that eight minutes of abdominal crunches burn only 25 calories, while eight minutes of walking burns 70," says Dr. Olson.

**CELLULITE ON BUTTOCKS AND THIGHS**  Most women are all too familiar with the lumpy look of cellulite. Those lumps are made by pockets of fat, separated by bands of tissue, explains Dr. Humphreys. Popular hangouts for cellulite include the buttocks and outer thighs. And despite all the lotions and gadgets that claim to erase cellulite forever, just about every woman alive still has plenty. "Certain things can reduce the lumpiness, but cellulite cannot be eliminated altogether," says Dr. Humphreys.

"In fact, when women lose weight—particularly a lot of weight—they can end up with very loose skin, making cellulite look even worse than it did before," says Dr. Olson. So be sure to add the appropriate strength training to your exercise program. Here are some steps you can take.

**Build up your legs.** If you develop your leg muscles, they will press out on the skin and smooth the look of cellulite, says Dr. Olson. Work each area—inner thighs, backs, outer legs, and quads—three times a week, doing three sets of 10 to 15 repetitions of each exercise. In addition to the exercises recommended for baggy knees on page 503, Dr. Olson suggests you try these moves.

- Dumbbell squats: Stand in front of a chair, with your feet shoulder-width apart. Hold a dumbbell in each hand, with palms toward you and arms hanging straight at your sides. Keeping your back straight, slowly bend from your knees and hips as though you were sitting down; stop bending just before your bottom touches the chair seat. Use your leg muscles to push yourself back to a standing position.
- Lateral (side-to-side) lunges: These moves will tighten your outer legs. Stand with your feet slightly apart and hands on hips. Keep

your back straight and shoulders square throughout the move. Take a big step to the side with your right foot. Shift your weight onto your right leg, and bend your right knee and ankle as you slowly lower your torso toward your right foot. Keep your left leg straight and bend your right knee at a 90-degree angle. Push with your right foot to raise yourself back to the starting position. Repeat with your left leg.

- Leg curls: These will help shape the backs of your legs. Lie facedown on a weight bench, positioning your legs under the weight bar so that the bar pad rests at the base of your calf muscles. With your right leg, slowly lift the weight toward your buttocks as far as you can, holding on to the bench for support. Then slowly lower your right leg. Repeat with the left leg.

**Get a deep massage.** Localized massage to cellulite-prone areas can produce a temporary smoothing effect. "It probably works by improving lymphatic drainage, but results are not permanent," says Dr. Humphreys.

**HEAVY THIGHS** Women tend to carry the most weight on their hips and thighs. "This pattern of female fat distribution evolved so that a woman would have enough fat to support a pregnancy during times of famine," says *Jana Klauer, M.D.,* research fellow at the New York Obesity Research Center at St. Luke's-Roosevelt Hospital Center at Columbia University. Try these moves to thin your thighs.

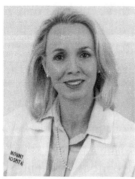

*Blame it on evolution: Women store a lot of fat on their hips and thighs to ensure the ability to support a pregnancy, explains Jana Klauer, M.D.*

- Lunges: "Resistance training will stimulate the muscles in the thighs and give legs an attractive shape," says Dr. Olson. Use the resistance of your own body by doing the walking lunges advised to help shape up baggy knees. (See opposite page.)
- Leg raises: Strap on 3- to 5-pound ankle weights while you perform this move. Lie flat on your back, with your legs straight out in front of you and arms at your sides. Raise your right leg so that it forms a 90-degree angle with the floor. Slowly lower your leg back to the floor. "Do three sets of 15 raises," advises Dr. Olson. Repeat with your left leg. In addition, try the exercises recommended for combating cellulite and baggy knees.

**FLABBY INNER THIGHS** Many women need to strengthen and develop the quadricep muscles of their inner thighs, says Dr. Olson. To perform this muscle-building exercise, you will need an exercise ball (available at sporting-goods and national department stores). Lie faceup on the floor, with your arms at your sides. Place your feet flat on the floor so that your thighs form a 90-degree angle with your body. Place the exercise ball between your knees. Squeeze your legs as hard as you can against the ball and hold for three seconds. Do three sets of 10 to 15 repetitions.

**BAGGY KNEES** Like plumped-up arms, baggy knees are caused by decreased skin elasticity and excess weight, says Dr. Olson. Follow her advice to send those bags packing.

**Shade your legs.** Use sunscreen with an SPF of at least 30 to prevent further skin damage.

**Build your quads.** "Strength-training exercises tone muscles in the knee area, and more developed muscles push out more on the skin to give it a smoother appearance," explains Dr. Olson. Leg-extension exercises and walking lunges work the lower quadricep muscles that attach to the knees. Dr. Olson suggests you do three sets of 10 to 15 repetitions of each leg exercise below.

- Leg extensions: You may need to perform this move at a gym, since leg extensions require a weight bench. Sit at the end of the bench and place both legs under the padded weight bar so that the pads rest on your shins, just above your ankles. Grasp the bench behind you for support and raise both legs until they are straight in front of you. Drop the left leg to the floor. Use your right leg to slowly lower the weight about 45 degrees and then lift it to the starting position. Repeat with the left leg to complete one repetition.

- Walking lunges: Stand with your feet together and your arms hanging straight at your sides. Grasp a dumbbell in each hand, with your palms facing your thighs. Take a big step forward with your right leg and plant your right foot, not letting your knee extend beyond your toes. Keeping your weight centered, slowly lower your left knee toward the floor until your right knee is bent at a 90-degree angle. Keep your back straight as you push yourself up to a standing position. Repeat with your left leg. Take a step forward each time you switch legs. If you don't have room to take 10 or 15 giant steps, stand in place.

# *Health* Magazine's
# 10-Week Weight-Loss Plan

Persistence and patience are key to any successful weight-loss plan. You didn't put on those excess pounds overnight, and they're not likely to go away any faster. Those "miracle" products that promise instant results are little more than hype—and some are downright dangerous. Experts agree that the healthiest way to lose weight is gradually, one pound at a time.

With each small change you make, you're building skills and learning new habits that will enable you to reach and maintain your desired weight. Let each little triumph motivate you to continue toward success.

We developed this easy-to-follow, 10-week weight-loss plan with the help of *Susan Burke, M.S., R.D., C.D.E.,* director of nutrition services at eDiets.com. It follows the three-legged structure of attitude, dietary changes, and exercise described in this chapter.

Tailor this plan to your needs, adding new lifestyle changes to your weight-loss regimen each week.

## WEEK 1: TAKING STOCK
### ATTITUDE
**Gear up mentally.** Realize that you are not on a diet. Rather, you have chosen to make fundamental lifestyle changes in order to lose weight and improve your health. If you maintain a positive attitude and stay motivated, you'll enjoy moving toward a trimmer and healthier you. Acknowledge that you won't be transformed overnight. A healthy weight loss is no more than 2 pounds each week.

### DIETARY CHANGES
**Keep a journal.** For at least three days, including one weekend day, write down everything you eat and drink. *Everything*—no fudging! Also note the time of day you eat, where you eat, and how you feel at the time. This will help you identify your eating patterns and emotional triggers that cause you to reach for food you don't need for fuel. Use this food-and-activity journal throughout your weight-loss journey to help you stay on track.

**Do your homework.** Your journal will help pinpoint which aspects you need to change to have a healthier diet. For example, you may need to limit simple carbohydrates, such as those in white breads and refined cereals, in favor of the complex carbs in such foods as whole grains. Or perhaps you should replace butter and other saturated fats with healthier fats, such as olive oil. Identify your trigger foods and aim to eliminate them first; at the least, cut back on them. Then start to add healthier alternatives. Personalized weight-loss Web sites, such as eDiets.com, can also provide assistance. For best results, though, consult a registered dietitian. For estimates of calories and nutrients in specific foods, visit your local library or bookstore for an appropriate reference book. Or check out the following online references.

- www.nal.usda.gov/fnic/cgi-bin/nut_search.pl
- www.foodcount.com (Click on "Food Finder.")
- www.caloriecontrol.org/calcalcs.html
- www.nhlbi.nih.gov/about/oei/index.htm (Click on "Menu Planner.")

### SUCCESS CHECK

**Assess where you are now.** Talk to your doctor to determine how much weight you need to lose. For additional advice, join a weight-loss group; you can attend meetings in person or go online. Your body mass index, or BMI (see chart, page 479), and waist measurement can also guide you to a healthy weight range for your height.

## WEEK 2: GETTING STARTED

### ATTITUDE

**Target one small change.** Focus on changing just one habit that has contributed to your weight gain. For example, if you normally have four soft drinks a day, cut down to two. If you usually eat sweets after both lunch and dinner, reserve your treat for evening only—it will give you something to look forward to. It takes a reduction of 3,500 calories to lose one pound, so you need to reduce your daily intake by at least 500 calories to lose a pound per week.

**Celebrate.** Congratulate yourself for each positive step you took in Week 1. Take note of what seems to work well—and what doesn't—so that you can carry those actions forward.

### DIETARY CHANGES

**Make a plan.** Decide which will work better for you: three square meals a day plus a small snack or two, or five or six minimeals scattered throughout the day. Based on your meal plan, make a shopping list.

**Go to market.** Take your new outlook to the grocery store. Choose fruits, vegetables, and whole-grain breads that you haven't tried before. Check out the health-food section for fat-free, low-calorie, low-sodium soups, chilis, and cereals. As you shop for the items on your list, take time to look at nutrition labels. The calories and fat listed for what appears to be an individual portion might actually apply to only a half or third of the product.

### EXERCISE

**Get moving.** Where you start your exercise program depends on your present level of fitness. If you're not a regular exerciser, check with your doctor before you initiate a fitness regimen. Then you might begin with a 5- to 10-minute walk or bike ride each day. Slowly increase the time you spend exercising each week. If you're already a regular exerciser, add minutes to your current routine or try a new activity.

### SUCCESS CHECK

**Set yourself up to succeed.** Aim for a realistic and maximum weight loss of 2 pounds a week. Focus on that weekly goal rather than on your target weight. If you stick to your plan, you're likely to lose 2 pounds or more per week in the first few weeks, as your body adjusts to fewer calories and more activity.

## WEEK 3: MOVING FORWARD

### ATTITUDE

**Get satisfaction.** Eating healthfully doesn't have to leave you feeling deprived. If healthier food choices aren't giving you the pleasure and taste you want, think about what you can do to feel more satisfied, while still following a healthy eating plan. If you crave sweets, for example, treat yourself to a fat-free ice-cream sandwich after dinner. It's okay to indulge the occasional yen if you make the necessary modifications in your food choices for that day.

**Continue to make small changes.** Keep working on building weight-reducing habits. This week, you might focus on eliminating fried foods and switching to fat-free condiments, such as mustard and sliced tomato, instead of mayonnaise.

## DIETARY CHANGES

**Partition your plate.** This tip allows you to eat more and still lose weight: Picture your plate as a clock face. Then fill two-thirds of it—from 12 to 8 o'clock—with vegetables, fruits, and whole grains. That leaves only one-third free for protein foods. Which lunch would you prefer: A burger and fries? Or a fat-free turkey sandwich, loaded with veggies, on a whole-grain bun, plus a cucumber-and-tomato salad and strawberries for dessert? The second choice is healthier, filling, and takes longer to eat. What satisfaction!

**Substitute water.** Cut down on or eliminate soft drinks, sweetened teas, fruit juices, and high-fat milk. Opt for water instead. Metabolism, the rate at which you burn calories, is a chemical process that requires plain ol' water. Plus, drinking water flushes out toxins that inhibit weight loss and helps prevent the constipation that sometimes results when you eat more fiber.

**Mind your fiber.** You have many choices in meeting your daily quota of 25 to 35 grams fiber each day. Add chickpeas to salads or kidney beans to spaghetti sauce. Select cereals that have at least 5 grams fiber per serving and whole-grain breads that contain at least 3 grams per serving.

**Try something new.** Instead of reaching for an apple, give your taste buds a thrill with a papaya or kiwifruit. Bok choy and artichokes are interesting alternatives to green beans and broccoli. Variety is likely to help keep you enthusiastic about your eating plan.

**Restaurant tip:** If you have dessert, take three or four bites—just enough to feel satisfied—then call it quits. To help you succeed, share your sweet with a dining partner or ask your server to remove the plate. After the first few bites of any rich food, the flavor fades with each consecutive bite anyway.

## EXERCISE

**Count your steps.** On your daily walk, wear a pedometer to tally your strides. Then increase that number by 100 steps each day for a week. At week's end, total the steps you've taken. Then congratulate yourself for such progress.

**Bump it up.** If you walked for 15 minutes each day last week, make it 20 minutes per day this week. Your goal should be to reach 30 to 60 minutes a day of aerobic exercise on most days of the week. But don't get bogged down by numbers. You're doing your body good any time you get moving, even if it's just for a few minutes.

**Work out stress.** Many women overeat in response to stress, so it's wise to add a stress-buster to your fitness routine. For this week's innovation, try yoga, tai chi, or meditation. Buy an instruction book or video, or consider attending a class. Start with 15 to 20 minutes a day, three days a week. You might try all three techniques and then pick the one that works best for you.

### SUCCESS CHECK

**Skip the scale.** From now on, check your weight loss only once a week.

**Take it slow.** Make sure you're not losing weight too quickly. Remember, you're aiming to shed no more than 2 pounds a week. You may lose a bit more in the first weeks as your body adjusts to your new efforts. But if you're consistently losing more, you may be cutting too many calories too rapidly.

## WEEK 4: STICKING WITH THE PLAN

### ATTITUDE

**Give a cheer.** Assess the benefits you've reaped so far. Perhaps you have more energy or less heartburn. Maybe your clothes are looser or your skin is clearer. Look beyond the weight loss and give yourself a hearty hurrah for each new healthy action and positive feeling.

### DIETARY CHANGES

**Eat breakfast every day.** Fuel your body with a high-fiber cereal and fruit.

**Make more small changes.** For a change of pace, snack on something different this week. You might replace your after-dinner ice cream with a cup of sugar-free hot chocolate. Add a sliced Granny Smith apple for a delicious combination of sweet and tart.

**Eat less, more often.** Try to eat a little every three to four hours. Take such healthy snacks as whole-grain crackers or low-fat cheese to work to nibble on.

**Try psyllium to increase fiber.** Psyllium is available at health-food stores and drugstores as a powder, capsules, and chewable wafers. You must take it with water (follow the manufacturer's directions). *Amanda McQuade Crawford,* a medical herbalist and author of *Herbal Remedies for Women,* recommends taking 1 to 2 teaspoons psyllium seed before each meal to help you quickly feel full. Psyllium can interfere with some medications, so consult with your doctor or pharmacist before taking it.

**Restaurant tip:** Ask your server to remove the bread and butter from the table so that it won't tempt you. Request that all dressings and sauces be served on the side so that you can limit the amount you use.

## EXERCISE

**Take it up a notch.** Add another five minutes to your exercise routine this week. Also try to increase your daily walks by another 100 steps a day.

**Start strength training.** If you've never lifted weights—or it's been a few years—start with 5-pound dumbbells. If that's too easy, use 10-pound ones. Do three sets of 10 to 15 repetitions of each exercise described in the arms section of "Tackling Problem Spots and Trouble Zones," page 498.

## SUCCESS CHECK

**Take a good look.** If you're still keeping a food journal, use it to assess how your eating patterns have changed since Week 1. Which foods have you eliminated or added? How often have you slipped into an old habit? What changes do you need to make? Maybe you've eliminated some empty carbohydrates, but you still need to add more fiber to your diet. Incorporate new goals into your meal plan and shopping list for the coming week.

# WEEK 5: MAKING PROGRESS

## ATTITUDE

**Think of your health.** You're losing weight and, thus, you look and feel better. An added bonus: As your waistline shrinks, so does your risk of heart disease, diabetes, and a host of other ailments.

## DIETARY CHANGES

**Stay energized.** Your muscles need protein to work efficiently. Now that you are exercising aerobically and have added weights, you need to be sure you get sufficient protein. Check the recommendations for your weight on page 488.

**Fight afternoon slump.** Space out meals to every three to four hours to maintain your energy and mood. For instance, instead of having a cup of yogurt with lunch, eat it later in the day with a piece of fruit.

**Restaurant tip:** Never super-size. If you must occasionally succumb to a fast-food craving, order the smallest drink, burger, and fries.

## EXERCISE

**Keep up with stress relief.** Continue with the stress-relieving technique—yoga, meditation, or tai chi—that works for you. Practice your chosen method at least 15 to 20 minutes a day, three days a week.

**Tough it out.** Add another 5 to 10 minutes a day to your workout. Try interval training, described on page 497.

**Get stronger.** To build up your strength-training program, do the thigh exercises recommended on page 502.

## SUCCESS CHECK

**Rate your fitness.** Performing aerobic exercises should now be easier than in the beginning. You've come a long way. Exercise will continue to be more comfortable for you.

# WEEK 6: STAYING ON TRACK

## ATTITUDE

**Don't be discouraged.** Stay focused on your goal. Good health is your true aim—a slimmer body is just icing on the cake. Remember that moderation is key to success; you don't have to deprive yourself. There are no forbidden foods, just forbidden portions.

## DIETARY CHANGES

**Go fish.** If you're like most Americans, you don't eat enough heart-healthy fish. Eat seafood three to four times this week. Have a tuna sandwich for lunch. Or enjoy grilled salmon for dinner. Think it's too expensive? Consider what you save by shunning fast food. Besides, you're worth it. You can eat a satisfying serving of shrimp and consume relatively few calories—and what a treat! Just make sure the shrimp is steamed, baked, or broiled (without butter), instead of fried. Many large grocery stores will steam fish or shellfish for you while you shop. If you want to learn to prepare fish at home, a cookbook that highlights fish recipes is a sound investment.

**Restaurant tip:** Swear off greasy appetizers. An order of loaded nachos can serve up more than 800 calories; and a plate of buffalo wings has more than 500 calories. Opt for shrimp cocktail, instead.

## EXERCISE

**Stick with aerobic exercise.** Continue doing 30 minutes of aerobic exercise, five days a week. Each day, keep trying to take more steps. If you're bored with walking, reinvigorate your workouts with swimming, biking, or using an elliptical machine at the gym.

**Round out your regimen.** Pump up your strength training by adding the abdominal crunches described on page 501.

### SUCCESS CHECK

**Note your successes.** Make a list of dietary changes you've made, healthy habits you've adopted, and unhealthy behavior you've discarded. Also record how much exercise you've built up to each day, as well as how much weight you've lost.

**Rediscover clothes.** Try on some clothes you haven't been able to wear in a while. You'll love how your favorite jeans fit now. Notice where they're loose. That extra room is proof that your efforts are paying off.

# WEEK 7: LOOKING AHEAD

## ATTITUDE

**Freshen up your menu.** Give your meals a boost with new low-fat recipes from magazines and cookbooks. The more varied your menu, the more likely you are to stay motivated to stick with the program.

## DIETARY CHANGES

**Bulk up.** Enhance your recipes with vegetables or fruits. Any casserole or pasta dish will contain fewer calories and more fiber if you replace some of the starch with nonstarchy vegetables. Pizza tastes terrific garnished with broccoli and mushrooms—and less cheese. Top your cereal with fresh fruits.

**Enjoy sweet success.** Pineapple contains bromelain, an enzyme that helps your body digest proteins and fats. Enjoy pineapple fresh or canned in juice rather than syrup.

**Restaurant tip:** Drizzle balsamic vinegar on your salad instead of ladling on blue cheese or ranch dressing. You'll save as many as 300 calories.

## EXERCISE

**Extend your exercise.** Increase your daily aerobic workout to 45 minutes, five days a week, following the interval format. You might look into rebounding, a weight-bearing exercise that involves bouncing on a miniature trampoline. Add another 100 steps daily to your walks.

**Alternate your routines.** Do three days of strength training, alternating arm, leg, and abdominal exercises.

## SUCCESS CHECK

**Ask your doctor.** At this point, you should be seeing results from your hard work. If your weight hasn't gone down at all, see your physician to rule out an underlying medical problem.

# WEEK 8: CARRYING ON

## ATTITUDE

**Reward yourself.** You've worked hard, so you deserve a treat. Indulge in a movie or manicure—whatever activity or event that makes you feel pampered.

**Keep up your journal.** Continue to record the dietary changes you've made, healthy habits you've adopted, and unhealthy behavior you've discarded. Also track how much exercise you've built up to each day, as well as how much weight you've lost.

**Relish compliments.** People are bound to praise your new healthier appearance. Each time you receive a compliment, silently give yourself one as well.

## DIETARY CHANGES

**Vary your fruits and veggies.** The more fruits and vegetables you eat, the better. Variety keeps you interested and motivated to get your five-a-day. Try passionfruit, pomegranates, and kumquats. Experiment with eggplant, rhubarb, and watercress.

**Introduce a friendly fat.** Crawford recommends taking 1,000 to 3,000 milligrams evening primrose oil each day to boost your intake of essential fatty acids. This supplement aids digestion and assists the immune system.

**Restaurant tip:** Watch your protein portion, even if you order chicken or fish, since restaurants tend to bulk up all their portions. Too much of even a good thing adds up to excess calories.

## EXERCISE

**Go farther.** Increase your walk by another 100 steps a day. You're really covering some ground now! Keep up 45 minutes a day of aerobic exercise, five days a week (preferably in the interval format). If you're feeling ambitious, try working out 60 minutes a day, six days a week.

**Build up.** Do the same strength-training routine as last week but add a few repetitions to each set.

# WEEK 9: GOING THE DISTANCE

## ATTITUDE

**Find a role model.** Note the habits of people who appear to be healthy eaters and routine exercisers. How do they manage to stay on track? Modeling some of their techniques and attitudes can help move you toward your goal.

## DIETARY CHANGES

**Every little bit helps.** Weight loss is a step-by-step process, so you'll benefit from every small change. This week, be mindful of superfluous calories you take in with such embellishments as sugar in coffee or tea, jelly on toast, or ketchup on a sandwich. Eliminate at least one sugary additive a day—you may not even miss it.

**Spice things up.** Add flavor to your cooking with aromatic herbs and spices, such as basil, rosemary, and cinnamon. For a twist, add ground fenugreek to casseroles, marinades, soups, and baked goods. A staple of North African and Middle Eastern cuisine, fenugreek's flavor is similar to that of maple syrup or brown sugar.

**Restaurant tip:** A large baked potato may contain more than 300 calories, and that's without toppings. If you're served an exceptionally large potato, eat only half or share it with a friend.

## EXERCISE

**Keep counting.** Give your strength training a boost by increasing the repetitions of each move until you reach failure point.

## SUCCESS CHECK

**Assess where you are now.** Determine how much weight you've lost since embarking on your weight-loss journey. Also check your BMI and waist circumference, then congratulate yourself on the results. Take note of how you've built up your fitness through exercise.

# WEEK 10: EYEING THE PRIZE

By now, you should have put a real dent in your weight-loss goal. Continue to practice healthy habits, including aerobic exercise, strength training, and pedometer-measured walking.

# Index

514

Crohn's disease.
*See* Inflammatory bowel
disease (IBD).
Cryosurgery. *See* Freezing
therapy.
CT scan. *See* Computed
tomography scan.
Cushing's disease, 23
Cutler, Winnifred B., Ph.D.,
416, 417, 429
Cyclic fibrocystic changes, 55
Cyclophosphamide, 217
Cyclosporine, 30
Cysts, breasts, 55
aspiration, 56
treatments, 56, 57

**D**alton, Gail, M.D., 157,
162
Daly, Anne, R.D., C.D.E.,
135
Dandruff. *See* Hair.
Darvocet (propoxyphene), 39
Dawson-Hughes, Bess, M.D.,
20, 24, 29
Debt, coping with
acceptance, 224
curbing spending, 225
discarding credit cards, 225
and low-interest credit
cards, 225
paying off credit cards, 224
and scams, 225
and spending plan, 224
using cash, 225
Decléor's Micro-Exfoliating
Face Gel. *See* Acne.
Deglycyrrhized (DGL)
licorice. *See* Ulcers.
Dehydration. *See* Diarrhea.
Dehydroepiandrosterone
(DHEA), 50, 240
Delsym, 206
Deltasone (prednisone), 89
Demerol (meperidine), 318
Denavir (penciclovir), 321
Dental dams. *See* Sexually
transmitted diseases (STDs).
Depression
causes
emotional difficulties,
285
genetics, 285
hormones, 285

illness, 285
neurotransmitter
imbalance, 285
and chronic fatigue
syndrome (CFS), 130
Mother Nature, M.D., 290
One Woman's Story, 286
and Parkinson's disease, 53
symptoms, 285, 288
treatments
and alcohol, 292
antidepressants, 287
and birth control pills,
292
changing outlook, 293
cognitive behavioral
therapy (CBT), 287
diet, 291
exercise, 289
humor, 293
journaling, 292
and routines, 290
and sleeping habits, 291
stress-relieving
techniques, 293
support groups, 279,
288
therapy, 287, 289
de Roos, Nicole M., M.Sc.,
Ph.D., 192
Desenex, 165
Designer estrogens, 32
Evista (raloxifene), 34
Nolvadex (tamoxifen), 34
risks, 35
Desipramine. *See* Norpramin.
Detrol (tolterodine), 474
Dexamethasone elixir.
*See* Canker sores.
DEXA scan. *See* Dual-energy
X-ray absorptiometry scan.
DGL (deglycyrrhized) licorice.
*See* Ulcers.
DHEA. *See*
Dehydroepiandrosterone.
Diabetes
and exercise, 135
and feet, 158
and nail discoloration,
328
and osteoporosis, 23
as risk factor
for cataracts, 145
for celiac disease, 100

for heart attack, 135,
188
with influenza
immunization, 205
types, 134
Diamond, Merle, M.D.,
336
Diarrhea
bloody diarrhea
and colitis, 93
and diverticulitis, 93
and dysentery, 94
and inflammatory bowel
disease (IBD), 93
and severe infection, 93
causes
artificial sweeteners, 94
caffeinated beverages,
95
dairy products, 94
excess magnesium, 95
excess vitamin C, 95
lactose intolerance, 94
menstrual cramps,
273
description, 93
fatty diarrhea
and celiac sprue, 93
and pancreatic disease,
93
symptoms, 93
and hemorrhoids, 98
and medications
Imodium (loperamide),
94
Lomotil (diphenoxylate
and atropine), 94
magnesium overdose,
274
treatments
bland and binding
foods, 94
fluids, 95
probiotics, 94
watery diarrhea
and food poisoning,
93
and intestinal infection,
93
and medications, food,
or drink, 93
and stomach flu, 93
and viral infection, 93
Dicyclomine. *See* Bentyl.

Jacknin, Jeanette, M.D.,
446, 448, 451
Jaliman, Debra, M.D., 450
Jealousy
symptoms, 297
treatments
and assumptions, 298
and envy, 297
and jealousy, 298
Johnson, Yvonne, O.D.,
143, 150, 152
Joint
and celiac disease, 100
description, 37
and osteoarthritis, 38
and rheumatoid arthritis,
40
Jones, Kornelia, 168
Joslyn, Sue, Ph.D., 62

Katz, Lawrence C., Ph.D.,
244
Kava extract, 123
and liver toxicity, 284
Kaye, Susan, M.D., 3, 65
Keflex (cephalosporin), 467
Kegel, Arnold, M.D., 425
Kegel exercises, 425, 472
Kennedy, Alexandra, M.A.,
227, 230
Kenney, Kim, 130
Keratin protein, 170
Ketoconazole. See Nizoral.
Ketotifen. See Zaditor.
Kidney damage, and
diabetes, 135
Kidney diseases
and influenza
immunization, 205
and nail discoloration,
328
Kidney energy, 123
Kidney stones
description, 475
and diet, 477
and genetics, 476
preventing recurrences
Aloprim (allopurinol),
476
Aquatensen (thiazide),
477
Esidrix (thiazide), 477
Polycitra-K (potassium
citrate), 476

Zyloprim (allopurinol),
476
remedies
diet, 477
liquids, 477
symptoms, 475
treatments
extracorporeal shock-
wave lithotripsy
(ESWL), 475
percutaneous
nephrolithotomy, 476
ureteroscopy, 476
Kitchin, Beth, M.S., R. D.,
25, 31
Klauer, Jana, M.D., 486,
488, 502
Klein, Lorrie J., M.D., 191
Kleinman, Dushanka,
D.D.S., M.Sc.D., 349
Kleinsmith, D'Anne, M.D.,
456
Knee pain
causes
high-heeled shoes, 351
microtears in cartilage,
351
osteoarthritis, 351
weak muscles, 350
treatments
cortisone and other
therapies, 351
exercises, 351
glucosamine and
chondroitin, 352
knee brace, 351
physical therapy, 351
and weight, 353
Koenig, Christina, 225
Kopf, Rebecca, 129
Kowalski, Carol, P.T., 331
Kunin, Audrey Gottlieb,
M.D., 3, 447

Lactobacillus acidophilus,
89, 94, 97, 374, 427
Lactose intolerance
and celiac disease, 100
description, 97
and hydrogen breath test,
97
and lactase deficiency,
97
and race, 97

remedies
food-and-symptoms
diary, 98
lactase-fortified
products, 98
and prepared foods, 98
soy products, 98
symptoms, 97
Lamisil (terbinafine), 329
Lansoprazole. See Prevacid.
L-arginine, 470
Lark, Susan, M.D., 46, 380,
385
LaRoche, Loretta, 280
Laser in-situ keratomileusis
(LASIK), 153
costs, 154
description, 153
questions, 155
risks, 154
Laser resurfacing. See Aging
skin.
LASIK. See Laser in-situ
keratomileusis.
Lauersen, Niels, M.D., 264
LDL (low-density lipopro-
teins). See Cholesterol.
Lecithin, 85
Lee, Cyndi, 301
LEEP. See Loop electrosurgi-
cal excision procedure.
Leimyomas. See Uterine
fibroids.
Lethargy. See Fatigue.
Leuprolide. See Lupron.
Levine, Suzanne M., D.P.M.,
158, 160, 161, 164
Levobunolol. See Betagan.
Levsin (hyoscyamine), 71, 73
Libido, 417
Ligation. See Surgery.
Lindberg, Jill S., M.D., 475
Lipitor (atorvastatin), 77,
178, 181
Lipski, Elizabeth, Ph.D.,
C.N.N., 69, 73, 74, 77,
82, 83, 87, 89, 90, 94, 96
Liver
and hepatitis, 212
and nail discoloration, 328
L-Lysine, 320
Lomotil (diphenoxylate and
atropine), 94
Lonsdorf, Nancy, M.D., 274

Plaque. *See* Heart disease.
Plaquenil (hydroxychloro-
quine), 42
PMDD. *See* Premenstrual
dysphoric disorder.
PMS. *See* Premenstrual
syndrome.
Poirier-Solomon, Laurinda,
M.P.H., R.N., 137
Polycitra-K (potassium
citrate), 476
Polycystic ovary syndrome
(PCOS)
and amenorrhea, 275
description, 381
and fertility, 391
and genetics, 383
hair and skin problems
medical treatments, 382
removal methods, 382
treatments
diet, 383
exercise, 384
and insulin, 383
oral contraceptives, 384
and weight, 383
Positron emission
tomography (PET), 413
Postnasal drip. *See* Sinusitis.
Postpartum depression.
*See* Depression.
Post-traumatic stress
disorder (PTSD)
description, 295
symptoms, 296
treatments
combating anxiety, 296
therapy strategies, 296
Potassium citrate.
*See* Polycitra-K.
Power, Deborah Jane, D.O.,
36
PPIs. *See* Proton pump
inhibitors.
Prather, Charlene M., M.D.,
70, 97
Pravachol (pravastatin), 77,
178
Pravastatin. *See* Pravachol.
Prednisolone (prednisone),
89
Prednisone, 42, 89. *See also*
Deltasone, Orasone,
Prednisolone.

Pregnancy
and age, 391
and backache, 361
and endometriosis, 385
and hemorrhoids, 98
and indigestion and
heartburn, 363
and infertility, 389
and insomnia, 366
morning sickness, 358
and polycystic ovary
syndrome (PCOS), 382
pregnancy mask, 443
preparation for, 357
uterine fibroids, 379
and varicose veins, 367
Pregnenolone, 48
Premarin. *See* Estrogen,
Estrogen replacement
therapy (ERT), Hormone
replacement therapy (HRT).
Premenstrual dysphoric
disorder (PMDD), 266
and serotonin, 272
and serotonin reuptake
inhibitors (SSRIs), 272
versus premenstrual
syndrome (PMS), 272
Premenstrual syndrome (PMS)
and abnormal bleeding,
267
and calcium, 271
causes, 264
charting symptoms, 266
and depression, 266, 285
and diuretics, 270
endometriosis, 267
journaling, 270
and menstrual cramps, 273
minimizing
and caffeine, 269
and chocolate, 269
and salt, 269
and premenstrual
dysphoric disorder
(PMDD), 266, 272
and progesterone, 271
Should I See a Doctor?,
267
symptoms, 264
treatments
and blood sugar, 268
calcium supplements,
271

exercise, 268
gamma-linolenic acid
(GLA), 269
vitamins and minerals,
269
Yasmin, 272
Prempro. *See* Estrogen,
Estrogen replacement
therapy (ERT), Hormone
replacement therapy (HRT).
Presbyopia
eye exams, 147
glasses, 147
Should I See a Doctor?,
147
symptoms, 147
Preston, Leslie, 286
Prevacid (lansoprazole), 80
Price, Deborah R., Au.D.,
110
Prilosec (omeprazole), 80
Primary dysmenorrhea.
*See* Menstrual cramps.
PRK (photorefractive keratectomy). *See* Laser in-situ
keratomileusis (LASIK).
Probiotics
*Bifidobacterium*, 89, 94
*Lactobacillus acidophilus*,
89, 94
*Saccharomyces boulardii*,
89
Pro-Gest, 235
Progesterone
description, 48, 255, 258
and menopause, 235
and mouth diseases, 308
natural hormone replace-
ment therapy (nHRT),
258
and premenstrual
syndrome (PMS), 271
as risk factor
for menopausal
depression, 242
for uterine fibroids,
379
and testosterone, 246
and wild yam creams,
259
Progressive muscle
relaxation, 339
Promethazine. *See* Phenergan.
Propoxyphene. *See* Darvocet.